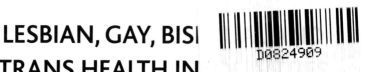

LESBIAN, GAY, BISI
TRANS HEALTH IN

International perspectives in social work

Edited by Julie Fish and Kate Karban

First published in Great Britain in 2015 by

Policy Press
University of Bristol
1-9 Old Park Hill
Bristol BS8 1SD
UK
t: +44 (0)117 954 5940
pp-info@bristol.ac.uk
www.policypress.co.uk

North American office:
Policy Press
c/o The University of Chicago Press
1427 East 60th Street
Chicago, IL 60637, USA
t: +1 773 702 7700
f: +1 773-702-9756
e:sales@press.uchicago.edu
www.press.uchicago.edu

British Library Cataloguing in Publication Data
A catalogue record for this book is available from the British Library

Library of Congress Cataloging-in-Publication Data
A catalog record for this book has been requested

ISBN 978 1 44730 968 0 paperback
ISBN 978 1 44730 967 3 hardcover

The right of Julie Fish and Kate Karban to be identified as editors of this work has been asserted by them in accordance with the 1988 Copyright, Designs and Patents Act.

Cover design by Qube Design Associates, Bristol
Front cover image: istock
Printed and bound in Great Britain by CMP, Poole
Policy Press uses environmentally responsible print partners

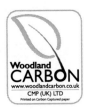

To Sue Wilkinson

Contents

List of tables, figures and photographs

Tables

Figures

Photographs

List of abbreviations

AIDS	acquired immune deficiency syndrome
ASO	AIDS service organisation (Canada)
BME	black and minority ethnic
CASW	Canadian Association of Social Workers
CASWE	Canadian Association for Social Work Education
CAUT	Canadian Association of University Teachers
CDA	critical discourse analysis
CIHR	Canadian Institutes of Health Research
CLA	critical language awareness
CLAS	Culturally and Linguistically Appropriate Services
CP	critical pedagogy
CRHC	Canadian Rainbow Health Coalition
EoLC	end of life care
EU	European Union
FGDM	family group decision making
GBA	gender-based analysis
GLBTIQ	gay, lesbian, bisexual, trans, intersex and queer (North American usage)
GLSEN	Gay, Lesbian, and Straight Education Network
GP	general practitioner
GSA	gay–straight alliance
HIV	human immunodeficiency virus
HSRB	Human Subject Review Board
IASSW	International Association of Schools of Social Work
IFSW	International Federation of Social Workers
IPC	Indian Penal Code
ISTAT	Italian National Institute of Statistics
LGB	lesbian, gay and bisexual
LGBT	lesbian, gay, bisexual and trans
LGBTQ	lesbian, gay, bisexual, trans and queer
LHIN	Local Health Integration Network (Canada)
MSM	men who have sex with men
NAAC	National Assessment and Accreditation Council (India)
NACO	National AIDS Control Organisation (India)
NASS	National Asylum Support Service (UK)
NASW	National Association of Social Workers (US)
NEoLCP	National End of Life Care Programme (UK)
NGO	non-governmental organisation
NSF	National Service Framework

NTCP	narrative therapy and community practice
PAGFB	persons assigned gender female at birth
PFLG	Parents and Friends of Lesbians and Gays
PUCL-K	People's Union for Civil Liberties – Karnataka (India)
RHO	Rainbow Health Ontario (Canada)
SDoH	social determinants of health
SRS	sex reassignment surgery
UAI	unprotected anal intercourse
UDHR	Universal Declaration of Human Rights
UGC	University Grants Commission (India)
UK	United Kingdom
UKBA	UK Border Agency
UN	United Nations
US	United States
VOYPIC	Voice of Young People in Care (Northern Ireland)
WG	Welsh Government

Glossary

Biphobia is a source of discrimination against bisexual people, it is based on stereotypical assumptions and unfounded fear.

Bisexual: someone who is bisexual may describe themselves as emotionally, physically or sexually attracted to men and women. Bisexual may describe people's identity, behaviours or desire.

Cisgender is the term to denote that an individual's gender matches the sex they were assigned at birth and is a complementary definition to transgender.

Cisnormativity is the assumption that cisgenderism is the norm.

Coming out describes the process of acknowledging one's sexual orientation as lesbian, gay or bisexual to oneself or other people. It is commonly assumed that this is a one-off event, but it is best conceived of as a process that involves a number of stages and may take many years. The term 'come out' is an abbreviation for 'come out of the closet'.

Gay: The word 'gay' was introduced in the early 20th-century to serve as an alternative to the clinical (and often pejorative) term 'homosexual'. Gay was originally used as a noun by both men and women but from the 1980s it was replaced by the terms 'gay man' (predominantly) and 'gay woman'. The word 'lesbian' is more commonly used to describe women who have romantic, sexual or emotional connections to other women.

Gender typically refers to a Western binary model of being male or female, and this binary model is constricting for people who are trans or transgender. Gender describes the cultural significance of sex and refers to the social roles associated with being male or female.

Gender-based analysis (GBA) is an analytical tool that integrates a gender perspective into the development of policies, programmes and legislation, as well as planning and decision-making processes. Key proponents of this approach include Public Health Canada, but it has also been used to implement Equality Impact Assessments as part of the Equality Act 2010 in the UK. GBA helps to identify and clarify the differences between women and men, boys and girls, and demonstrates how these differences affect access to, and interaction with, social policy initiatives.

Gender-creative children identify and express their gender in ways that differ from what others may expect. They are also sometimes referred to as gender non-conforming, gender variant, gender independent or transgender.

Gender dysphoria describes the discomfort or distress a person experiences because there is a mismatch between their biological sex and gender identity. The term is used by psychiatrists as a diagnosis in the Diagnostic and Statistical Manual (DSM-V) and replaces the term previously used, 'gender identity disorder'. There is some controversy about the term as it medicalises people's experiences and feelings, but the diagnosis also provides access to treatment and care.

Gender identity refers to an individual's personal and subjective experience of being male, female or gender creative

Gender-transgressive *see* **Gender-creative**

Guru: the head of the *hijra* household who initiates a new entrant (*chela* or disciple) into the *hijra* community through different rituals. The *guru–chela* [mentor–disciple] relationship is an important aspect of the social organisation of the *hijra* community.

Heteronormativity is a term used by social and cultural theorists to refer to institutions, policies and commonly held assumptions that promote heterosexuality as the norm and preferred sexual orientation.

Heterosexism is a construct or way of thinking that privileges heterosexuality as inherently normal and superior to homosexuality. It is based on the assumption that everyone is, or should be, heterosexual. In contrast to homophobia, which refers to individual fears and prejudice, heterosexism describes a system, in common with other forms of oppression, such as sexism, racism and disablism which intersect with each other.

Heterosexual describes an individual who is emotionally, physically or sexually attracted to people of the opposite sex to themselves. People who are heterosexual often do not describe their sexual orientation in this way, but often think of it as *natural* or *normal*.

Homophobia: the term is derived from the Greek word *phobia* meaning fear. It has often been used to describe the discrimination experienced by LGB people

Homosexual: This term is used infrequently in everyday language by LGB people as it has historically been associated with approaches in psychiatry or medicine which sought to cure or convert LGB people to heterosexuality. Its use often implies pathology.

Hijra: A local language term in India used to refer to a specific trans identity in India with sociocultural, religious connotations. A *hijra* is usually a person who is assigned the male gender at birth (rarely a person with intersex variation), but identifies with the characteristics, roles and behaviours conventionally associated with the female gender. They cross-dress and live their life as a woman or may identify as belonging to a 'third gender'. They may or may not undergo castration and often live in a group with their *guru*. Most *hijras* earn a living through sex work, begging or dancing during festivals and auspicious occasions.

Intersectionality is a term first coined by Kimberle Crenshaw in *Critical Race Theory* in 1989 and is increasing in its popular usage. Intersectionality describes the conjunctions or meeting points of different forms of oppression. The term recognises that people occupy multiple, not singular identities, and they may consequently have different experiences and outcomes. For example, a Black lesbian's experiences of poverty and unemployment may differ from those of a white lesbian; she may have had fewer educational advantages, access to fewer financial resources and less social capital. It is likely she will experience both racism and heterosexism.

Intersex is variation in sex characteristics including chromosomes or genitals that do not allow an individual to be distinctly identified as male or female. Such variation may involve genital ambiguity or different combinations of chromosomes other than XY-male and XX-female.

Kothi is in common usage across India and refers to men who take a feminine role in same-sex relationships.

La Pasión is a model used with Spanish-speaking gay men in Canada which social workers can adopt for intervening in HIV prevention knowledge.

Lesbian is a woman who is romantically, sexually or emotionally attracted to other women and is derived from the name of the Greek island of Lesbos in recognition of the writings of the poet Sappho. Some women prefer the words 'queer' or 'gay' to describe themselves.

Men who have sex with men is the term used to categorise men who engage in sexual behaviours with other men regardless of how they identify themselves and it can describe gay, bisexual and heterosexual men. The term was created by epidemiologists in the 1990s to identify the prevalence and transmission of HIV.

Minority stress is a conceptual framework developed by Ilan Meyer (2003) to explain how stigma, prejudice and discrimination create a social environment which may cause mental health problems

Persons assigned gender female at birth: This term is used in India and reflects the understanding that none of us is born with a ready-made gender; gender is assigned to us at birth based on the traditional conflation of sex, in particular external genitalia. This assigned gender may or may not match our own sense of our gender. (See **Trans** and **Gender-creative** for comparable terms.)

Pride is an event, born out of activism against discrimination and invisibility of LGBT people, which is often held annually in June to commemorate the Stonewall riots in New York in 1969 which led to Gay Liberation Movements of the 1970s. More recently, Pride has become a celebration of LGBT rights and positive identities, but there is recognition that in many countries worldwide, being LGBT is illegal and may be punishable by imprisonment or death.

Queer was a term of abuse in the late 19th century and by the early 20th century it had been reclaimed and redefined. In the 1990s it became a popular term to describe a radical theory and politics. Queer theory rejects the notion of fixed and stable identities and a number of queer theorists were heterosexual (eg Eve Kosofsky-Sedgwick). Other queer theorists, (Judith Butler, Jack Halberstam) argued that gender is a performance and that it is socially constructed.

Social capital describes the personal and collective resources that improve one's educational, economic and social position.

Trans and **transgender** are terms which describe a person who does not conform to the traditional binary presentation of what it means to be male or female. Trans includes a range of different identities and behaviour and refers to an individual's own sense of self and not who they are attracted to. Trans people may be heterosexual, lesbian, gay, bisexual or asexual. It is an umbrella term to denote people who are transsexual, transgender or transvestite. Some trans people may seek gender reassignment surgery including genital reconstruction, others may take hormonal treatments to change their body form while others, blend their gender presentation (see also **Gender-creative**).

Transition(ing): the process of changing one's gender from that assigned at birth to one which accords with an individual's internal sense of gender. A **trans woman** (or **trans man**) is someone who is going through (or has completed) the process of changing the gender they were assigned at birth to their perceived gender. Their new gender is the 'opposite' to that assigned at birth.

[Note, however, that the meaning of 'transition' in Chapter Five refers to a process or period of changing from one state to another (in this case transition out of the public care).]

Transphobia describes the discrimination expressed towards people who do not conform to society's traditional expectations about gender.

Yogyakarta Principles: These principles form a charter or universal guide to LGBT human rights which was drawn up by a group of lawyers who met in Yogyakarta, Indonesia in 2007. They have since informed the United Nations formal recognition of LGBT rights as human rights in 2012 in the document *Born Free and Equal*.

Notes on contributors

Kathryn Almack is a senior research fellow in the School of Health Sciences at the University of Nottingham, UK. She is a sociologist whose research interests encompass the dynamics and diversity of people's friendship and family lives. Kathryn is leading a two-year, UK-wide project (2012–14) entitled 'Last outing: exploring end of life experiences and care needs in the lives of older LGBT people', funded by the Marie Curie Cancer Care Research Programme, and pilot research exploring bisexual ageing.

Tyler M. Argüello is an assistant professor in the Division of Social Work at California State University, Sacramento, USA. His chapter is based on his research for his doctoral dissertation on identities, sex/uality and the 'logic of objects' in the production and prevention of health disparities. Currently, Tyler is studying HIV historical trauma, intergenerational divides and queer populations. He is a diplomate in clinical social work and is a licensed clinical social worker.

Louis Bailey is a research fellow in health inequalities in the Centre for Health and Population Sciences at Hull York Medical School, UK. He is a medical sociologist specialising in the lifecourse, ageing and end of life. His research explores the cumulative impact of health inequalities on marginalised and minority populations as well as the interaction of gender identity, disembodiment and (social) death.

Gerardo Betancourt is a PhD student in the Factor–Inwentash Faculty of Social Work at the University of Toronto, Canada. He is also an AIDS community educator at the HIV Prevention Program at the Centre for Spanish Speaking Peoples. Current interests include community-based research in sex and gender health disparities, health interventions, intersectionality, HIV prevention and immigrants' health.

Elizabeth Breshears is an associate professor of social work at California State University, Stanislaus, USA. Her research uses a strengths perspective to explore societal changes that can help to address social inequalities. She focuses on the oppression of marginalised and vulnerable populations, particularly children and lesbian, gay, bisexual and trans (LGBT) older people. Recent publications include an article (co-authored with Valerie Leyva) 'Assessing the efficacy of LGBT cultural competency training for aging services providers in California's Central Valley' in (2014) *Journal of Gerontological Social Work* 57, 2–4.

Nicola Carr is a lecturer in the School of Sociology, Social Policy and Social Work at Queen's University Belfast. She has been chair of EPIC, a national organisation in the Republic of Ireland representing young people with care experience. She is a co-author of the first national study on LGBT mental health and wellbeing in the Republic of Ireland – *Supporting LGBT lives* (Mayock et al, Gay and Lesbian Equality Network and BeLonG To Youth Services, 2009).

Andy Dunlap is an assistant professor of social work at Elizabethtown College in Elizabethtown, PA, USA. He is a clinical social worker specialising in late adolescence and early adulthood and he teaches social work practice classes. His research focuses on understanding the coming-out process for LGBT people and how it has changed over time.

Diane E. Elze is an associate professor of social work at the University at Buffalo, NY, USA, where she also directs the Master of Social Work Program. She has spent most of her professional career working with and on behalf of LGBT young people. Her research and publications have focused on risk and protective factors for, and service delivery to, lesbian, gay, bisexual, trans and queer (LGBTQ) young people.

Julie Fish was joint convener (with Kate Karban) between 2010 and 2014 of the Social Work and Health Inequalities Network, an association of over 300 social work academics and practitioners from 25 countries worldwide, who seek to combat the causes and consequences of socially created physical and mental health inequalities. She has conducted research in LGBT health and social care inequalities for 18 years, recently completing an Economic and Social Research Council (ESRC) knowledge exchange project (RES-192-22-0111) with Macmillan and Breast Cancer Care. In 2012, her book *Social work and lesbian, gay, bisexual and trans people: Making a difference* was published by Policy Press. She is Director of the Mary Seacole Research Centre.

Kate Karban is a senior lecturer in social work at the University of Bradford, UK. She was a co-author of *Confronting prejudice: Lesbian and gay issues in social work education* (Logan et al, Ashgate, 1996) and has written and researched about mental health and interprofessional learning. She was joint convenor of the Social Work and Health Inequalities Network, with Julie Fish, between 2010 and 2014.

Andrew King is a lecturer in sociology at the University of Surrey, UK. He is a sociologist whose research interests are in the intersection of ageing, sexuality, gender and citizenship. He has conducted research funded by the ESRC to enable service providers to find ways to improve services for older LGBT people. He has published widely in this research area.

Hans Knutagård has served as a senior lecturer in social work at Kristianstad University, Sweden since 2011. He has been working for 30 years as both a social work practitioner and a theoretician. His current research revolves around social work, sexualities and health inequalities, especially for LGBT people, focusing on areas such as male rape, male sex work, HIV/AIDS, honour-related violence and hate crime.

Valerie Lester Leyva is an associate professor of social work at California State University, Stanislaus, USA. Active research areas include the needs of older LGBT people in residential care, trans young people and civilian reintegration of military veterans. A recent article, with Elizabeth Breshears – 'Assessing the efficacy of LGBT cultural competency training for aging services providers in California's Central Valley' – has been published in (2014) *Journal of Gerontological Social Work* 57, 2-4.

Tracey Maegusuku-Hewett is a senior lecturer in social work at Swansea University, UK. Her research interests include sexuality and equality; child welfare and rights; and the social work response to immigration and asylum. Tracey and colleagues at Swansea University have recently completed a study examining the provision of inclusive and anti-discriminatory services to older lesbian, gay and bisexual-identifying people in residential care environments in Wales.

Kimberley Ens Manning is associate professor of political science at Concordia University, Montreal, Canada. She is principal investigator of a Canadian Social Sciences and Humanities Research Council team research project designed to develop new research and community resources in support of gender-creative children and their families. She also teaches and conducts research related to gender and politics in the People's Republic of China.

Bridget Moss is education and research director at St Helena Hospice, Colchester, UK. Her research interests include the impact of health and illness on LGBT relationships, including children, and how this relates to the changing landscape of health and social care. Bridget is a nurse and a teacher by background and has held positions within clinical practice and education.

Nick J. Mulé is an associate professor in the School of Social Work at York University, Canada. His research interests include the social inclusion/exclusion of LGBTQ populations in social policy and service provision. He also engages in critical analysis of the LGBTQ movement and the development of queer liberation theory. A queer activist, Nick is currently the founder and chairperson of Queer Ontario. Additionally, he is a psychotherapist serving LGBTQ populations in Toronto.

Andrea Nagy is a PhD candidate in educational sciences at the University of Innsbruck, Austria and research assistant in social work at the Free University of Bozen/Bolzano, Italy. Her research areas include access to social services, care leavers, LGBT issues in social work and regional lesbian feminist culture.

Urban Nothdurfter is a PhD candidate in comparative social work at the University of Trento, Italy and research fellow at the Free University of Bozen/Bolzano, Italy. His research interests lie mainly in the interface between social policy development and professional social work practice. He also works on social work history and on LGBT topics.

John Pinkerton is professor of child and family social work at Queen's University Belfast, UK. He was the principal investigator in a government-funded Northern Ireland baseline study of young people leaving state care in the early 1990s and has continued to write and undertake research on the subject since then. He is a founding member of the International Research Network on Transitions to Adulthood from Care (INTRAC).

Annie Pullen Sansfaçon is an associate professor of social work at the Université de Montréal, Canada. She obtained her PhD at De Montfort University in the UK, where she specialised in ethics and social action. In her work, she has applied social action methodologies as a tool for ethical practice, with various oppressed populations, including families of trans young people.

Michele Raithby is a senior lecturer in social work at Swansea University, UK. After practising as a generic social worker, she specialised in adult care, then the regulation and inspection of residential care settings before undertaking further research and moving into social work education. Her research interests include social work with older people, sexuality in adult social care, and reflective practice in social work education.

Ketki Ranade is assistant professor at the Centre for Health and Mental Health, School of Social Work, Tata Institute of Social Sciences, Mumbai, India. She is member of LABIA (www.labiacollective.org), a queer feminist LBT collective in Mumbai. Ketki has worked for a decade within the mental health service sector and has also conducted research studies on the use of reparative/conversion treatments for homosexuality by healthcare providers, understanding gay-affirmative approaches to counselling LGBTQ clients and familial responses to same-sex sexuality of a family member.

Mitchell Rosenwald is an associate professor of social work at Barry University, Florida, USA. His practice experience includes working with LGBTQ young people, child welfare and mental health. He is the co-author of *Advocating for children in foster and kinship care* (with Beth N. Riley, Columbia University Press, 2010). Currently, Mitchell is the president of the National Association of Social Workers, Florida Chapter.

Susan Saltzburg is an associate professor of social work at Ohio State University, USA. Her clinical and community work with LGBTQ young people and families has been instrumental in shaping scholarship and teaching. Her areas of interest are family adjustment to coming out, LGBT young people, preparing students for LGBT practice, and narrative therapy. Susan currently serves as co-chair of the Council on Sexual Orientation and Gender Identity of the Council on Social Work Education (CSWE).

Ala Sirriyeh is a lecturer in sociology in the School of Sociology and Criminology at Keele University, UK. Her research is centred in the field of migration and refugee studies, particularly with reference to children, young people, gender, identities and personal relationships.

Her recent book *Inhabiting borders, routes home: Youth, gender, asylum* (Ashgate, 2013) explored young refugee women's narratives of home and transitions to adulthood.

Tes Smith is business development manager for Essex Carers, UK. Her research interests include how people manage long-term conditions and access care services and the responsiveness of care providers to differing needs of the community. A social worker by background, Tes has held a variety of positions in adult social care and as national social care lead, most recently as the social care programme manager for Macmillan Cancer Support.

Yiu-Tung Suen is assistant professor in the Department of Sociology at the Chinese University of Hong Kong, Hong Kong. His research examines the lived experiences of sexual minority groups, noting the influences of *historical time*, with his research on older gay men, and *space*, studying LGBT issues in care homes and universities. His sites of research currently include the UK and Hong Kong.

Sue Westwood has qualifications in gerontology, law, and gender, sexuality and human rights. A freelance trainer, researcher, organisational consultant and occasional tutor in the Law School at Keele University, UK, Sue is also completing a PhD in law. Her research explores equality issues in relation to ageing, gender and sexuality from a feminist socio-legal perspective.

Paul Willis is a senior lecturer in social work at Swansea University, UK. His practice experience includes supporting LGBQ young people in counselling and community development roles in rural Tasmania. His research interests include sexuality and care, sexuality and ageing, and the social identities and wellbeing of LGBQ young people. Paul is co-chair of the UK Sexuality in Social Work Interest Group.

Elizabeth A. Winter is a clinical assistant professor of social work in the Child Welfare Education and Research Programs at the University of Pittsburgh, USA. She previously worked in the human services provider community and still maintains a clinical practice. Her interests include LGBTQ people in child welfare, child welfare workforce development, the treatment of addictions and traumatic stress.

Foreword

Gary Bailey

I am delighted to have been asked to write the foreword for this book, *Lesbian, gay, bisexual and trans health inequalities: International perspectives in social work*, especially because I have lived my life as an openly gay male of African descent in the United States. Over the years I have had the opportunity to watch the emergence of the lesbian, gay, bisexual, trans and queer (LGBTQ) community from the shadows, while at the same time participating in the work needed to ensure that globally all LGBTQ people are able to live out their lives safely, healthily and openly.

Recent anti-LGBTQ actions in India, Russia and Uganda, as well as heated protests and resistance in France as the government there moved to make same-sex marriage legal and allow same-sex couples to adopt, show that there is still work to be done. According to an article that appeared in *The Guardian* newspaper in November 2013, currently 41 out of 53 Commonwealth countries have laws that allow for discrimination of LGBTQ people and more importantly this topic is not on their agenda (Davidson, 2013).

The primary mission of the social work profession is to enhance human wellbeing and help to meet the basic human needs of all people, with particular attention to the needs and empowerment of people who are vulnerable, oppressed and living in poverty. A historic and defining feature of social work is the profession's focus on individual wellbeing in a social context and the wellbeing of society. Fundamental to social work is attention to the environmental forces that create, contribute to and address problems in living.

As professional social workers we know that individuals who are lesbian, gay, bisexual or trans are members of every community. LGBT people are diverse, come from all walks of life and include people of all races, ethnicities and ages, they are from all socioeconomic statuses and they exist in all parts of the globe.

In addition to considering the needs of LGBT people in programmes designed to improve the health of entire communities, there is also a need for culturally competent medical care and prevention services that are specific to this population. Social inequality is often associated with poorer health status, and sexual orientation has been associated with multiple health threats. Recent research shows that members of the LGBT community are at an increased risk for a number of health threats when compared to their heterosexual peers. Differences in sexual behaviour account for some of these disparities, but others are associated with social and structural inequities, such as the stigma and discrimination that LGBTQ populations experience. The unique perspectives and needs of LGBTQ people should be routinely considered in public health efforts to improve the overall health of every person and eliminate health disparities. At the same time, we must also take into account that many of us exist in the intersection of competing 'isms' and systemic racism and the glaring contradiction that, globally, women and black and minority ethnic people continue to face means that they linger behind the progress made by the larger LGBTQ community in areas such as income, education and training.

In 2011, in the book *Social determinants and mental health* (Bährer-Kohler, 2011), I wrote:

> The social determinants of health are viewed by many as the conditions into which people are born, grow, live, work and age, including the health system. In large part these circumstances are shaped by the distribution of money, power and resources at global, national and local levels, which are themselves influenced by policy choices. The social determinants of health are mostly responsible for health inequities – the unfair and avoidable differences in health status seen within and between countries. (Bailey, 2011, p 12)

Erich Fromm (1955, p 27), in his classic book, *The sane society*, proposed that:

> [H]ealth in a comprehensive sense, and free and full development of human potential seem unattainable in the existing social context … when people are forced to adjust to an insane reality which frustrates their material, social, and psychological needs, they tend to develop various forms of ill health and to defend themselves by escaping or by acting aggressively … the insanity of the current social context is insane.

The World Health Organization (WHO), responding to increasing concern about these persisting and widening inequities, established the Commission on Social Determinants of Health (CSDH) in 2005 to provide advice on how to reduce them. The commission's final report was launched in August 2008, and contained three overarching recommendations:

- improve daily living conditions;
- tackle the inequitable distribution of power, money, and resources;
- measure and understand the problem and assess the impact of action (CSDH, 2008, p 2).

The International Federation of Social Workers' (IFSW) policy statement on health asserts that:

> Health is an issue of fundamental human rights and social justice and binds social work to apply these principles in policy, education, research and practice. All people have an equal right to enjoy the basic conditions which underpin human health. These conditions include a minimum standard of living to support health and a sustainable and health promoting environment. All people have an equal right to access resources and services that promote health and address illness, injury and impairment, including social services. IFSW demands and works towards the realization of these universal rights through the development, articulation and pursuit of socially just health and social policies. (IFSW, 2008)

Sometimes we are confronted by poor outcomes and just scratch our heads and reflect on the negatives associated with the data. One wonders whether we truly expect the outcome to change if we continue to do things the same way. Wasn't it Albert Einstein who said: 'Insanity is doing the same thing over and over again and expecting different results'?

As professional social workers we promote social justice and social change with and on behalf of our clients and the communities in which they live and circumstances in which they exist. The term 'clients' is used inclusively to refer to individuals, families, groups, organisations and communities. We are challenged to be aware of and sensitive to cultural and ethnic diversity and strive to end discrimination, oppression, poverty and other forms of social injustice. These activities may be in the form of:

- direct practice;
- community organising;
- supervision;
- consultation;
- administration;
- advocacy;
- social and political action;
- policy development and implementation;
- education;
- research and evaluation.

As social workers we seek to enhance the capacity of people to address their own needs. We also seek to promote the responsiveness of organisations, communities and other social institutions to individuals' needs and social problems.

> Human rights condenses into two words, the struggle for dignity and fundamental freedoms which allow the full development of human potential. (IFSW, 1996)

IFSW as an organisation is an advocate for the recognition of LGBTQ individuals' human rights. It has continuously articulated its support for the rights of lesbians and gay men to have families, and to keep their own children, and its support for their rights to adoption. It has supported same-sex marriage and endorsed long-term partners' rights to the same benefits afforded to those in so-called traditional marriages.

The Reverend Dr Martin Luther King, Jr once said: 'Injustice anywhere is a threat to justice everywhere. We are caught in an inescapable network of mutuality, tied in a single garment of destiny. Whatever affects one directly, affects all indirectly. (Letter from Birmingham jail, 16 April 1963, available from: http://abacus.bates. edu/admin/offices/dos/mlk/letter.html). The journey to equal justice continues ... so in the spirit of Martin Luther King's letter from Birmingham jail, I would encourage us to take what action we can as there is work for us all to do

This new book presents the reader with exciting opportunities to develop international theoretical and practice perspectives about the contribution of social work to reducing LGBT health inequalities.

References

Bährer-Kohler, S (ed), 2011, *Social determinants and mental health*, Hauppauge, NY: Nova Science Publishers

Bailey, P, 2011, 'Social determinants and mental health – an international perspective', in S. Bährer-Kohler (ed) *Social determinants and mental health*, Hauppauge, NY: Nova Science Publishers, 9-14

CSDH (Commission on Social Determinants of Health), 2008, *Closing the gap in a generation: Health equity through action on the social determinants of health* (Marmot review), Geneva: World Health Organization, http://whqlibdoc.who.int/publications/2008/9789241563703_eng_contents.pdf

Davidson, H, 2013, 'Homosexuality illegal in 41 out of 53 Commonwealth countries – report', *The Guardian*, 10 November, www.theguardian.com/world/2013/nov/10/homosexuality-illegal-in-41-out-of-53-commonwealth-countries-report

Fromm, E, 1955, *The sane society*, New York, NY: Rinehart

IFSW (International Federation of Social Workers), 1996, 'Human rights', http://ifsw.org/policies/human-rights-policy/

IFSW, 2008, 'Health', www.ifsw.org/p38000081.html

In solidarity,
Gary Bailey
Professor of Practice at Simmons College School of Social Work and Simmons College School of Nursing & Health Studies, Boston, MA, USA
President, International Federation of Social Workers, 2010–14

Introduction: social work's contribution to tackling lesbian, gay, bisexual and trans health inequalities

Julie Fish and Kate Karban

The international mandate for social work's role in tackling health inequalities

The social conditions of people's lives have a cumulative impact on their health and wellbeing. A child born in Sierra Leone may live to the age of 40, while a child born in Japan can expect to live to 83 years (Bywaters et al, 2009). Such differences in life expectancy are known as health inequalities; these 'lost' years of life are a consequence not solely of poor health services, but also of people's social and material circumstances (for example, diet, education, the quality of housing and the nature of employment).

Health inequalities emerged as a global concern in the early 21st century, notably in the work of Marmot (for example, CSDH, 2008; Marmot, 2010) and Wilkinson and Pickett (2009). However, social work's contribution to addressing them has been only recently acknowledged, for example in the Rio Declaration 2011 – a commitment by 125 governments worldwide to take action against health inequalities – and in the Global Agenda for Social Work and Social Development - in which over 3,000 social work practitioners, educators and researchers launched a global movement to meet joint aspirations for social justice (IFSW et al, 2012). Together with the International Federation of Social Workers' (IFSW) policy statement on health (IFSW, 2008), social work practice and education have made explicit commitment to the highest attainable standard of health as a fundamental human right and a matter of social justice. Mitigating the impact of poverty and social disadvantage is a core concern of social work around the globe; supporting people to manage the tasks of daily living and maintain their family and support networks makes a key contribution to their social care outcomes and, consequently, to their health. As the IFSW statement articulates, social workers 'in all settings are engaged in health work whether in creating the conditions for improved health chances or working alongside people to manage the impact of poor health on themselves or those close to them' (IFSW, 2008).

But it is not only the material conditions of people's lives that influence their physical health and mental wellbeing; the effects of discrimination and oppression arising from people's social position, including their gender, ethnicity, age or disability, are recognised as having a profound impact on their quality of life. Prejudice and discrimination limit the lives of lesbian, gay, bisexual and trans (LGBT) people and contribute to unequal health outcomes; this book explores how social work can address LGBT health inequalities and promote positive social care outcomes.

In the next section of this introductory chapter, we consider six conceptual frameworks commonly used to theorise about, or as an approach to inform research in, health inequalities. Taking each in turn, we examine the implications of the approach in understanding LGBT health inequalities. In the third section, we discuss the nature, role and purpose of social work intervention with LGBT people and illustrate how social work contributes to the six Marmot policy objectives and to tackling LGBT health inequalities. In the final sections we put forward some implications for social work education and research, conclude this chapter and outline the structure of this book.

Understanding LGBT health inequalities through six conceptual frameworks

A population-based approach to health inequalities

Population-based research, as its name implies, aims to improve the health of populations. Commonly utilised in the field of public health, it is an approach that typically draws on large-scale data to illustrate differences, between groups of people, in their health experiences (people's access to healthcare or susceptibility to ill-health) and health outcomes (the likelihood of living a long and healthy life). The example at the start of this chapter illustrates disparities in longevity between people in different social classes and societies. Population-based approaches have compared the health status of LGBT people with that of their heterosexual counterparts; studies reveal an increased likelihood of mental distress, self-harm and suicidal behaviour, substance misuse and increased prevalence of certain cancers (for example, Conron et al, 2010; Alvy et al, 2011; Hagger-Johnson et al, 2013).

In several countries, population-based studies have been influential in policy making in LGBT health and social care. In the United States (US), Healthy People 2020 – the federal government's prevention agenda for increasing the health of the nation – includes LGBT people as a priority group; and in the UK, the Public Health Outcomes Framework includes an LGBT companion document, which sets out priority health needs (Williams et al, 2013). Elsewhere, the Australian state of Victoria implemented an action plan to tackle LGBT health inequalities (McNair, 2003) and there have been similar initiatives led by Rainbow Health Ontario in CanadaOntario – a programme designed to improve access to services and promote the health of Ontario's LGBT communities. Although population studies provide important evidence about LGBT health, particularly in the US, in the UK and other countries there are a limited number of large-scale or government surveys that include LGBT people in their datasets. Consequently, in many countries worldwide, population-based approaches are still in their infancy for LGBT health and social care.

The social determinants of health

The social determinants of health (SDoH) approach has been promoted by the World Health Organization (CSDH, 2008). It offers a 'good fit' with social work because the conceptual framework recognises the relatively limited role of medical care in reducing mortality and the broad range of factors that lead to poor health outcomes (Moniz, 2010, p 310). Social work is committed to tackling the complex social problems that lie at the heart of health inequalities and is dedicated to rooting out the social injustice that gives rise to them. The SDoH approach acknowledges the multiple factors influencing health and wellbeing, including 'government policy, social and economic conditions, societal norms and values, social position, social cohesion, psychosocial behaviours and access to health care' (CSDH, 2008, p 43).

Although the model acknowledges that social position (for example, gender, race and ethnicity) has an influence on the distribution of health and wellbeing, sexual orientation and gender identity are not recognised (Logie, 2012). This is a serious omission; social factors have a determining influence on the everyday lives of LGBT people and limit their ability to live a flourishing life. These factors include:

- the sociopolitical context in their home country, including the lack of policy initiatives for LGBT health and social care;

- the cultural and societal norms and values that privilege heterosexuality;
- incidents of homophobic bullying in schools, which affect young LGBT people's educational attainment;
- material circumstances, including social exclusion and homelessness.

In Chapter One, Mulé examines social work's contribution to tackling the impact of social 'problems' on health, through the profession's implicit recognition of social determinants, including homelessness, survival sex work, suicidality, depression, substance use and the human immunodeficiency virus (HIV).

An intersectional approach to LGBT health inequalities

As discussed earlier, population-based approaches have established the construct of LGBT health inequalities by revealing that LGBT people's health experiences and outcomes differ from those of their heterosexual counterparts. But in doing so, the focus on intergroup differences (that is, between LGBT people and their heterosexual counterparts) has obscured intragroup differences (that is, the differences within LGBT communities, for example in terms of race, disability and age). The effect has been to constitute LGBT communities as homogenous and may potentially re-inscribe pathology (Terry, 1999). For example, although levels of smoking and drinking are proportionately higher among some LGBT communities than among heterosexual communities, not everyone who is LGBT is a smoker.

By contrast, intersectionality recognises that people do not occupy singular identities; instead, it draws attention to the multiple social positions that people occupy simultaneously. It recognises the interconnections of gender, race and class, which require a nuanced understanding of health experiences in relation to complex social identities. While white gay and bisexual men are more likely to have attempted suicide, evidence suggests that black and minority ethnic (BME) gay and bisexual men are less likely to have done so (King et al, 2003). This difference may be explained by cultural or religious taboos about suicide, by the relatively small proportions of BME gay and bisexual men in the study or by different attitudes towards suicide by LGBT people from BME communities. An intersectional approach seeks to understand the protective factors for LGBT people from BME communities and explore their health beliefs and behaviours (Fish, 2008). Race, disability, class and gender have an impact on people's experiences of discrimination and access to social capital, that is, the personal and collective resources that improve one's educational, economic and social position (Makadon, 2011). Intersectional approaches in LGBT health research uncover distinctive experiences within LGBT communities – for example, in secondary analysis of the Canadian Community Health Survey of 90,310 people, bisexual people are more likely to report fair/poor health than heterosexual people (Veenstra, 2011) – and greater barriers to healthcare (Conron et al, 2010). In Chapter Four, Maegusuku-Hewett and colleagues use the intersectional approach to discuss the impact of mental distress in lesbian, gay and bisexual (LGB) people living in rural communities in Wales. Although the intersectional approach has not been used widely in social work, it offers a useful perspective and its theoretical underpinnings are informed by social justice.

Minority stress

'Minority stress', a conceptual framework developed by Meyer (2003), recognises the impact of discrimination in creating a hostile environment, which affects the mental health and wellbeing of LGBT people. For LGBT people there is potentially a toxic combination of the actual experience of prejudice and their own internal response to that stress and this is sometimes described as internalised homophobia, where negative social attitudes contribute to:

• feelings of shame and low self-esteem;
• perceived stigma;
• expectations of rejection;
• discrimination, including differential treatment and violence.

While being careful to avoid linking poor mental health with any intrinsic characteristic of being LGBT, as has been evident historically in the inclusion of 'homosexuality' as a diagnostic category in both the *Diagnostic and statistical manual of mental disorders* (DSM) published by the American Psychiatric Association *and the International classification of diseases and related health problems* (ICD) published by the World Health Organization, there remains an element of risk associated with the minority stress framework in overstating the subjective component of the model, leading to an overemphasis on supporting individuals to 'adjust' their personal coping strategies in order to counteract the adverse circumstances in which they find themselves. However, there is recognition that LGBT people develop resilience and strategies for survival, often through involvement in social groups in the wider LGBT community where they may find support and affirmation.

In Chapter Two, Nagy and Nothdurfter propose that if the mechanisms of oppression based on sexual orientation and gender identity are not recognised by residential care workers, a looked-after child may experience minority stress and their mental and physical health may be damaged. The concept of 'minority stress' is also explored by Carr and Pinkerton in Chapter Five, who argue that it offers something of a corrective to individualised accounts of mental distress among *some* LGBT people. They contend that sexual minority and gender identity status is not solely associated with vulnerabilities and that LGBT young people display considerable resilience in forging positive identities.

An ecosocial approach

An ecosocial approach to health inequalities recognises multiple spheres of influence on individuals, including families, communities and society: 'political economy, political ecology, history class, race/ethnicity and other unjust social relations (for example, involving sexuality, immigration status, disability and geographic location)' (Krieger et al, 2012, p 257). The approach includes the concept of 'embodiment', where the trauma, discrimination and disadvantage of the material world accumulate and are incorporated in the body. The everyday incidents of discrimination experienced by LGBT people can impact on their overall physical and mental wellbeing. The approach has influenced the work of campaigning groups:

- in developing community networks for older people to reduce social isolation, for example, the Queensland Ageing Action Group in Australia;
- in working to challenge homophobic hate crime in Honduras;
- in improving the health of LGBT people, such as the work of the Rainbow Health Campaign in Birmingham and the MindOut Mental Health Project in Brighton and Hove, both in the UK.

A human rights approach

Drawing on the 1948 United Nation's (UN) *Universal Declaration of Human Rights* (UDHR), this approach recognises that fundamental entitlements – including fair and dignified treatment, freedom from discrimination, freedom of expression and the right to peaceful assembly – underpin good health and social wellbeing. Almost 65 years after the declaration, the human rights of LGBT people were recognised by the UN in a ground-breaking document entitled *Born free and equal* (UN, 2012). The document sets out the core legal obligations that all member states must implement and identifies five entitlements and protections for LGBT people. However, the five protections fall short of the 29 rights outlined in the Yogyakarta Principles, a universal guide to LGBT human rights, including social protection and the right to health, which constitute a global charter for LGBT human rights (International Service for Human Rights, 2007).

A human rights approach brings an international perspective to social and political injustices that impact on people's health. In many countries, LGBT people do not enjoy the rights and freedoms contained in the UDHR. In 76 UN member states, consensual same-sex behaviour among adults is criminalised, leading to imprisonment; moreover, in five countries, same-sex behaviour is punishable by the death penalty. A human rights approach recognises that the absence of entitlements, fundamental to humanity, has a detrimental impact on health and wellbeing (Fish and Bewlay, 2010). The approach has relevance for social work by protecting people's entitlement to respect for family and private life, their right not to be treated in a degrading way, their freedom to have control over their lives and their right to fair and equal services from public bodies (Fish, 2009, 2012).

In Chapter Three, Ranade analyses the impact of human rights violations in India. She highlights the role of LGBT non-governmental organisations (NGOs) in human rights campaigns to recognise LGBT people as legitimate citizens of the Indian state. She documents human rights abuses in the form of blackmail, extortion, threats, beatings, sexual assault of gay men, *hijras*,[1] *kothis*[2] and other trans people by the police prior to a 2009 judgment that repealed section 377 of the Indian Penal Code, which criminalises LGBT relationships and identities, but which was subsequently overturned by the Supreme Court in 2013.

Each of these theoretical approaches provides a different lens for identifying and conceptualising LGBT health inequalities. The following section examines the practical ways in which social work can contribute to tackling LGBT social and health inequalities.

Using Marmot's six policy objectives to examine how social work can address LGBT health inequalities

When a social worker intervenes to protect an LGBT young person from homophobic bullying at school or when in care, when a social worker enables a disabled LGBT service user to have a greater ability to manage their own life or when a social worker recognises an older LGBT person's social isolation and identifies strategies to ameliorate it, they are addressing social and health inequalities and contributing to improving quality of life. In everyday practice, these interventions could be described as 'bread and butter' for the profession, but social workers have often been unaware of the benefits for people's health in mitigating the impact of social inequalities (Fish and Karban, 2013).

Understanding that their role with service users not only improves social outcomes, but also contributes health benefits, is not well recognised in social work. This is partly because the existing conceptual frameworks have been developed in the field of public health and their relevance to social work as a discipline is not readily accessible. For this reason, the following six subsections adopt the model identified in a UK review of health inequalities (Marmot, 2010), which builds on social work principles and shares some commonalities with international conceptual frameworks. The seeds for the six objectives were identified in the SDoH model (CSDH, 2008). In the subsections we discuss some examples of the ways in which social workers can address health and social outcomes through preventive interventions for LGBT people across the lifespan.

Giving every child the best start in life

What happens during the early years of a child's life has long-term effects on their health and wellbeing, including their mental health, educational attainment and future economic status. Social work plays a key role in these formative years through family support and early intervention (as a UK example, through initiatives such as the Sure Start, Home-Start and Think Family programmes); safeguarding children from harm and supporting them in public care. Social workers can give children the best start in life by widening the pool of potential substitute parents. Several countries have recently welcomed LGBT people in fostering and adoption services for children who have had a poor start in life or are estranged from their birth family. Research reveals that outcomes for children adopted by LGBT people are positive: they are just as likely to thrive as those adopted by heterosexual couples (for example, Mellish et al, 2013).

In Chapter Two, Nagy and Nothdurfter explore the assumptions of residential social workers towards a young lesbian in their care who believed that she was experimenting sexually and that that this was just a phase. Nagy and Nothdurfter contend that the education of social workers is a potential starting point for a debate on LGBT issues in Italian social work.

Through family support and early intervention initiatives, social workers practise alongside families to support children and young people who are questioning their sexual orientation or are gender non-conforming. Pullen Sansfaçon and Manning discuss social work advocacy for gender-creative children in Chapter Thirteen. As increasing numbers of children and young people transition (i.e undergo the process of changing their gender), social workers will be called on to support and educate parents, teachers and medical providers, and children and young people themselves. Pullen Sansfaçon and Manning found that 'many [gender-creative] children do not get access to care ... because their primary caregivers do not understand what is happening or are too frightened to seek help' (p 226).

Social work makes a key contribution to ensuring that LGBT children and young people receive the best start in life by supporting them to develop positive LGBT identities. Furthermore, social workers play a central role in placing children with adoptive families or in foster care and the process of matching children with families should recognise the skills and abilities of carers whatever their sexual orientation or gender identity.

Enabling young people and adults to maximise their capabilities and have control over their lives

Maximising capabilities and supporting people to have control over their lives is fundamental to social work practice. As a global profession, social workers play a key role in ensuring that adults with physical or learning disabilities, people in mental distress, women fleeing domestic violence or older people wishing to remain in their own homes are able to have choice and control over the care they receive. Social work principles of empowerment aim to support people to make a difference in their own lives.

Enabling young LGBT people to reach their potential is a key social work role. Social workers may act in loco parentis to positively support them to achieve full personhood and accommodate feelings of being different. Young LGBT people may be at greater risk of bullying and victimisation than other young people and may suffer from low self-esteem, truant from school, have lower attainment levels and leave education early. The long-term effects may include poor mental health, risk of self-harming behaviour and suicide. The presence of gay–straight alliances in progressive schools in Canada and the US function as a protective resource particularly for LGBT children and young people who are in receipt of services through community-based social workers (Walls et al, 2010). Successful interventions, where social workers and teachers collaborate, which build on or develop the young person's social support networks, provide affirmative support for LGBT young people (Mishna et al, 2009).

In Chapter Five, Carr and Pinkerton explore how social workers can contribute to helping young LGBT people leaving care to realise their full potential through a rights-based approach that acknowledges a young person's sexual orientation. To achieve this, they argue, a young person's in-care experience needs to be thought of as part of an individually 'lived life' in a way that connects it to pre-care and after-care experiences and to a range of emotions and relationships, past, present and future.

Increasingly, social workers in palliative care are called on to enable LGBT people to have some measure of control over their dying: a 'good death' acknowledges their personal and social relationships and enables them to choose the place of their dying and funeral arrangements. In Chapter Ten, Almack and colleagues discuss how LGBT people may have particular support needs following the loss of a partner. They argue that the full extent of their grief and loss may not be acknowledged, which they describe using the concept of 'disenfranchised grief'. When a heterosexual spouse dies, the surviving partner has a recognised social role of widow/er, which carries a certain social status and a permissible range of emotional expression. These kinds of 'privileges' may be denied a same-sex partner.

Mental health inequalities are the focus of two chapters. In Chapter Fourteen, Leyva calls for the development of service delivery systems and evidence-based practice models that take account of the distinctive needs of older LGBT adults in order to improve mental health outcomes. Taking a different approach to understanding mental health inequalities, in Chapter Four, Maegusuku-Hewett and colleagues report on findings from a mixed-method study conducted in Wales. Shaun, one of their study participants, expressed his concern about the lack of support to enable him, as a young LGBT person, to maximise his capabilities and live independently on leaving care: "I was in care all my life and when I came out at 16, the only people who were around me were like social workers and support workers, and I always say like that there's no support for young people who are coming out" (p 90). Shaun's subsequent mental distress may have been reduced had he been able to talk about his sexual orientation to his social worker when he left care.

In Chapter Sixteen, Knutagård considers the impact of the untreated experience of male rape, which prevents men's rightful access to health services, social inclusion and justice. The experience of rape often triggers a destructive trajectory for men, especially in the area of sexual health behaviour. Knutagård argues that men's vulnerability is potentially compounded by lack of recognition and social workers and health services have failed to reach out to this potential service user group. Supporting men to regain a sense of control over their lives following such a trauma is a crucial contribution that social workers can make.

Service users are more likely to achieve good physical and mental health if they are not passive recipients of care but instead are actively involved in decision making about and planning for their own care needs. Maximising outcomes and empowering people to have control over their own lives are underpinning principles of effective social work.

Creating fair employment and good work for all

Being in employment is protective of health; by contrast, adverse working conditions can damage health. Pending protective legislation, in many states of the US and in other countries worldwide it is possible for an LGBT person to be dismissed from employment simply on the grounds that they are LGBT. Unemployment is more common among gay and bisexual men than among heterosexual men. Bisexual people, taking into account their education and employment, are more likely to live in poverty (Conron et al, 2010). Research has revealed that discrimination in the workplace impacts on the productivity and continuation of service of LGBT employees (Ng et al, 2012). A UK workplace poll of LGBT social workers found that four out of 10 said that homophobia was a problem and some had left the profession because of it (*Community Care*, 2012). Tackling workplace cultures and practices is key to creating fair employment for LGBT employees.

Although none of the chapters in this book addresses this Marmot objective, creating fair employment is relevant for both the providers and users of social work services. Stonewall, a UK LGB NGO, has contributed to changing the working environment for LGBT people in the public, voluntary and private sectors through its recently launched global Diversity Champions programme. It recognises that being comfortable about their identities at work can impact positively on staff performance and build the emotional resilience needed in this challenging profession. Strategies include:

- building a strong public commitment;
- creating employee networks;
- role models;
- support groups;
- policies and monitoring;
- embedding equality and diversity so that they cover every aspect of an organisation in order to create a positive workplace culture.

Stonewall's requirement of engaging in local communities means that local authorities, such as Bristol City Council's fostering and adoption team, attend LGBT Pride events to promote their services (Guasp and Balfour, 2009). A number of local authorities and social care organisations are included in Stonewall's current list of 100 top UK employers and this is likely to extend to organisations internationally.

Social workers have a role in supporting service users, including people with mental health problems, to develop the skills necessary to stay in employment and ensuring that informal carers are not financially disadvantaged and supporting people. Social workers also provide support for people with learning disabilities to develop skills for employment and prepare for job applications (Dickson and Gough, 2008). Recognising that LGBT people may be included within these service user groups is essential to achieving this policy objective for all communities.

Ensuring a healthy standard of living for all

The minimum income for healthy living must provide for nutrition, housing, transport, healthcare and maintaining social networks. Having insufficient income is a significant cause of health inequalities. A common myth about LGBT people is that they are wealthier than other social groups. However, studies in the US have found that children in gay- and lesbian-coupled households have poverty rates twice those of children in heterosexual married–couple households (Albelda et al, 2009). Furthermore, the effects of poverty are compounded for LGBT people living in rural areas and for BME gay men living with children (Badgett et al, 2013). Social workers have a pivotal role in making sure that service users have an adequate standard of living for good health and social wellbeing, by:

- supporting them to calculate benefit entitlements;
- signposting them to appropriate support organisations;
- supporting their use of credit unions;
- advising about managing debt.

Access to a healthy standard of living is a key issue for most users of social work services: ill-health may have led to unemployment or poverty or low income may have exacerbated an existing health problem. In Chapter Six, Winter and colleagues examine the impact of homelessness, and in Chapter Eleven, Karban and Sirriyeh consider asylum seekers; both circumstances have a negative impact on the living standards of LGBT people.

For LGBT young people, homelessness often occurs as a consequence of an unsupportive reaction from parents to their coming out. Being homeless undermines LGBT young people's opportunity to become healthy and independent adults and it increases their risks of mental health problems, substance abuse, risky sexual behaviour and the likelihood of being victimised (Rice et al, 2013). In Chapter Six, Winter and colleagues draw attention to the over-representation of LGBT young people in the child welfare system in the US. Ensuring safety and placement stability poses a challenge for social workers as LGBT young people placed out of home risk victimisation because of their sexual orientation or gender identity and are more likely to run away. Winter and colleagues reveal that many LGBT young people report feeling 'safer' on the streets than in group care or in foster homes.

In Chapter Eleven, Karban and Sirriyeh draw attention to the global phenomenon of asylum and expose the destitution experienced by LGBT asylum seekers. They contend that effective social work practice requires sustainable and trusting relationships with local organisations to support partnership working. Developing human rights-based social work practice may entail challenging restrictive immigration legislation and its accompanying ethos.

Creating and developing sustainable places and communities

Good neighbourhoods make a significant difference to the quality of people's life and health; social support within communities is vital in reducing social isolation and preventing loneliness. But LGBT communities are communities of interest, rather than geographic entities. As an alternative to the lack of cultural competence in mainstream services, the voluntary sector plays an essential role in promoting LGBT health and wellbeing (Smith, 2005). Governments in Canada, the UK and beyond recognise that the sector offers a fundamental mechanism in bringing about citizen engagement and the delivery of social care services (Smith, 2005). In Chapter Three, Ranade illustrates that the voluntary social care sector in India has been instrumental in challenging discriminatory legislation and human rights abuses and thereby in improving people's health; while in Chapter One, Mulé highlights the role of NGOs in tackling LGBT health inequalities in Canada.

In the UK, London has the most established LGBT voluntary social care sector, documented in an annual almanac (Kairos in Soho, 2012), which aims to:

- promote LGBT equality and human rights;
- challenge oppression and discrimination;
- build self-determining communities;
- address LGBT needs, specifically health and social care and housing;
- promote an agenda of social change;
- influence law and policy.

The range of issues addressed by the sector (specifically in London, but also in Brighton, Birmingham and Manchester) include:

- violence, safety and hate crime;
- mental health;
- substance misuse;
- domestic violence;
- health, wellbeing and HIV;
- coalition against racism;
- helplines and counselling support;
- housing;
- the social support that is critical to physical and mental wellbeing for specific identity, cultural, religious and ethnic groups within LGBT communities.

In Chapter Eight, Westwood and colleagues illustrate that interventions that provide social support and community links for older LGBT people – including outreach projects such as Opening Doors in London (Knocker, 2012) and Sage in New York (Kling and Kimmel, 2006) – are a necessary means of mitigating the negative health effects of social isolation and enhancing wellbeing. They argue that had support been in place before Gary, the service user in one of the chapter's case studies, became confused, social care professionals may have responded to his deteriorating mental state sooner and advocated on his behalf. In light of Gary's circumstances, social work with older LGBT people should seek guidance and support from older LGBT networks.

In Chapter Seven, Breshears and Leyva document the work of the San Joaquin County Roundtable in California, a collaborative project led by a social worker, which aimed to inform the delivery of culturally competent services for trans older people. Although San Joaquin is only 160 miles from San Francisco, often regarded as the gayest city in the US, for most participants the training was their first introduction to considering the experiences and needs of older LGBT people.

The current contraction of the social care sector in the UK, and in other countries worldwide, may thus have a disproportionate negative impact on the health and wellbeing of LGBT individuals, families and communities because they represent an important social and rights-based resource for LGBT people.

Strengthening the role and impact of ill-health prevention

While the five previous policy objectives aim to tackle the causes of health and social inequalities, this final objective is aimed at addressing unhealthy behaviours. The health behaviours that often lead to long-term conditions – for example cancer and cardiovascular disease – include smoking, alcohol consumption, drug misuse, lack of physical activity and poor diet. These health behaviours are a core concern of social work because they are often a response to, or coping behaviour for, adverse life conditions: people who experience poverty and disadvantage are more likely to smoke (ONS, 2013). Social workers thus play a key role in preventing ill-health by providing targeted interventions for people with chronic conditions.

Substance misuse

The nature and extent of substance misuse in LGBT communities have been a cause for concern over the last 20 years. Alcohol consumption is linked to a number of chronic conditions, including liver disease, increased risk of heart attack and adult-onset diabetes. Smoking increases the risk of lung cancer, is associated with cervical cancer and hastens the onset of acquired immune deficiency syndrome (AIDS) for people living with HIV. Findings from the previously named British Crime Survey (now called the Crime Survey for England and Wales) indicate that substance misuse is higher in LGBT populations in comparison with the general population (Hoare, 2010). Possible explanations for the increased prevalence include minority stress, perhaps leading people to self-medicate their psychological distress with cigarettes or alcohol. An alternative explanation is that young LGBT people may socialise in recreational spaces where cigarettes and alcohol are easily available or where peer norms encourage engagement in these behaviours (Hagger-Johnson et al, 2013).

Cancer

For LGBT people, cancer inequalities exist in relation to:

- early diagnosis, information and support;
- the dignity and respect with which they are treated;
- the management of pain (DH, 2012).

They may have an increased risk for some cancers, specifically anal and breast cancer, and have a lower quality of life in survivorship (DH, 2012). Macmillan social workers and other staff engaged in a collaborative project to develop professional knowledge about LGBT cancer service users identified four ways of promoting recovery in these users:

- understanding the distinctive needs of LGBT cancer service users;
- understanding the attitudes and assumptions of cancer professionals;
- improving access to information and support;
- developing the wider team (Fish, forthcoming).

HIV/AIDS

Social care and social work have made important contributions in the fight against HIV/AIDS. Since the early 1980s, knowledge about the disease, activism to raise public and political awareness and the provision of social support have been achieved largely through LGBT social movements. Since the introduction of effective anti-retroviral therapy, HIV is no longer a death sentence but is now a chronic lifelong condition.

New diagnoses of HIV in 2012 were higher among men who have sex with men than their heterosexual peers; reducing the risk of sexual transmission of the disease remains a social and health priority (CDC, 2013). Being HIV positive is a cancer risk factor, for both AIDS-associated (Karposi's sarcoma, non-Hodgkin lymphoma and invasive cervical cancer) and non–AIDS-associated cancers (lung, vaginal, liver, anal, colorectal and renal cancers) (Burkhalter et al, 2011).

In Chapter Seventeen, Argüello discusses new guidelines for combating HIV, published by the US Centers for Disease Control and Prevention, which recommend that people get smart about HIV, reduce their risk, get tested and start talking about the virus. These efforts prioritise surveillance, early prevention and increased access to linkage to care. Such strategies de-emphasise socioeconomic conditions, environmental conditions and cultural factors that impact on communities' abilities to prevent and/or cope with HIV. Argüello argues that social work is an optimal site to decentre the power and privilege of the HIV industry. Through social welfare research, we can begin asking the obvious question of how we as professionals might, in fact, be contributing to the enduring epidemic.

In Chapter Nine, Betancourt proposes a model, known as *La Pasión*, which social workers can adopt for intervening in HIV prevention knowledge, self-regulation and decision making, and these factors influence whether safe-sex behaviours are present or absent.

HIV specialist social workers provide vital support for people living with AIDS, for example:

- providing help with accessing disability and housing benefits;
- talking to service users about the importance of managing their treatment and taking their medication;
- monitoring service users' wellbeing, recognising that people often experience psychological and emotional distress;
- being aware of the financial impact of HIV in people's lives: people with HIV often experience high levels of poverty.

Many services for men who have sex with men exist in the LGBT voluntary social care sector, for example the Naz Project in London, which provides sexual health and HIV prevention and support services to selected BME communities in the capital.

Implications for social work education and research

Recognising the 'privileged' position that professionals, including social workers, can have with regard to reducing health inequalities, the Marmot review for the World Health Organization (CSDH, p 189) called on schools of social work to incorporate training on the social determinants of health. In Chapter Twelve, Saltzburg contends that the inclusion of curricula content on sexual orientation and gender identity requires a pedagogy for unpacking heterosexist and cisgender bias. She explores how critical self-reflection, narrative therapy and community practice enable students to engage with culturally affirmative LGBT social work practice.

Acknowledging the gaps in research in social work and LGBT health inequalities, in Chapter Fifteen Dunlap discusses a recent study entitled 'Changes in the coming-out process over time' and explores some of the conceptual and practical issues in optimising participation from across sexual minority communities.

Conclusion

We believe that this book makes an important contribution to the development of theory by using relevant conceptual frameworks and models to inform understanding of health inequalities on the grounds of sexual orientation and gender identity. The book brings together two fields of study that hitherto have not been considered together: social work *and* LGBT health inequalities Social work's contribution to reducing health inequalities (in general) is itself an emerging discipline; moreover LGBT service users have often been marginalised in social work. Although health inequalities have been previously considered through a public health lens for sexual minorities (Meyer and Northridge, 2007), for gay and bisexual men (Wolitski et al, 2008) and for LGBT people (Makadon, 2011), no previous publication has taken a social work perspective or been international in scope: this text includes contributory chapters from eight countries worldwide aiming to disrupt assumptions that theory and practice in LGBT health and social care are solely concerns of English–speaking countries.

The structure of the rest of the book

The chapters that follow are organised into three parts.

Part One develops an understanding of the theoretical or policy context surrounding social work with LGBT people from the perspective of the country of location of the contributors: Canada (Chapter One), Italy (Chapter Two), India (Chapter Three) and Wales (Chapter Four).

Part Two addresses practice issues across a broad range of service user groups. Each of the chapters is introduced by a case example and the contributors discuss developments in service delivery or practice that seek to provide equitable services for LGBT people as users of social work services. These involve:

- work with young LGBT people, including those in the care system (Chapters Five and Six);
- work with older LGBT people (Chapters Seven and Eight);
- work with Latino gay male migrants in Canada (Chapter Nine);
- end of life care (Chapter Ten);
- work with LGBT asylum seekers (Chapter Eleven).

Part Three examines some key challenges in embedding sexual orientation and gender identity in education and research. Chapters Twelve and Fourteen, based on the experience in the US of the respective contributors, highlight the shortfall in current social work education curricula regarding LGBT health inequalities. Chapter Thirteen argues that social action research in Canada can achieve good outcomes for and with gender-creative children. Chapters Fifteen to Seventeen offer new approaches to research on LGBT health inequalities. Chapter Fifteen, based on research using internet surveys, offers a positive response to the challenges of accessing a population that can be both difficult to access and hard to define. Chapter Sixteen, based on research with gay and bisexual men who have been raped by men, draws attention to experiences that previously have been invisible, emphasising the need to develop greater understanding of the issues involved and the help and support that may be required. Chapter Seventeen brings together queer theory, visual culture and applied practice, informed by critical communication methodologies, in order to examine approaches to HIV prevention and the implications for self-reflexivity in practice. In the concluding chapter, we reflect on the under-recognised role of social work in tackling social and health inequalities and making a key contribution to equality for those most marginalised in societies across the globe. We anticipate that the book will offer new and creative ideas, to stimulate and inspire the continuing development of social work practice to address LGBT health inequalities, wherever they may live, informed by social justice and human rights

Taken together, the book makes a unique contribution to theory, research, education and practice in social work that seeks to address LGBT health inequalities, promoting narratives of strength, resilience and agency and identifying strategies and approaches that are sensitive to the concerns of LGBT people in many countries worldwide.

Notes

General note on terminology: Terms defined in the glossary appear in **bold** the first time they are used in the main chapters of the text.

[1] See definition of *Hijra* in the glossary.

[2] See definition of *Kothi* in the glossary.

References

Albelda, R, Badgett, MVL, Schneebaum, A and Gates, GJ, 2009, *Poverty in the lesbian, gay and bisexual community*, Los Angeles, CA: The Williams Institute, University of California

Alvy, LM, McKirnan, D, Du Bois, SN, Jones, K, Ritchie, N and Fingerhut, D, 2011, Health care disparities and behavioral health among men who have sex with men, *Journal of Gay & Lesbian Social Services*, 23, 4, 507-22

Badgett, MVL, Durso, LE, Kastanis, A and Mallory, C, 2013, *The business impact of LGBT-supportive workplace policies*, Los Angeles, CA: The Williams Institute, University of California

Burkhalter, JE, Hay, JL, Coups, E, Warren, B, Li, Y and Ostroff, JS, 2011, Perceived risk for cancer in an urban sexual minority, *Journal of Behavioural Medicine*, 34, 157-69

Bywaters, P, McLeod, E and Napier, L (2009) (eds) *Social work and global health inequalities*, Bristol: Policy Press.

CDC (Centers for Disease Control and Prevention), 2013, HIV in the United States: At a glance, www.cdc.gov/hiv/statistics/basics/ataglance.html

Community Care, 2012, Four in ten social workers say homophobia is 'problem in the profession', *Community Care*, 31 July, www.communitycare.co.uk/2012/07/31/four-in-ten-social-workers-say-homophobia-is-problem-in-the-profession/#.UoDJejNFCM9

Conron, KJ, Mimiaga, MJ and Landers, SJ, 2010, A population-based study of sexual orientation identity and gender differences in adult health, *American Journal of Public Health*, 100, 10, 1953-60

CSDH (Commission on Social Determinants of Health), 2008, *Closing the gap in a generation: Health equity through action on the social determinants of health* (Marmot review), Geneva: World Health Organization, http://whqlibdoc.who.int/publications/2008/9789241563703_eng.pdf?ua=1

DH (Department of Health), 2012, National Cancer Patient Experience Survey Programme, London: DH, https://www.gov.uk/government/uploads/system/uploads/attachment_data/file/212860/Cancer-Patient-Experience-Survey-National-Report-2011-12.pdf

Dickson, K and Gough, D, 2008, Supporting people in accessing meaningful work: Recovery approaches in community based adult mental health services, London: SCIE, www.scie.org.uk/publications/knowledgereviews/kr21.asp

Fish, J, 2008, Navigating Queer Street: researching the intersections of lesbian, gay, bisexual and trans (LGBT) identities in health research, *Sociological Research Online*, 13, 1, www.socresonline.org.uk/13/1/12.html

Fish, J, 2009, All things equal? Social work and lesbian, gay and bisexual global health inequalities, in P, Bywaters, L, Napier and E, McLeod (eds) *Social work and global health inequalities: Policy and practice developments*, Bristol: Policy Press, 144-9

Fish, J, 2012, *Social work and lesbian, gay, bisexual and trans people: Making a difference*, Bristol: Policy Press.

Fish, J and Bewley, S, 2010, Using human rights based approaches to conceptualise lesbian and bisexual women's health inequalities, *Health & Social Care in the Community*, 18, 4, 355-62

Fish, J and Karban, K, 2013, Health inequalities at the heart of the social work curriculum, *Social Work Education*, online, doi: 10.180/02615479.2012.742502

Fish, J, forthcoming, Co-producing knowledge about lesbian and bisexual women with breast cancer: messages from a knowledge exchange project, under submission

Guasp, A and Balfour, J, 2009, *Peak performance: Gay people and productivity*, London: Stonewall

Hagger-Johnson, G, Taibjee, R, Semlyen, J, Fitchie, I, Fish, J, Meads, C and Varney, J, 2013, Sexual orientation identity in relation to smoking history and alcohol use at age 18/19: cross-sectional associations from the Longitudinal Study of Young People in England (LSYPE), *BMJ Open*, 3, e002810

Hoare, J, 2010, Annex 2: nationally representative estimates of illicit drug use by self-reported sexual orientation, 2006/07-2008/09 BCS data tables, in J, Hoare and D, Moon (eds) *Drug misuse declared: Findings from the 2009/10 British Crime Survey*, Home Office Statistical Bulletin 13/10, London: Home Office

IFSW (International Federation of Social Workers), 2008, Health, http://ifsw.org/policies/health/

IFSW, International Association of Schools of Social Work and International Council on Social Welfare, 2012, *The Global Agenda for Social Work and Social Development: Commitment to action*, Berne, Switzerland: IFSW, http://ifsw.org/get-involved/agenda-for-social-work/

International Service for Human Rights, 2007, The Yogyakarta Principles: Principles on the application of international human rights law in relation to sexual orientation and gender identity, www.yogyakartaprinciples.org/principles_en.pdf

King, M and McKeown, E, 2003, *Mental health and social wellbeing of gay men, lesbians and bisexuals in England and Wales*, London: Mind

Kling, E and Kimmel, D, 2006, SAGE: New York City's pioneer organization for LGBT elders, in D, Kimmel, T, Rose and S, David (eds) *Lesbian, gay, bisexual and transgender aging*, New York, NY: Columbia University Press, 265-76

Knocker, S, 2012, *Perspectives on ageing lesbians, gay men and bisexuals*, York: Joseph Rowntree Foundation

Krieger, N, Dorling, D and McCartney, G, 2012, Mapping injustice, visualizing equity: why theory, metaphors, and images matter in tackling inequities, *Public Health*, 126, 256-8

Logie, C, 2012, The case for the World Health Organization's Commission on the social determinants of health to address sexual orientation, *American Journal of Public Health*, 102, 7, 1243-6

Makadon, H, 2011, *The health of lesbian, gay, bisexual, and transgender people: Building a foundation for better understanding*, Washington, DC: Institute of Medicine

Marmot, M, 2010, *Fair society, healthy lives: The Marmot review: Strategic review of health inequalities in England post-2010*, The Marmot Review, www.instituteofhealthequity.org/projects/fair-society-healthy-lives-the-marmot-review

Mellish, L, Jennings, S, Tasker, F, Lamb, M and Golombok, S, 2013, *Gay, lesbian and heterosexual adoptive families*, London: British Association for Adoption and Fostering

Meyer, IH, 2003, Prejudice, social stress, and mental health in lesbian, gay, and bisexual populations: conceptual issues and research evidence, *Psychological Bulletin*, 129, 5, 674-97

Meyer, IH and Northridge, ME, 2007, *The health of sexual minorities: Public health perspectives on lesbian, gay, bisexual, and transgender populations*, New York, NY: Springer

McNair, RP, 2003, Lesbian health inequalities: a cultural minority issue for health professionals, *Medical Journal of Australia*, 178, 643-5

Mishna, FA. Newman, PA. Daley, A and Solomon, S, 2009, Bullying of lesbian and gay youth: a qualitative investigation, *The British Journal of Social Work*, 39, 8, 1598-614

Moniz, C, 2010, Social work and the social determinants of health perspective: a good fit, *Health and Social work*, 35, 4, 310-12

Ng, ESW, Schweitzer, L and Lyons, ST, 2012, Anticipated discrimination and a career choice in nonprofit: a study of early career lesbian, gay, bisexual, transgendered (LGBT) job seekers, *Review of Public Personnel Administration*, 32, 4, 332-52

ONS (Office for National Statistics), 2013, *Opinions and Lifestyle Survey, Smoking Habits Amongst Adults*, Newport: ONS, www.ons.gov.uk/ons/dcp171776_328041.pdf

Rice, E, Barman-Adhikari, A, Rhoades, H, Fulginiti, A, Astor, R, Montoya, J, Plant, A and Kordic, T, 2013, Homelessness experiences, sexual orientation, and sexual risk taking among high school students in Los Angeles, *Journal of Adolescent Health*, 52, 6, 773-8

Smith, M, 2005, Diversity and identity in the non-profit sector: lessons from LGBT organizing in Toronto, *Social Policy & Administration*, 39, 5, 463-80

Terry, J, 1999, Agendas for lesbian health: countering the ills of homophobia, in AE, Clarke and VL, Olesen (eds) *Revisioning women, health and healing: Feminist cultural and technoscience*, New York, NY: Routledge, 325-42

UN (United Nations), 1948, *Universal Declaration of Human Rights*, Geneva: UN

UN, 2012, *Born free and equal: Sexual orientation and gender identity in international human rights law*, Geneva: United Nations, Office of the High Commissioner on Human Rights

Veenstra, G, 2011, Race, gender, class, and sexual orientation: intersecting axes of inequality and self-rated health in Canada, *International Journal for Equity in Health*, 10, 3, 1475-9276

Walls, NE, Kane, SB and Wisneski, H, 2010, Gay–straight alliances and school experiences of sexual minority youth, *Youth & Society*, 41, 3, 307-32

Wilkinson, R and Pickett, K, 2009, *The spirit level: Why more equal societies almost always do better*, Harmondsworth: Penguin

Williams, H, Varney, J, Taylor, J, Fish, J, Durr, P and Elan-Cane, C, 2013, *The Lesbian, Gay, Bisexual and Trans Public Health Outcomes Framework companion document*, Manchester: The Lesbian and Gay Foundation, www.lgf.org.uk/policy-research/the-lgbt-public-health-outcomes-framework-companion-document/

Wolitski, RJ, Stall, R and Valdiserri, RO (eds), 2008, *Opportunity: Health disparities affecting gay and bisexual men in the United States*, New York, NY: Oxford University Press

PART ONE

Key issues in social work with LGBT people

ONE

Much to be desired: LGBT health inequalities and inequities in Canada

Nick J. Mulé

Introduction

Canada is commonly seen as a progressive country with its multicultural model, its tolerance for diversity and its sensitised human rights legislation (Elliot and Bonauto, 2005). Although Canada can be commended for the progress it has made in each of these areas, one need only scratch the surface to expose the inequalities and inequities that lie beneath.

Lesbian, **gay**, **bisexual** and **trans** (LGBT) populations are a clear example of a people who were once unrecognised culturally, neither tolerated nor accepted socially, and completely devoid of inclusion in human rights legislation and its ensuing protections in Canada. The last 45 years have seen momentous shifts in each of these areas, so much so that it has produced a near utopian veneer that serves to mask continuing forms of oppression and micro-aggressions that simmer from below. Despite the elevation of Canada's LGBT communities as a recognised population that makes up part of the multicultural fabric of the land, with near full recognition of human rights protection in legislation, LGBT people fall woefully behind the general population with regard to health and wellbeing. HIV/AIDS continues to be the illness-based focus that the Canadian state gives varying degrees of support to, barely recognising the broader health and wellness issues, needs and concerns that affect LGBT Canadians.

Two models have informed health policy in Canada (with international influence), which have progressively focused on diversity, given the multicultural make-up of the country, with varying success:

- the world-renowned 'Health Promotion' model (Government of Canada, 1974), which focused on achieving a healthy lifestyle;
- the internationally regarded Population Health model (Health Canada, 1998, 2001), which more explicitly identifies diverse

populations and attempts to address the social determinants of health (SDoH) (Public Health Agency of Canada, no date).

Neither have completely addressed LGBT people as a population that experiences health inequalities: the former was critiqued for its lack of attention to structural differences; and the latter fell short, due to its over-emphasis on determinants of health at the expense of 'social' aspects – becoming mired in unsatisfactory notions of 'health cause and effects' (Orsini, 2007). Victim blaming becomes the focus in a responsibilisation paradigm backed by social and political forces that, for example, can easily attach responsibility on an individual for becoming infected with HIV, who is presumed armed with information to protect themselves, yet the system pays far less attention to access and understanding of such information, proper use of safe drug-use kits, faulty condoms, 'heat of the moment' behaviours and risky behaviour engaged in by one of the partners, among other complex scenarios. Underscoring such foci is the influence of neoliberalism (Duggan, 2003), which places responsibility squarely on the shoulders of individuals (Lupton, 1999; Petersen and Brunton, 2002), absolving the state of its responsibility (Foucault, 1979; Murray, 2007) to promote and accommodate a healthy citizenry. What is lost in the individualisation of such a concern as health is the welfare state's role in its collective redistribution that is overwhelmingly **cisgendered** and **heteronormatively** framed.

Since the early 2000s, Health Canada – the government department responsible for the national health policy – has attempted to implement a policy development method known as **gender-based analysis** (GBA) (Health Canada, 2003, pp 6-7) or gender mainstreaming. This approach takes **gender** into consideration in all aspects of policy making, including that of policy choices and how they will affect women, even when seemingly gender neutral. Although initially located in Health Canada and influencing the establishment of the Public Health Agency of Canada, GBA, more recently updated to sex-and-gender-based analysis, was also intended to affect all federal policy making (Health Canada, 2010). To date this has not been the case, nor has it taken on a more nuanced understanding of gender, particularly from the perspectives of *gender identity* or gender expression. Despite increased state attention to diversity, including that of gender in health policy throughout the 2000s, simultaneously there was and is a systematically narrowed gaze, if any, given to LGBT health issues.

Most often referenced, when it comes to LGBT health, is HIV/AIDS, which from its crisis-induced emergence in the early

1980s, predominantly affected gay men more so than other groups. Recently, the health issues of trans people have also arisen within healthcare discourses, as several provinces debated the funding of sex reassignment surgery (SRS) and hormone therapy among other publicly funded medical treatments for these populations. Aside from these issues, usually taken up within health circles, there has been little public discussion in Canada regarding the distinctive health needs of LGBT people. Yet, increasingly research has highlighted the extent to which the social location of LGBT communities along with the discrimination and stigmatisation experienced by these populations influence health outcomes. Examples of health disparities, amenable to social work intervention, include:

- higher rates of certain cancers (Fish and Wilkinson, 2003);
- alcohol, drug (Senreich, 2010) and tobacco use;
- reproductive health issues;
- (dis)abilities (Shildrick, 2004);
- specific mental health concerns (Hooghe et al, 2010; Volpp, 2010);
- young people's issues (Toomey and Richardson, 2009);
- older people's issues (Concannon, 2009).

Also, there are larger systemic issues such as barriers to accessing social work and healthcare, professionals' lack of knowledge about and erasure of LGBT people from public health structures and initiatives and so on (Mulé, 2007; Mulé et al, 2009, pp 20-1; Lehavot and Simoni, 2011).

Research into such matters was often spurred by the LGBT community itself who undertook a number of community-based studies as early as the 1990s, then throughout the 2000s increasingly calling attention to their broad health and wellbeing issues (CRHC, 2013; Rainbow Health Ontario, 2013a). Prior to and during this time, non-profit organisations sprung up offering broad health and wellness services, information and coordination apart from the highly established AIDS service organisation (ASO) structures. Yet such LGBT research and organising with regard to broad health and wellness concerns for these populations fly largely under the radar of formalised policy structures (Smith, 2007). The existence of LGBT people in society is marked with marginalising effects by their absentia in public policy. Implications of such erasure can be felt materially due to a lack of funding, programmes and services (Carabine, 2004a; Mulé, 2005). In essence, this has heteronormalising implications in which heterosexuality, by its very presence and acknowledgement in public policy, is reified as the norm, casting notions of abnormality on sexualities that fall outside such narrowed discourse (Carabine, 2004b).

This chapter explores the hidden lacunae, highlighting the paradox of Canada's commitment to health policy templates that purport population-based health and SDoH matters, and the state's lack of substance in considering the broad health issues of LGBT people. A brief description of how public health is administered in Canada is provided, followed by how such broad LGBT health issues are taken up in light of the continued dominant focus on HIV/AIDS regarding health issues and LGBT communities. Variances in approaches across a number of Canadian provinces and municipalities are reviewed. How social work is implicated by the governance of these issues both by the Canadian state and by the profession's governance structure in Canada and internationally is discussed. An argument is then made, based on a critical analysis of Canada's surface consideration of LGBT people, for a more substance-driven alignment with health policy templates that would provide meaningful health and social care benefits.

Structural landscape of public health administration in Canada

In Canada, federal health policy discourse and action are governed by federal departments Health Canada as well as the Public Health Agency of Canada, respectively charged with overseeing and providing guidelines for health and public health. These federal bodies are responsible for national discourses, perspectives and models that shape conceptualisations of health and healthcare in Canada, which have and continue to wield international influence. While the federal government does not engage in direct delivery of health services to most Canadians, it plays a lead role in developing and disseminating macro-level discourse, healthcare strategies and funding that influence healthcare delivery at the provincial/territorial level where healthcare is administered. The focus of this chapter, for the most part, is at the national level and the influence the Canadian federal government has on addressing the health issues of LGBT populations, while also featuring how a number of provinces and communities are innovating to address the same.

An illness-based HIV/AIDS focus – broader LGBT health issues overshadowed

Since 1990, the Canadian government has spent millions of dollars on numerous AIDS strategies and initiatives (CIHR, 2008). Over the years, government attention to the illness has resulted in a highly structured system of ASOs at the federal, provincial/territorial and municipal levels attempting to contain the spread of the virus and provide supports for those affected. Although Canada has benefited greatly from anti-retroviral drugs that have essentially changed the dynamics of the virus from a terminal illness to a chronic illness managed with medications (CATIE, 2013), HIV/AIDS continues to dominate the LGBT health focus. While the Canadian AIDS initiative has become so established and essentialised, broader health and wellness concerns of the LGBT communities have been neglected for years and continue to struggle to get governmental support.

Simultaneously, Canadian LGBT communities also established non-governmental organisations (NGOs) at the national, provincial/territorial and local levels, advocating for a broader agenda of LGBT health and wellbeing. One such national organisation is a case in point. The Canadian Rainbow Health Coalition (CRHC), established in 2001, has undertaken a range of broad-based LGBT health and wellness initiatives. Yet, it has suffered of late in not being able to access state funding, due to a non-HIV/AIDS focus and a conservative federal government generally unsupportive of the LGBT populations. Nevertheless, the CRHC website contains a wealth of material on LGBT health and wellness (CRHC, 2013).

Provincial administration of health services to the LGBT communities is uneven, with varied approaches across Canada. In British Columbia and Ontario, the Vancouver Coastal Health (2013) and Rainbow Health Ontario (RHO) (RHO, 2013a) respectively offer information and referral resource programmes for LGBT people. Additionally, RHO provides a comprehensive website, LGBT training for healthcare providers and liaises with LGBT community outreach workers in each of the 14 Local Health Integration Networks (LHINs) in Ontario. Similarly, Nova Scotia's Capital Health provides 'prideHealth' – a health initiative for gay, lesbian, bisexual, trans, **intersex**[1] and **queer**[2] (GLBTIQ) people, offering resource and referral information primarily in the Halifax region (Capital District Health Authority, Nova Scotia, 2013).

By contrast, in Québec, a major policy initiative was undertaken with the release of its *Québec policy against homophobia* (Justice in Québec,

2009). This is a comprehensive policy that acknowledges the existence of **homophobia**, with a wide-reaching set of strategic guidelines to address it within the provincial public sector. One such guideline is to promote wellbeing, with strategic choices such as:

- providing support for victims of homophobia;
- promoting the adaptation of public services;
- providing support for community action.

For example, victim services in social work/social care are urged to become sensitised to and develop interventions for LGBT-targeted bashings. Québec is the only province in the country to take such a unique approach – a macro systemic perspective on addressing homophobia in public services via a sweeping provincial policy. This strategy goes beyond sole-based provincial coordination services with limited funding to embedding anti-homophobia measures structurally within the Québec government and its ensuing policies, services and programming.

Funded services at the municipal level across Canada include the following, which have all been active in addressing LGBT health issues through provincial health delivery systems:

- Avenue Community Centre for Gender and Sexual Diversity Inc. in Saskatoon, Saskatchewan;
- PTS in Ottawa, Ontario;
- QMunity in Vancouver, BC;
- Rainbow Resources Centre in Winnipeg, Manitoba.

Both the Rainbow Health Network located in Toronto and The Well in Hamilton are grassroots advocacy groups that address LGBT health issues and provide public education without any state support, except for occasional project-based funding (Rainbow Health Network, 2013; The Well, 2013).

Many of these groups and organisations have developed due to community-based research, sometimes funded by the federal government. Their sporadic existence throughout the country highlights the few voices doing ongoing advocacy work, and the political demands for formal structural recognition in health policy making and delivery. Such NGOs have taken on responsibility for providing services to tackle health inequalities that have not been provided through mainstream services.

Critical implications for social work

Social work practice

Social workers play a prominent role in the provision of health and social care related services to the LGBT populations, whether they be government funded or not, within mainstream services or specialised (including many described in the previous section), illness-based such as HIV/AIDS or broader. In contrast to biomedical interventions, which focus primarily on addressing downstream health issues such as the mental and physical effects of health problems (for example, homelessness, survival sex work, suicidality, depression, substance use, HIV and other sexually transmitted infections), social work is well positioned to take an upstream role via the SDoH towards the mitigation and prevention of such problems. The social worker can carry out such practice via means of recognising, acknowledging, ensuring representation of and prioritising such issues specific to LGBT people in social and health systems that overlook them. For example, social workers can intervene by providing support for same-sex parenting, advocating for supports for LGBT young people, responding appropriately to domestic abuse in LGBT communities and promoting independence among older LGBT people.

Social workers can play an influential role in mainstream as well as specialised LGBT health and social care services and society in general. Such a role can be varied, whether it be through direct practice with individuals, couples, families, groups or communities, public education and/or advocacy, policy design, development, implementation, review and/or evaluation, or via research and education. By providing accessible, inclusive, sensitive and equitable services to LGBT communities, the social worker would be engaging in transformative practice, contributing to an upstreaming of health and wellbeing (Mulé et al, 2009). The implications of such practice have emancipatory potential for the LGBT people who are served by the profession and transformative potential for the systems involved, the profession and society in general.

Social work education

Professional associations, ethics and principles

It is noteworthy that the lack of structural recognition of LGBT people in governmental policy is mirrored in formal Canadian social work structures. Nationally, the Canadian Association of Social Work Education (CASWE), the Canadian Association of Social Workers (CASW) and the Canadian Association of University Teachers (CAUT) have no statistics, documents, research or reports on LGBT social work educators and social work practitioners. The same is the case for Canadian provincial and territorial social work regulatory bodies and associations. If LGBT information exists in accreditation and/or self-study reports for individual faculties and schools of social work, they are inaccessible as they are not on the public record. Internally, CASWE has a Queer Caucus that along with other social location-based caucuses is fighting to get a formal voice on the board, CAUT has an LGBT Working Group that similarly is struggling for a legitimised voice within its structure and CASW has no equivalent internal body.

Social work as a profession is premised on its unique set of values, beliefs, principles and standards of practice. CASW has a *Code of ethics* (CASW, 2005a) and *Guidelines for ethical practice* (CASW, 2005b), both of which stipulate that social workers do not tolerate discrimination or discriminate on the basis of sexual orientation. Despite naming sexual orientation along with numerous other characteristics as grounds that should not be discriminated against, neither documents provide any further discussion on this matter and gender identity and gender expression are absent from both. The latter *Guidelines* (2005b) discuss demonstrating cultural awareness and sensitivity, but provide no definition for 'culture', despite having a glossary. More inclusive is CASWE's (2012) *Standards for accreditation* (2012), which refer to gender and sexual identities in the standards' principles guiding accreditation of social work education programmes. Internationally, the International Federation of Social Workers and the International Association of Schools of Social Work in their joint *Statement of ethical principles* (IFSW and IASSW, 2012) iterate that social workers are to challenge negative discrimination on the basis of sexual orientation. Here too, gender identity and gender expression are absent. Although all of these professional associations include sexual orientation in their documents, only CASWE mentions gender diversity, demonstrating an ongoing need to educate and sensitise within on the breadth and depth of gender and sexual diversity issues (Mulé, 2006). Furthermore, none of the above documents addresses the **intersectionality** of LGBT people in that for many, their sexual orientation and/or gender identity intersects with social locations, among others race, ethnicity, age, (dis)abilities, religion and class.

Policy implementation?

Although we should be under no illusions that having LGBT people explicitly named in formal policy, be it governmental or in the social work profession, will necessarily provide material responses to the recognition that LGBT people seek, I argue that there is still relevance to having LGBT people named rather than not. With regard to the former, when governmental agencies absent LGBT people from named inclusion in health and social care policy it wilfully releases them from being accountable to LGBT people's social and health issues, needs and concerns. I use the term 'wilfully' because it is not as though the Canadian government is not aware of the health issues, given its funding of numerous community-based LGBT research studies and lobbying by the likes of CRHC. A recent study reviewing the recognition of LGBT people in current federal health and social policy not only revealed a major lacunae, but also that by the very nature of premising such policies on population health and the SDoH, in the absence of corresponding funding and programming this results in such extenuating policies having little influence on service provision including that of social work practice (Mulé and Smith, forthcoming). For example, little if any federal funding is extended to LGBT health issues, outside of HIV/AIDS.

The implication for social work academics is that our research is seen as 'too specialised' or based on 'special interests' and thus does not warrant attention, and LGBT people in social work are often perceived to be a marginal community and not as a group central to social work practice. While the government was forced to allocate HIV/AIDS funding, some might argue that this was more to do with the so-called threat to the general population rather than to protect the health of gay and bisexual men. Discourses of risk and illness were the factors that have shaped and continue to shape its response. Similarly, the inconsistent recognition of sexual orientation, gender identity and gender expression in national and international social work professional bodies demonstrates a disconnect between the administrative structures of the profession and the scholarship and practitioner-based work specialising in LGBT health concerns that is not properly reflected in their policies. The incongruence between the professional bodies, social work scholars in LGBT issues and the training of students to address these issues undermines the very principles and values of the profession. For social work practitioners, material supports such as funding, programmes and services are only minimally available in large urban centres, limiting their capacity to combat homophobia,

heterosexism and cisgenderism in other social work and healthcare settings that social workers work in. In the end it is LGBT people in need of accessible, equitable and sensitive services who suffer.

Limits of equality, aspirations for equity, desire for liberation

Given the sheen of acceptance and equality for LGBT people in Canada, I challenge government at all levels and social work as a profession to drill down deeper if they are to meaningfully address the broad health and wellbeing issues of these populations. The rights claims battle that has dominated the mission of the Canadian LGBT movement over the last 20 years, or more, has produced the limiting effects of equality, in which LGBT people are supposedly elevated to the same level as cisgendered heterosexuals within cisgendered heterosexual models in a cisgenderist and heteronormative society. Alternatively, queer liberationists understand the need to attain equality as one mere step in the process. Beyond equality is to aspire to equity in which the specific and unique health and wellbeing issues and concerns that affect LGBT people is recognised. The ultimate desire for liberation is to then develop and shape health and social care services to be sensitive to their needs as they define them and not based on cisgenderist heterosexist norms. In essence, the inclusion of sexual orientation and increasingly gender identity (and gender expression) in human rights legislation and social work professional associations' policy must not be iterated as a mere additive, but rather be meaningfully positioned with material outputs.

Material outputs, such as explicit policies, core funding (outside of or in addition to illness-based HIV/AIDS funding), specialised LGBT health and social services and focused LGBT programming in mainstream health and social services, are uneven and sporadic across Canada's vast landscape. Large urban centres benefit most in being able to provide direct healthcare services obviously in response to the larger number of LGBT people who have formed communities in these cities. Nevertheless, their funding is far from adequate, nor guaranteed. For all the Canadian legal justice recognition of LGBT people (Daley, 2005), what about LGBT people in smaller urban or rural settings? The provincial resource and referral model begins to address this, but falls short. What about the right of LGBT people in smaller more rural settings to accessible, meaningful and sensitised frontline health services? In many of these types of remote settings in Canada the only resource that LGBT people have for health or social support services is an ASO. With the social stigma associated with HIV/AIDS, imagine turning to this kind of an organisation for broad health issues, as it may be the only one that is LGBT sensitised. It is not uncommon that broad healthcare services for LGBT people are drawn from HIV/AIDS funding, because there is very little funding outside this illness-based envelope. What broad health and wellbeing LGBT funding can be attained is usually project focused or very limited outside of this. This makes for a precarious broad health and social care service delivery system for LGBT Canadians.

Others and I have argued elsewhere that the broad health and wellbeing needs of the LGBT populations need to be recognised as part of the SDoH model (Jackson et al, 2006; Mulé et al, 2009) and although I maintain this position, given Canada's weak commitment to actual implementation of health model templates, more needs to be done to infuse health policy with the material outputs to address social exclusion that the templates are premised on. This is where the social work profession can play a role. Given that social justice figures prominently in social work ethics (CASW, 2005a; IFSW and IASSW, 2012), practice (CASW, 2005b) and curriculum standards (CASWE, 2012), as social workers we need to think about macro frameworks that feature structural systems that are inclusive of LGBT people. Furthermore, we need to advocate not only for their inclusion, but also for the receipt of social and wellbeing benefits that will generate a more sustainable level of service provision that would rightfully address the numerous, complex, ongoing, broad health issues, needs and concerns of LGBT people and redress the precarious health service provision currently available to LGBT people in Canada. From an international comparative perspective, Canada has most certainly made progress, yet from a queer liberationist perspective that values diversity and recognises the unique social and health issues of LGBT people, Canada still leaves much to be desired.

Internationally, health inequalities have become a major concern, and the World Health Organization has provided a conceptual framework that identifies their causes (CSDH, 2008). These include differing experiences of groups regarding conditions, support and options available to them in response to external variables such as disease, environmental conditions, employment and class. Also, social stratification and related inequities based on societal biases, norms and values, both economic and social policy and governance processes. The conceptual framework captures social positionings such as education, occupation, income, gender and race/ethnicity, yet completely ignores sexual orientation. Although the World Health Organization's SDoH

(WHO, 2008) justifiably place an emphasis on women, due to power imbalances in society, similar power imbalances are not recognised in relation to gender variance. This is most unfortunate, because what I am arguing in this chapter is that if a country like Canada, whom in its own right has made attempts to recognise LGBT people through legal justice (human rights legislation), yet continues to fall far short on the social justice front (recognition in health and social care among others), it becomes most apparent that LGBT people are a highly vulnerable population the world over with obvious health implications due to their unequal social position. The World Health Organization chose its social determinants based on a combination of 'conceptual plausibility, availability of supporting empirical evidence, and consistency of relationship between and among populations – and the demonstration that these determinants were amenable to intervention' (WHO, 2008, p 42). There is an extensive and growing literature as cited in this chapter and others in this anthology, regarding the health and wellbeing of LGBT people, all of which calls for interventions. Given the existence of this extensive empirical evidence, the question arises as to why the World Health Organization's Commission on Social Determinants of Health could not plausibly conceptualise sexual orientation and gender identity and expression as determinants of health?

Conclusion

Canada's innovative social and health policy templates coupled with increasingly sensitised human rights legislation have created a public impression of a progressive country that makes room for numerous minority and disenfranchised groups, inclusive of LGBT people. Although progress has been made, I have drilled down beneath the surface and critically questioned to what extent current Canadian social and health policy is addressing the broad health and wellbeing issues, needs and concerns of the LGBT populations with any material and substantive outputs. What is revealed is:

- a concerning unevenness that contributes to precarious service provision to Canadian LGBT people based on a contentedness with mere additive representation (albeit inconsistent) of these populations in human rights legislation, health and social work policy;
- lack of recognition of health issues outside of HIV/AIDS;
- a geographical stance whereby large urban centres are privileged.

The contradiction that the macro image presents at both governmental and social work professional levels needs to be exposed, examined and change advocated for, if we are to meaningfully address the social and health issues of LGBT people and uphold the social justice frameworks that these larger structural governance bodies claim to support.

What we know about this already

- Canada is perceived to be one of the most progressive countries in the world.
- Canada has contributed a number of health policy templates with international influence.
- Human rights legislation includes sexual orientation across Canada and gender identity (and gender expression) increasingly so.

What this chapter adds

- It provides an understanding of the limitations of additive representation of 'sexual orientation' and 'gender identity' to legislation and policy.
- It shows that having such 'inclusions' masks the lack of infusion of LGBT people in health policy.
- It highlights that there is a lack of funding, programming and services that provide meaningful healthcare to Canadian LGBT people.

How this is relevant for social work and LGBT health inequalities

- The unevenness of health services to LGBT people creates precarious healthcare delivery to these populations.
- Both the Canadian state and the social work profession fall short of adequately addressing the healthcare issues, needs and concerns of LGBT people.
- Social work has a crucial role to play in advocating on a macro level for meaningful material outputs regarding health services for LGBT people based on social justice principles.

Notes

[1] Intersex refers to those born with ambiguous genitalia and for which binary sex such as male or female is not apparent or easily applied.

[2] Queer in this context refers to those with a politicised sense of self based on their sexual orientation and/or gender identity or expression, usually non-heterosexual and/or cisgender.

References

Capital District Health Authority, Nova Scotia, 2013, prideHealth, www.cdha.nshealth.ca/pridehealth

Carabine, J, 2004a, 'Personal lives, public policies and normal sexualities', in J, Carabine (ed) *Sexualities: Personal lives and social policy*, Bristol: Policy Press, 159-73

Carabine, J, 2004b, 'Sexualities, personal lives and social policy', in J, Carabine (ed) *Sexualities: Personal lives and social policy*, Bristol: Policy Press, 1-48

CASW (Canadian Association of Social Workers), 2005a, *Code of ethics*, Ottawa: CASW

CASW, 2005b, *Guidelines for ethical practice*, Ottawa: CASW

CASWE (Canadian Association for Social Work Education), 2012, *Standards for accreditation*, Ottawa: CASWE-ACFTS

CATIE (Canadian AIDS Treatment, Information and Exchange), 2013, *A practical guide to HIV drug treatment for people living with HIV*, Toronto: CATIE, www.catie.ca/en/treatment

CIHR (Canadian Institutes for Health Research), 2008, *HIV/AIDS research initiative strategic plan 2008-2013*, Ottawa: CIHR, www.cihr-irsc.gc.ca/e/37801.html

Concannon, L, 2009, 'Developing inclusive health and social care policies for older LGBT citizens', *The British Journal of Social Work*, 39, 3, 403-17

CRHC (Canadian Rainbow Health Coalition), 2013, 'Links to GLBT health and wellness documents', www.rainbowhealth.ca/english/documents.html

CSDH (Commission on Social Determinants of Health), 2008, *Closing the gap in a generation: Health equity through action on the social determinants of health*, Geneva: World Health Organization

Daley, A, 2005, *Lesbian and gay health issues: OUTside of the health policy arena*, Critical Social Policy, 26, 4, 794-816

Duggan, L, 2003, *The twilight of equality? Neoliberalism, culture politics, and the attack on democracy*, Boston, MA: Beacon Press

Elliot, RD and Bonauto, M, 2005, 'Sexual orientation and gender identity in North America: legal trends, legal contrasts', *Journal of Homosexuality*, 48, 3/4, 91-106

Fish, J and Wilkinson, S, 2003, 'Understanding lesbians' healthcare behaviour: the case of breast self-examination', *Social Science & Medicine*, 56, 2, 235-45

Foucault, M, 1979, 'On governmentality', *Ideology and Consciousness*, 6, 5-22

Government of Canada, 1974, *A new perspective on the health of Canadians*, Ottawa: Minister of Supply and Services Canada

Health Canada, 1998, *Taking action on population health*, position paper for Health Promotion and Programs Branch Staff, Ottawa: Health Canada

Health Canada, 2001, *The population health template: Key elements and actions that define a population health approach*, Ottawa: Health Canada, Population and Public Health Branch, Strategic Policy Directorate

Health Canada, 2003, *Exploring concepts in gender and health*, Ottawa: Health Canada

Health Canada, 2010, *Health portfolio sex and gender-based analysis policy*, www.hc-sc.gc.ca/hl-vs/pubs/women-femmes/sgba-policy-politique-ags-eng.php

Hooghe, M, Claes, E, Harell, A, Quintelier, E and Dejaeghere, Y, 2010, Anti-gay sentiment among adolescents in Belgium and Canada: a comparative investigation into the role of gender and religion, *Journal of Homosexuality*, 57, 3, 384-400

IFSW and IASSW (International Federation of Social Workers and International Association of Schools of Social Work), 2012, *Statement of ethical principles*, http://ifsw.org/policies/statement-of-ethical-principles/

Jackson, B, Daley, A, Moore, D, Mulé, N, Ross, L, Travers, A, Montgomery, E, 2006, *Whose public health? An intersectional approach to sexual orientation, gender identity and the development of public health goals for Canada*, Toronto: Rainbow Health Network and Coalition for Lesbian and Gay Rights in Ontario, www.rainbowhealth.ca/documents/english/whose_public_health.pdf

Justice in Québec, 2009, *Québec policy against homophobia: Moving together towards social equality*, Québec: Government of Québec

Lehavot, K and Simoni, JM (2011) 'The impact of minority stress on mental health and substance use among sexual minority women', *Journal of Consulting and Clinical Psychology*, 79(2), 159-170.

Lupton, D, 1999, *Risk*, London: Routledge

Mulé, NJ, 2005, 'Beyond words in health and wellbeing policy: "sexual orientation" – from inclusion to infusion', *Canadian Review of Social Policy*, 55, 79-98

Mulé, NJ, 2006, 'Equity vs. invisibility: sexual orientation issues in social work ethics and curricula standards', *Social Work Education*, 25, 6, 608-22

Mulé, NJ, 2007, 'Sexual orientation discrimination in health care and social service policy: a comparative analysis of Canada, the UK and USA', in L Badgett and J Frank (eds) *Sexual orientation discrimination: An international perspective*, New York, NY: Routledge, 306-22

Mulé, NJ and Smith, MC, forthcoming, Invisible populations: LGBTQs and federal health policy in Canada, *Canadian Public Administration*

Mulé, NJ, Ross, LE, Deeprose, B, Jackson, BE, Daley, A, Travers, A and Moore, D, 2009, 'Promoting LGBT health and wellbeing through inclusive policy development', *International Journal for Equity in Health*, 8, 18, www.equityhealthj.com/content/8/1/18

Murray, KB, 2007, 'Governmentality and the shifting winds of policy studies', in M Orsini and M Smith (eds) *Critical policy studies*, Vancouver: University of British Columbia Press, 161-84

Orsini, M, 2007, 'Discourses in distress: from health promotion to population health to "you are responsible for your own health"', in M, Orsini and M, Smith (eds) *Critical policy studies*, Vancouver: University of British Columbia Press, 347-63

Paterson, S, 2010, 'What's the problem with gender-based analysis? Gender mainstreaming policy and practice in Canada', *Canadian Public Administration*, 53, 3, 395-416

Petersen, A and Brunton, R, 2002, *The new genetics and public's health*, London and New York, NY: Routledge

Public Health Agency of Canada, no date, 'What determines health?', www.phac-aspc.gc.ca/ph-sp/phdd/determinants/index.html#determinants

Rainbow Health Network, 2013, 'About us', www.rainbowhealthnetwork.ca/about

Rainbow Health Ontario, 2013a, About us, www.rainbowhealthontario.ca/about/whoWeAre.cfm

Rainbow Health Ontario, 2013b, Resource database, www.rainbowhealthontario.ca/resources/database.cfm

Senreich, E, 2010, 'Differences in outcomes, completion rates, and perceptions of treatment between White, Black, and Hispanic LGBT clients in substance abuse programs', *Journal of Gay and Lesbian Mental Health*, 14, 3, 176-200

Shildrick, M, 2004, 'Silencing sexuality: the regulation of the disabled body', in J Carabine (ed) *Sexualities: Personal lives and social policy*, Bristol: Policy Press, 123-57

Smith, M, 2007, 'Queering public policy: a Canadian perspective', in M, Orsini and M, Smith (eds) *Critical policy studies*, Vancouver: University of British Columbia Press, 91-109

The Well, 2013, 'History', www.thewellhamilton.ca/about-us/history/

Toomey, RB and Richardson, RA, 2009, 'Perceived sibling relationships of sexual minority youth', *Journal of Homosexuality*, 56, 7, 849-60

Vancouver Coastal Health, 2013, 'LGBT2SQ', www.vch.ca/your_health/lesbian_gay_bisexual_transgendered_twospirited/

Volpp, SY, 2010, 'What about the 'B' in LGB: are bisexual women's mental health issues same or different?', *Journal of Gay and Lesbian Mental Health*, 14, 1, 41-51

WHO (World Health Organization), 2008, *Social determinants of health*, Geneva: WHO, http://whqlibdoc.who.int/publications/2008/9789241563703_eng.pdf?ua=1

Between public neglect and private needs: conceptualising approaches to LGBT issues in Italian social work

Andrea Nagy and Urban Nothdurfter

The social and political background

A discussion about lesbian, gay, bisexual and trans (LGBT) issues in social work needs to take account both of the wider context, which has an impact on the lives of LGBT people and also of public debates, which construct social perceptions about them. In this sense, before focusing on LGBT issues in Italian social work, the rest of this section gives an overview of the current social and political context in Italy. Also, both the legislative and policy background and the development of the Italian LGBT movement are briefly addressed.

From a comparative perspective, Italy is often depicted as a conservative country, mainly due to the strong impact of a conservative religious commitment in Italian politics (Ginsborg, 2001; Giorgi, 2013) and due to its familialistic welfare tradition (Ferrera, 1996; Saraceno, 2003). With respect to the legal treatment of **homosexuality**, it is worth mentioning that the decriminalisation of homosexuality occurred in 1889 (a relatively early date in comparison with some other European countries) through the enactment of the Zanardelli Penal Code, which also introduced the concept of 'equal age consent' for heterosexual and homosexual activity (Dall'Orto, 1998). However, today, Italy is the only one among the founding countries of the European Union (EU), and one of 12 countries of today's EU 28, without any legal recognition of same-sex partnerships. Despite several legislative proposals for civil partnerships, for example the 'PACS' Bill in 2002 and the 'DICO' Bill in 2007, none of them has ever been accepted by the National Parliament. This complete lack of legal recognition has a variety of consequences on the level of legal benefits, obligations and responsibilities of same-sex partnerships. They are not recognised in taxation, pension and housing tenancy rights. A same-sex partner is not even recognised as next of kin in hospital, in inheritance or in immigration and asylum rights. For the Italian state, and thus for its social and family policies, same-sex partnerships do not exist.

However, there have been some recent signals that have brought about hope for some change. The 2011 national Census made it possible for the first time to indicate the status of a same-sex relationship. In 2010 and again in 2013, the Constitutional Court urged the National Parliament to legislate in matters of the legal recognition of same-sex partnerships and in 2012 a sentence by the Court of Cassation stated that 'same sex couples have the same right to a family life as married straight couples' (*Corte di Cassazione, sentenza* 4184/2012). However, so far, no progress in legislation has been made and same-sex partnerships continue not to be recognised at all.

The only anti-discrimination Act on sexual orientation appears in Legislative Decree 216/2003, which has transposed the European Directive 2000/78/CE and explicitly prohibits discrimination on the basis of sexual orientation in employment. With regard to transgender rights, Statute Law 164/1982 allows for official gender identity change, but only after medically indicated sex reassignment surgery. Gender identity is not included in official anti-discrimination legislation. Furthermore, there is no explicit recognition of hate crimes on the grounds of sexual orientation and/or gender identity. Two Bills on homophobic hate crimes, introduced in 2009 and 2011, were rejected by the National Parliament. Currently, a new 'anti-homophobia' Bill is being discussed in the Parliament.

The beginnings of the Italian LGBT movement are closely linked to the efforts of single leading figures and their social impact as both activists and intellectuals (Barilli Rossi, 1999; Barbagli and Colombo, 2007). During the 1970s, the first gay and lesbian associations and social groups were established in the major urban centres, the most famous one being the association *FUORI!* (OUT!), founded in 1973 in Turin. During the 1980s, the movement gained more public visibility due to alarming reports of crime against gay people and to the new and growing AIDS crisis. In 1985, different local associations were united under the national umbrella organisation of ArciGay, which was divided into ArciGay/ArciLesbica in 1996, providing the gay and lesbian movement two distinct but allied national associations (Barilli Rossi, 1999). As to public visibility, the first official national Gay Pride march was held in Rome in 1994. In 2000, Rome hosted the World Gay Pride, which led to harsh critique from both the Vatican and from many representatives high up in the Italian political arena (D'Ippoliti and Schuster, 2011). Europride 2011 was also held in Italy, again in Rome. In 2011 the event was organised under the patronage of the city of Rome, with the official endorsement of many representatives from both the cultural and the political spheres.

Although Italy can be credited with a thriving LGBT movement, and although leading activists in the partisan landscape have also been elected to the National Parliament, success in terms of recognition of LGBT concerns by law and in public policies remains conspicuously absent (Scalfarotto and Mangiaterra, 2010; D'Ippoliti and Schuster, 2011).

LGBT issues in Italian social work

As to the presence of LGBT issues in the Italian academic debate in general, scholars complain of a resistance or delay in including gender identity and sexual orientation in academic curricula and scientific research (Trappolin, 2008; Ross, 2010; Operto, 2011; Ruspini, 2013). These issues are often seen as niche topics, as delicate and not conducive to successful academic careers (Ruspini, 2013). Moreover, the required interdisciplinary perspective of gender identity and sexual orientation studies is often at odds with the strict 'departmentalisation' of Italian academia and, thus, this field of studies often lacks an institutional home. However, in recent years there has been increasing research activity on LGBT issues in the Italian social sciences. Contributions often come from individual researchers and/or specific networks across disciplines and institutions having a strong foothold outside of traditional institutions and being informed by the LGBT movement (Ross, 2010). An overview of the state of the art of LGBT issues in the Italian social sciences (Ruspini, 2013) shows that, initially, they focused mainly on biomedical and pathological aspects of sexuality, but the focus has progressively expanded, taking into account both the broader dimension of social and cultural factors influencing the development of LGBT identities as well as the experiences of LGBT people in different spheres of everyday life (Saraceno, 2003; Barbagli and Colombo, 2007; Corbisiero, 2010, 2013). Moreover, it seems apparent that interest in more comprehensive conceptual work concerning LGBT issues and queer theory is growing (Pustianaz, 2011; Romania, 2013). In 2012, the Italian National Institute of Statistics (ISTAT) carried out a survey on LGBT people for the first time in Italy (ISTAT, 2012). There is also a discernible body of literature produced by legal scholars concerning the discrimination of LGBT people and the recognition of same-sex partnerships (Bilotta, 2008; D'Ippoliti and Schuster, 2011).

The fact that social work programmes in Italy have a limited academic tradition and therefore still lack recognition in academia (Campanini,

2007; Facchini and Tonon Giraldo, 2013) could perhaps explain why LGBT issues have been scarcely integrated into existing Italian social work programmes. However, social work's commitment to human rights and social justice (IFSW, 2000) should alert the profession to LGBT discrimination. The social work profession in Italy is distinguished by strict professional regulation and a strong identification with a Code of Ethics, at least at a formal level (Campanini, 2007). However, the Code of Ethics of Italian social workers does not refer explicitly to discrimination on the grounds of sexual orientation (CNOAS, 2009).

Historically, social work in Italy has been characterised by different periods. The beginnings of professional social work in Italy were closely linked to the processes of reconstruction and democratisation after fascism and the Second World War. During the 1970s, social movements such as the women's movement and the anti-psychiatry movement had a strong impact on the social work profession, which had been significantly involved in radical service reforms and in innovative social policy making (Diomede Canevini, 2005; Campanini, 2007; Fargion, 2008). However, the ensuing professionalisation process in Italian social work has been strongly oriented towards a traditionally acknowledged view of professionalism, aspiring to 'neutrality' and to a 'proper' area of competence within the micro dimension of the helping relationship (Nothdurfter, 2011). In her research on practitioners' representations of social work, Fargion (2008) shows that focusing on social aspects is rather linked to methodological and technical choices of interventions. Because this is 'not equally matched by a strong awareness of the structural nature of social problems and of the political dimension of the profession' (Fargion, 2008, p 212), she suggests that there is a lack of attention to issues of power, oppression and social justice in Italian social work practice.

But where can one find explicit accounts of LGBT issues within the field of Italian social work research and social work education? The following subsections present the findings of two pieces of work. First, an inventory aimed at outlining to what extent LGBT issues are addressed in Italian social work key journals and in social work curricula. Subsequently, an analysis of an exemplary case in the field of residential care illustrates that the inclusion of LGBT issues is not yet common in Italian social work practice.

Social work research

In order to assess the number of references to LGBT issues in the Italian literature, the authors undertook a systematic review of seven Italian social work journals covering the years from 2000 to 2012. The journals included can be considered the seven most important Italian social work journals, as they are national in scope, address a general spectrum of social work topics and are most likely to impact on social work education and practice.[1] Four of them are longstanding social work journals, the other three address wider topics of social welfare and social policy, but regularly address specific topics relating to social work practice and professional development. The review was performed using a systematic keyword search in two different Italian databases[2] combined with a supplementary hand-search in order to countercheck the findings. The review included only full articles. As Table 2.1 shows, the findings suggest that a debate on LGBT issues in Italian social work is practically non-existent. The percentage of articles concerning LGBT topics published over a period of 12 years was approximately 0.07%.

Table 2.1: Italian social work journals' inclusion of LGBT issues, 2000–12

Journal and number of issues	Number of titles in total	Number of full articles addressing LGBT issues and the article references
Animazione Sociale 10 issues per year	1,309	1 Molinatto and Rigliano (2001)
Autonomie Locali e Servizi Sociali 3 issues per year	606	1 Pietrantoni et al (2011)
La Rivista Di Servizio Sociale 4 issues per year	429	2 Pietrantoni et al (2000) Panico and Matarrese (2006)
Lavoro Sociale 3 issues per year	about 390	0
Prospettive Sociali e Sanitarie 22 issues per year until 2012 12 issues per year from 2012	1,344	0
Rassegna di Servizio Sociale 4 issues per year	about 450	0
Studi Zancan 6 issues per year	975	0

Social work education

In a first attempt to investigate the inclusion of LGBT issues in Italian social work education, the authors contacted the heads of social work programmes at Italian universities, asking them to respond to a short email questionnaire. The survey included the questions as to *whether or not the curriculum of their degree programme explicitly addresses the topic of LGBT people in social work and whether they thought that it was important or necessary for social work practice to address issues on gender and sexual orientation and to take into account the needs of LGBT people as social work clients.*

In 2012, there were 81 social work degrees at Italian universities, of which 64 programme directors could be contacted via email. As the response rate to the questionnaire was very low (responses were received from only 19 programmes), the findings do not allow for general statements about the effective inclusion of LGBT issues in Italian social work education. The survey does, however, produce interesting insights into reasons why a more explicit inclusion of LGBT issues in social work education is impeded. Some respondents argued that 'the curriculum does not allow a high degree of specialization'; others argued that, in their opinion, 'other minority issues have higher priority'. Some respondents also saw a risk of categorisation or 'labelling of LGBT people' when addressing the issues, or the danger of a 'reductionist focus on one dimension of identity' instead of a 'holistic view of a person'. By contrast, there was also the notion that LGBT issues are relevant and should be addressed, but, as one respondent stated, they are often 'forgotten'. These responses draw on discourses that construct:

- LGBT issues as specialised rather than LGBT people as a user group who are entitled to access social work services;
- LGBT people as a group who merit less attention than other disadvantaged groups.

The discourses also show respondents beliefs that by identifying LGBT as a population of interest, social work risks pathologising them by attaching a label; and that LGBT identities are somehow separate from the whole of a person's identity.

Social work practice

Through other research activities there was a contact between the authors, a girl who had been in care from 2010 to 2012 and the interdisciplinary team of care workers who had been caring for her at the time. The connection was used to conduct an interview with the residential youth care worker team about their work with this former client, who was a self-defined lesbian at the time she had been in care. The analysis of this social work practice example in children and young people's residential care shows that care workers, although not individually hostile towards lesbians or lesbianism, may not challenge common discourses about sexualities when they retrospectively discuss a case of a lesbian client. The residential social work team were asked *whether or not they thought that a former client's identification as a lesbian had had an impact on the care situation, and if so, how they would describe the impact.* The analysis is based on a view of a residential childcare setting as a certain 'field' (Lewin 1951), which structures the possible actions or the actors to some extent. In this sense, the residential childcare field seems to suggest the following interpretations of this case and of lesbian identity in general.

The residential social work team expressed that there are practical problems to address when someone in a group is gay. However, the following quote shows that these were thought about in terms of heterosexuality:

> 'I realise now where the topic was indeed an issue, when she requested to stay overnight with girlfriends ... and there we applied the standard procedure when someone in the group has a relationship. And I was always relieved, because we didn't have to think of contraception. That was practical.' (Care worker A)

'Heterosexuality' is the concept that shapes beliefs about romantic relationships and renders lesbianism unthinkable. In heteronormative constructs, every other relationship is a 'variation of' heterosexuality. The young lesbian's identity was seen only as a lesser risk, or, risk, for her sexual and reproductive health. The team members realised during the interview that their care planning practice did not include sexual *identity* in terms of emotional, social or physical wellbeing. Sexuality seemed to be addressed only in relation to sexual activity and the need for contraception.

In the discussion the team members 'trivialised' (Thompson, 2003)[3] the young lesbian's identity, reinforcing the prevailing stereotype that lesbianism is simply a phase, and that the girl might become heterosexual: "But I didn't take her seriously in that because I thought that she might just be experimenting a bit in her adolescence. For me this was not fixed yet [that she is a lesbian]" (care worker A). Furthermore, the team members assumed that lesbianism was less overtly sexual, less actively demanding than male homosexuality and would therefore not influence group dynamics as 'negatively'. This is evidence of the heteronormative construction of gender differences:

> 'I think it would have had another 'quality' if a boy would have proclaimed it so openly. I remember that X and Y, and yes Z [names of three boys in the care setting] toyed with being gay and this impacted heavily on the group dynamics in terms of disapproval.' (Care worker B)

> [*approval from the other team members*]

> 'That's right and there we started to listen attentively when we recognised that the boys performed games, sex-games in the house.' (Care worker A)

In these statements, the team members implied that boys and girls differed in their expression of sexuality; that is to say that boys were more active and obsessive in their sexuality and that girls were modest and moderate in their desires. As a consequence, the girl's identity as a lesbian and the group's reaction to her were ignored, whereas homo-erotic behaviour between the boys resulted in authoritative intervention, even though it was assumed that the boys were just joking. These are stereotypical views of gender roles, where men's sexuality is acknowledged and women's sexuality is not recognised. It is obvious through the contradictory statements made about the young woman's sexual assertiveness ("she did not express her sexuality openly" versus "she was very self-assertive and persistent in her sexual advances") that the care workers' perception of the case was constructed through knowledge based on their own personal experience. Only one care worker (C) who had been confronted with bisexuality in her own private surroundings perceived and acknowledged the girl's identity expression as a lesbian and reacted more sensitively to it. The young woman's self-definition as a lesbian was a subordinate issue: "And there were so many other urgent topics in her case, which were more important to address; the whole case was one big crisis management" (care worker B).

Even when love dramas were a daily issue[4] and self-harm and drug abuse were also issues, self-defined identity status was not considered relevant. But self-harm and drug abuse could very well have had to do with the girl's 'internalised oppression' (Elze, 2006, p 64) or **'minority stress'** (Elze, 2006, p 63) because of the discrimination of LGBT identities.

It would be possible to analyse some of the issues, which appeared in practice settings with the young lesbian, using existing anti-discriminatory and anti-oppressive concepts (see, for example, Thompson, 2003; Elze, 2006). In regard to the example of young people in residential care, it must be stated that the lack of knowledge of the issues resulting from the girl's self-definition as a lesbian and the lack of reflection on concepts of sexuality in general, might have caused the client to suffer and might also have hindered positive intervention. This is in contrast to the main policy goals defined for children and young people in care. The prevailing legal framework stresses the need to *reduce disadvantages* for young people in care and emphasises their rights to the *promotion of individual development* and to be *respected in their mental and body development*.[5] Disadvantages based on lesbianism cannot possibly be reduced if care workers do not know anything about lesbianism, do not take it seriously or do not critically reflect on the heterosexual norm. 'Minority stress' and 'internalised oppression' can even damage the young person's mental and physical health, if the mechanisms of oppression based on sexual orientation are not recognised by care workers.

Conceptualising approaches to LGBT issues in Italian social work

The evidence of a missing LGBT debate in Italian social work literature and the lack of inclusion of LGBT issues in social work education leads one to ask how LGBT issues could be introduced and theorised in Italian social work. Furthermore, the discussed practice situation has shown in an exemplary way, how operations and consequences of unchallenged structures of understanding about sexualities can result in mechanisms and, eventually, services that do not consider the circumstances and needs of LGBT people.

Thus, this section suggests a conceptualising approach for LGBT issues in Italian social work, which goes beyond 'mentioning LGBT too'. LGBT issues do not only represent minority issues, which can only be addressed in highly specialised social work education curricula. Approaching LGBT issues can rather make a valid contribution to the knowledge base of social work by 'a continuous and insistent interrogation of notions of the normal' (Hall, 2007, p 186). Queer theory, with its critical stance on heteronormativity (Hicks and Watson, 2003) offers a useful conceptual lens for challenging the construction of heterosexuality as the unproblematic norm, and its influence in shaping 'institutions, structures of understandings and practical orientations' (Berlant and Warner, 1998, p 548) that frame society as well as the accustomed knowledge base of professionals. The concept of 'heteronormativity', coined by queer theorist Michael Warner (1991), exposes the pervasive and invisible norm of heterosexuality embedded as a normative principle in social institutions and theories, which also determine processes of knowledge and understanding. As Weiss (2008) points out, the concept of 'heteronormativity'

> is useful in attempting to understand the assumptions upon which heterosexuality rests, and to show how and why deviations from heterosexual norms are subject to social and legal sanctions. For example, heteronormativity assumes a belief in dimorphic sexual difference (there are two sexes), biological essentialism (male and female functions are essentially different), and mimetic sex/gender relationship (psycho–social traits follow anatomy). Those who deviate from these assumptions by openly preferring romantic partners of the same sex, who change from one sex to another, or who violate heterosexual norms in other ways, are marginalised.

'Marginalisation' is the reason why the client's self-definition in the practice example was not seen as an important issue. As previously expressed by some social work programme directors, making *other* sexual orientations visible can lead to *categorisation* or *labelling* and the *risk of a reductionist focus on one dimension of identity*. Focusing instead on heteronormativity can help to theorise LGBT issues and expose invisibility as a structural problem.[6] 'Instead of detailing who is sexually different', Jeyasingham (2008, p 149) suggests that social work education 'should examine the operations and consequences of homophobia and heteronormativity'. In this way, it is not difference in itself, which is highlighted. In fact, the 'idea of making marginalised groups known through visibility (a logic of knowing through recognising how we appear) is at best a risky objective because images, whether positive or not, are one way in which we are turned into objects examined by those who do not themselves need to be defined in terms of difference' (Jeyasingham, 2008, p 141). Dealing with knowledge and ignorance and the construction of sexuality in social work education, Jeyasingham (2008, p 141) suggests instead to 'explore the system of knowledge that produces certain ways of knowing sexuality and its relevance'. The view that sexuality is only relevant in terms of contraception, as reported by the care workers in the practice example as well as their assumptions of *given* differences of men and women that pre-structured their perceptions, could be challenged on that basis. Queering social work not only helps students and social workers to challenge their personal attitudes towards LGBT people, but also enables them to see and to understand how heteronormativity works through structures and processes in society and, thus, contributes to mitigating heterosexist oppression (Foreman and Quinlan, 2008).

Fish (2008) discusses oppression in relation to sexuality. She shows how heterosexism is established through a system of beliefs that values heterosexuality as superior to homosexuality. Heterosexism is based on compulsory heterosexuality and it constitutes a complex system of oppression that intersects with other marginalised identities such as class and 'race' (Fish, 2008). An approach that challenges heteronormativity and illustrates the complex nature and form of sexuality oppression, shows that heterosexism is far from being trivial, but that institutions and practices maintain heterosexist oppression by rendering LGBT people invisible (or 'forgotten') while at the same time treating them unequally in many respects: legally, politically and socially but also morally and psychologically (Fish, 2008). As it has been shown, in the Italian context, that LGBT people continue to be oppressed and denied full citizenship status (Saraceno, 2012). Social work students should be educated to see these forms of disadvantage and oppression in order to develop approaches of emancipatory practice. As Fish (2008: 186) puts it, 'the family is a key site in which heterosexuality is maintained and where gender difference is constructed'. A sociological approach to 'family' is an important element of Italian social work curricula, and it could provide an excellent starting point in teaching about the heterosexual norm and related concepts. In this way, speaking about LGBT people in social work goes far beyond the constituency of yet another minority and holds a valuable potential for what is, ultimately, so important for social work in general; namely the better understanding of the complex process of developing identities in societal contexts with their institutionalised normativities (Otto and Ziegler, 2012).

The Code of Ethics of Italian social work states that social workers are obliged to challenge discrimination in all its forms. However, social work education and social work practice must go beyond such 'universal' formulas in order to recognise and to understand the many faces of discrimination and oppression. 'Heteronormativity' is a key concept in the understanding of oppression related to LGBT issues in social work, and must be introduced and handled in Italian social work education.

What we know about this already
- There is an international debate about LGBT issues in social work education and practice with varying impacts in different countries.
- The debate is informed by several theoretical concepts, which challenge inequalities and the oppression of LGBT people in health and social care.
- Knowledge on LGBT issues depends on normative systems of knowledge, which determine ways of (not) knowing about sexualities beyond heteronormative assumptions.

What this chapter adds
- It provides an overview of the social and political background of LGBT issues in Italy and a first exploration of the presence of LGBT issues in the context of Italian social work.
- A gives a rough sketch for a future debate on LGBT issues in Italian social work, suggesting that queer theory with its focus on heteronormativity is a useful approach to grasp the structural and political dimensions of sexual orientation and gender identity issues.
- It sets out the reasons why LGBT issues are not extra or niche topics, but rather provide a prime example for challenging the normative knowledge base of society and social work itself.

How this is relevant for social work and LGBT health inequalities
- Recognising LGBT issues as structural problems has the potential of revealing the social and health inequalities experienced by LGBT people, which have been neglected so far.
- An examination of consequences and operations of heteronormativity makes it possible to see and understand oppressions in relation to sexual orientation and gender identity, which should be challenged by social workers.
- The education of social workers is a potential starting point for a debate on LGBT issues in Italian social work.

Notes

[1] A similar, but much more articulated review on the coverage of gay and lesbian subject matter in social work journals has been carried out, for example, by Van Voorhis and Wagner (2001).

[2] Databases: *Centro Studi Gruppo Abele* (http://centrostudi.gruppoabele. org/?q=node/132) and *Associazione ESSPER periodici italiani di economia, scienze sociali e storia* (www.biblio.liuc.it/scripts/essper/default.asp).

[3] Thompson (2003, p 91) describes 'trivialization' as one possible 'process of discrimination' in which the relevance of an issue of discrimination is not accepted or made ridiculous. Also, the concentration on a minor aspect of the issue in order to distract from the more important aspects is described through this term.

[4] Care worker C, who had been confronted with bisexuality in her own private surroundings, said: "I think that it was really not right away when she arrived here, that she expressed openly her orientation. That came a little later, and then she was very self-assertive and persistent in her sexual advances and the issue developed quite intensively with lots of constructed romantic dramas, there were constantly dramas, romantic dramas. That was quite intense."

[5] There is a distinct national children's social policy in Italy that defines outcomes for children and young people in care. Due to the decentralisation of the welfare system and the autonomy of the province of Bolzano/Bozen, the main policy goals for children and young people in care are defined by the 'Guidelines for socio-pedagogical care for minors' on a provincial level (Autonome Provinz Bozen-Südtirol et al, 2013).

[6] Fish (2008) challenges the usual representation of invisibility as an individual choice whether or not to come out. '[I]nvisibility is structural in the absence of data and official statistics about the LGB [lesbian, gay and bisexual] population, the lack of social policies, the dearth of equality targets and monitoring systems, the paucity of published guidelines about sexuality and the lack of practice models and examples. Because improving access to services relies upon a visible, readily identifiable population, LGB people are often overlooked in developing service provision' (Fish, 2008, p 191).

References

Autonome Provinz Bozen-Südtirol, Abteilung Sozialwesen and Amt für Familie, Frau und Jugend, 2013, *Leitfaden sozialpädagogische grundbetreuung für minderjährige* [Guidelines for socio-pedagogical care for minors], Bozen: Landesdruckerei

Barbagli, M and Colombo, A, 2007, *Omosessuali moderni: Gay e lesbiche in Italia* [Modern homosexuals: Gays and lesbians in Italy], Bologna: il Mulino

Barilli Rossi, G, 1999, *Il movimento gay in Italia* [The gay movement in Italy], Milan: Feltrinelli

Berlant, L and Warner, M, 1998, 'Sex in public', *Critical Inquiry*, 24, 2, 547-66

Bilotta, F (ed), 2008, *Le unioni tra persone dello stesso sesso: Profili di diritto civile, comunitario e comparato* [Civil partnership for same sex couples: Profiles of civil, European and comparative law], Sesto San Giovanni, Milan: Mimesis

Campanini, A, 2007, 'Social work in Italy', *European Journal of Social Work*, 10, 1, 107-16

CNOAS (Consiglio Nazionale Ordine Assistenti Sociali), 2009, *Codice deontologico dell'assistente sociale* [Code of ethics for social workers], Rome.

Corbisiero, F (ed), 2010, *Certe cose si fanno: Identità, genere e sessualità nella popolazione LGBT* [Certain things you do: Identity, gender and sex in the LGBT population], Naples: Gesco Edizioni

Corbisiero, F (ed), 2013, *Comunità omosessuali: Le scienze sociali sulla popolazione LGBT* [Homosexual communities: Social sciences on the LGBT population], Milan: Franco Angeli

Dall'Orto, G, 1988, 'La "tolleranza repressiva" dell'omosessualità' ['The "repressive tollerance" of homosexuality'], in ARCIGAY nazionale (ed) *Omosessuali e Stato*, Bologna: Cassero, 37-57

D'Ippoliti, C and Schuster, A, 2011, *DisOrientamenti: Discriminazione ed esclusione sociale delle persone LGBT in Italia* [DisOrientations: Discrimination and social exclusion of LGBT people in Italy], Rome: Armando Editore

Diomede Canevini, M, 2005, 'Storia del servizio sociale' ['History of social work'], in M Dal Pra Ponticelli (ed) *Dizionario di servizio sociale* [Dictionary of social service], Rome: Carocci

Dunk-West, P and Hafford-Letchfield, T, 2010, *Sexual identities and sexuality in social work: Research and reflections from women in the field*, Farnham: Ashgate

Elze, DE, 2006, 'Oppression, prejudice, and discrimination', in DF Morrow and L Messinger (eds) *Sexual orientation and gender expression in social work practice: Working with gay, lesbian, bisexual and trans people*, New York, NY: Columbia University Press, 43-77

Facchini, C and Tonon Giraldo, S, 2013, 'The university training of social workers: elements of innovation, positive and critical aspects in the case of Italy', *British Journal of Social Work*, 43, 4, 667-84

Fargion, S, 2008, 'Reflections on social work's identity: international themes in Italian practitioners' representation of social work', *International Social Work*, 51, 2, 206-19

Ferrera, M, 1996, 'The southern model of welfare in Social Europe', *Journal of European Social Policy*, 6, 1, 17-37

Fish, J, 2008, 'Far from mundane: theorising heterosexism for social work education', *Social Work Education*, 27, 2, 182-93

Foreman, M and Quinlan, M, 2008, 'Increasing social work students' awareness of heterosexism and homophobia – a partnership between a community gay health project and a school of social work', *Social Work Education*, 27, 2, 152-8

Ginsborg, P, 2001, *Italy and its discontents: Family, civil society, state 1980-2001*, London: Penguin

Giorgi, A, 2013, 'Ahab and the white whale: the contemporary debate around the forms of Catholic political commitment in Italy', *Democratization*, 20, 5, 895-916

Hall, DE, 2007, 'Cluelessness and the queer classroom', *Pedagogy*, 7, 2, 182-91

Hicks, S and Watson, K, 2003, 'Desire lines: 'queering' health and social welfare', *Sociological Research Online*, 8, 1, www.socresonline.org.uk/8/1/hicks.html

IFSW (International Federation of Social Workers), 2000, *Definition of social work*, http://ifsw.org/policies/definition-of-social-work/

ISTAT, 2012, *La popolazione omosessuale nella società italiana* [*The homosexual population in Italian society*], Rome: ISTAT

Jeyasingham, D, 2008, 'Knowledge/ignorance and the construction of sexuality in social work education', *Social Work Education*, 27, 2, 138-51

Lewin, K, 1951, *Field theory in social science: Selected theoretical papers* (edited by D Cartwright), Oxford: Harpers

Molinatto, P and Rigliano, P, 2001,'Desiderio di un diverso e più ricco se stesso: riflessioni sull'essere donne e uomini, gay ed etero: intervista a Paolo Rigliano' ['Desire for another and richer self: reflections about being woman and man, gay and hetero: interview with Paolo Rigliano'], *Animazione Sociale*, 11, 3-10

Nothdurfter, U, 2011, 'Servizio sociale e politiche sociali: quali professionisti per quale welfare?' ['Social work and social policy: which professionals for which welfare?'], *Autonomie Locali e Servizi Sociali*, 34, 3, 521–34

Operto, S, 2011, 'L'osservazione indiscreta: uno sguardo sulle ricerche sociologiche riguardanti la sessualità e le sue trasformazioni' ['The indiscreet observation: a review of sociological reserach on sexuality and its transformations'], in M, Inghillieri and E, Ruspini (eds) *Sessualità narrate: Esperienze di intimità a confronto* [Sexuality narrated: Experiences of intimacy for comparison], Milan: Franco Angeli

Otto, H–U and Ziegler, H, 2012, *Das normativitätsproblem der sozialen arbeit: Zur begründung des eigenen und gesellschaftlichen handelns* [The problem of normativity in social work: On the foundation of self and society action], *Neue Praxis*, special issue 11

Panico, A and Matarrese A, 2006, 'Aids e società: tra esclusione e faticosi processi di integrazione' ['AIDS and society: between exclusion and hard processes of integration'], *La Rivista di Servizio Sociale*, 46, 3, 32–43

Pietrantoni, L, Prati, G and Saccinto, E, 2011, 'Bullismo e omofobia' ['Bullying and homophobia'], *Autonomie Locali e Servizi Sociali*, 34, 1, 67–79

Pietrantoni, L, Sommantico, M and Graglia, M, 2000, 'Anzianità impreviste: una ricerca su omosessualità e terza età' ['Unexpected retirement: a research on homosexuality and third age'], *Rivista del Servizio Sociale*, 40, 1, 31–42

Pustianaz, M (ed), 2011, *Queer in Italia: Differenze in movimento* [Queer in Italy: Differences on the move], Pisa: Edizioni ETS

Romania, V, 2013, *Queering social sciences: dall'epistemologia interazionista a quella del closet* [Queering social sciences: from the interactionist to the epistemology of the closet], *About Gender*, 2, 3, www.aboutgender.unige.it/ojs/index.php/generis/article/view/65

Ross, C, 2010, 'Critical approaches to gender and sexuality in Italian culture and society', *Italian Studies*, 65, 2, 164–77

Ruspini, E, 2013, 'Identità e sessualità LGBT: quali spazi offre la ricerca sociale in Italia?' ['LGBT identities and sexualities: which spaces does social research offer in Italy?'], in F, Corbisiero (ed) *Comunità omosessuali: Le scienze sociali sulla popolazione LGBT* [Homosexual communities: Social sciences on the LGBT population], Milan: Franco Angeli, 165–80

Saraceno, C (ed), 2003, *Diversi da chi? Gay, lesbiche, transessuali in un'area metropolitana* [Diverse of whom? Gay, lesbians, transsexuals in a city area], Milan: Guerini e associati

Saraceno, C, 2012, *Cittadini a metà: Come hanno rubato i diritti degli italiani* [Half citizens: How they stole Italians their rights], Milan: Rizzoli

Scalfarotto, I and Mangiaterra, S, 2010, *In nessun paese: Perchè sui diritti dell' amore l'Italia e fuori dal mondo* [In no country: Why in matters of rights for love Italy is outside of the world], Milan: Piemme

Thompson, N, 2003, *Promoting equality: Challenging discrimination and oppression*, Basingstoke: Palgrave Macmillan

Trappolin, L (ed), 2008, *Omosapiens 3: Per una sociologia dell'omosessualità* (Homosapiens 3: For a sociology of homosexuality], Rome: Carocci

Van Voorhis, R and Wagner, M, 2001, 'Coverage of gay and lesbian subject matter in social work journals', *Journal of Social Work Education*, 37, 1, 147-59

Warner, M, 1991, 'Introduction: Fear of a queer planet', *Social Text*, 29, 3-17

Weiss, JT, 2008, 'Heteronormativity', in *International encyclopaedia of the social sciences*, Encyclopedia.com, www.encyclopedia.com/doc/1G2-3045301024.html

Queering the pitch: a need for mainstreaming LGBTQ issues in professional social work education and practice in India

Ketki Ranade

Social work education in India and engagement with queer issues

Social work education in India predates the country's independence and can be traced back to the establishment of the Sir Dorabji Tata Graduate School of Social Work (now known as The Tata Institute of Social Sciences) in 1936. In its formative years, social work education in India was deeply influenced by American and European curricula and models. The focus was on developing professionals skilled at imparting welfare services through state and other philanthropic agencies (Bodhi, 2011). Over the last 75 years, several review commissions have been set up by the University Grants Commission (UGC) to review the social work curriculum in India. In 2001, the National Curriculum for Social Work was developed under the aegis of the UGC. A manual on the standards for social work education was developed in 2003 and was accepted by the National Assessment and Accreditation Council (NAAC) (Social Work Educators' Meet, 2011). The recommendations of the review commissions and discussions in formulating the curriculum focused on the necessity to move away from a welfare model of social work to an empowerment and transformative model with people's participation at the centre (UGC, 1980). Similarly, the need for social work education to be responsive to the context of globalisation, neoliberal political economies and the implications of the state–market nexus for the marginalised and vulnerable sections of the population has been highlighted (Alphonse et al, 2008).

As a result, social work education in India has moved away from the welfare, remedial approach and is engaging more with issues of structural oppression. Social structures of class, caste, patriarchy and the ways in which they cause structural inequalities find a central place in critical thinking in social work. Articulation of the 'rights discourse' that is critical of the 'benevolent' 'welfare state' and moves away from mere service provision to a discussion about entitlements is evident in the social work curriculum and practice. However, while there is a critical expression of inequalities and oppression that underlies poverty, caste discrimination and gender-based violence, this has not extended to interrogation of heterosexism, sexual hierarchies and gender binaries; some of the cornerstone ideas in queer theorising. Heterosexual privilege and the idea of compulsory heterosexuality (the assumption that everyone is heterosexual in their sexual orientation, identity and behaviour) that cuts across institutions of family, law, religion, education and science go un-noted in the curriculum (with some exceptions of programmes that are grounded in a feminist theoretical foundation). As a result, family studies as a discipline or practice remains restricted to heterosexual families. Similarly, curricula on human development or life-cycle studies continue to assume heterosexuality in all human beings while discussing adolescence as a period of 'emergence of sexuality' or while describing tasks of different life-cycle stages such as marriage or children.

Invisibility in the social work curriculum is reflected in practice too. Social workers have not been involved in developing affirmative approaches to work with lesbian, gay, bisexual, trans and queer (LGBTQ) people's health, mental health, education, livelihood, advocacy of rights with state actors such as police, campaigns for visibility and so on. As a result, services for LGBTQ people such as crisis centres, shelter homes, legal aid, police intervention in the context of violence and family interventions have not been developed in India. Moreover, the work carried out by queer movements in the country in areas such as legal reform, the articulation of human rights and addressing issues of stigma and discrimination has not been fully acknowledged and appreciated by social work educators in India. As a result, a significant people's resistance movement on issues of sexual and gender minorities has gone largely un-noted and un-integrated within the social work curriculum and practice in India.

In the area of HIV/AIDS, social work practitioners have partially dealt with issues of **men who have sex with men** (MSM) (that is, those who have sex with men, regardless of how they identify themselves, whether that be gay, heterosexual etc) and trans people as part of working with 'high-risk communities' for HIV. In the area of research and knowledge building, most of the contribution from social work has come in the area of sexual risk, HIV/AIDS and identifying barriers to care. The *Indian Journal of Social Work*, which has been in publication for 72 years, has a minority of articles that address LGBTQ concerns. The few articles that exist focus on sexual health risk.

In the last five years, student research within social work has shown some encouraging trends; student dissertations have been engaged with the human rights of LGBTQ, LGBT subcultures in urban India, and employment and livelihood concerns of *hijras/aravanis*.[1] Similarly, one of the schools of social work (Karve Institute of Social Service, Pune, India, December 2012), while celebrating its golden jubilee, held a conference entitled 'From exclusion to inclusion – issues, challenges and the road ahead' and dedicated a session to queer lives. However, this is more of an exception and probably one of the first schools of social work in India to include queer issues in a conference on exclusion and marginalisation. Social work education and practice, with their strong grounding in values of inclusion, human dignity and justice, are ideally placed to include queer issues, although it currently seems like a distant dream.

Outlining LGBTQ movements in India

LGBTQ movements in India are more visible and vibrant now than ever before, at least in urban India, with queer *Azaadi* (freedom) marches being organised in eight to ten cities, several film festivals, social and political events, an increasing number of books and magazines by queer writers and an increasing number of films by queer film makers being made. Several factors have influenced and provided impetus to the LGBTQ movement in the country and I discuss three such influences here.

The HIV/AIDS epidemic has been one such strong influence. The epidemic necessitated an open dialogue on the issue of sex and sexuality in an otherwise conservative culture; this meant commissioning research studies focusing on sexual practices and behaviours, conferences and seminars discussing strategies of sexual health promotion and awareness campaigns, resulting in visibility of a range of sexual practices that lay outside of the normative 'within marriage, heterosexual sex'. Interactions of Indian health practitioners, researchers, policy makers and functionaries of the state health department with stakeholders across the world, along with funding from national and international sources, led to an opening up of dialogue about groups such as gay men, MSM and trans people.

In the initial years of the epidemic, the National AIDS Control Organisation (NACO) was established under the Ministry of Health and Family Welfare, in 1986. Influenced by international aid agencies and global dialogue on HIV/AIDS, NACO eventually in its National Aids Control Program II (1999–2006) opened up to consider women in sex work, MSM as well as gay men as 'bridge populations' (Ramasubban, 2008). Thus, although seen as 'sexual deviants' and 'carriers of fatal infection' (to the heterosexual population), there was at least articulation in a state document about the existence of gay men and MSM in India. HIV/AIDS activists as well as gay activists played a crucial role over the years in shifting this position of NACO. NACO now runs separate targeted intervention programmes for MSM and trans people, including *hijras* and **kothis**[2]. Services under these programmes include not merely health services but also empowerment-based interventions. The national programmes encourage MSM and trans people to form their own local community-based organisations to carry out HIV/AIDS-related work. This has led to growth of several organisations led by MSM or trans people, advocating for HIV prevention as well as a broader agenda of sexual health and human rights. In fact, from the pathologising of MSM, gay men and trans people as 'bridge populations', the current national HIV/AIDS policy emphasises collectivisation, affirmative action and creating an enabling socio-legal and political environment for MSM and trans groups (NACO, 2007).

A nationwide campaign against the law criminalising homosexuality has been another influence on the LGBTQ movement. Homosexuality was branded as a criminal offence under section 377 of the Indian Penal Code (IPC) dealing with 'unnatural offences'. While Public Interest Litigation challenging section 377 was initiated in the court by one single non-governmental organisation – the Naz Foundation in 2001 – a demand for legal and political change was already being articulated within the LGBTQ communities in India. Community-based organisations led by gay men, MSM and trans people working on HIV and sexual rights, and lesbian women's groups organising in the wake of the violence and controversy surrounding the release of the film *Fire* (a Hindi-language film depicting a same-sex relationship between two middle-class Hindu women) (CALERI, 1999), were some factors that preceded the litigation against section 377 in the court. In 2006, several children's rights, women's rights and queer rights groups came together under the banner 'Voices Against 377' to plead against the violation of fundamental human rights of LGBT people (Voices Against 377, 2005). The litigation against section 377 proved to be a strong impetus for a larger collectivisation among LGBTQ groups all over the country and, simultaneously, public awareness and visibility campaigns were launched in different parts of the country (Ramasubban, 2008).

Another significant contribution to the vision of the LGBTQ movement in India came from queer feminists and their alignment with the women's rights movement. They enabled the framing of concerns of LGBTQ people within a broader framework of freedom from state and social repression of sexuality as well as patriarchal formulations of masculinity. Groups of lesbians, bisexual women and trans people have over the last decade made efforts to mainstream their issues within the women's movements in the country. They have been partially successful in integrating the issues within the network of services available for women in distress. For instance, services dealing with women facing domestic violence such as the Special Cell for Women and Children (a nationwide social work intervention service located within police stations) have started to cater for issues of LBT people in crisis.

Vulnerability and structural violence against LGBTQ people – impact on health and social wellbeing

In this section I will outline some of the common problems faced by the LGBTQ community in India and some areas for possible intervention. Needless to say, LGBTQ is not one uniform category of people and hence the issues faced by them are also not homogenous, but rather diverse. Some of the problems that I discuss in this section are directly related to physical and mental health. However, a range of problems such as human rights violations of LGBTQ people in public spaces, stigma and discrimination from a hostile environment and violence faced within the family are examples of adverse social factors that have an impact on an individual's overall quality of life, including health.

Human rights violations and the context of the criminalisation of LGBTQ people in India

As mentioned earlier, homosexuality was branded as a criminal offence under section 377 of the IPC dealing with 'unnatural offences', which was introduced in India in 1860 by the British colonial rulers. Based on Victorian norms of morality and Judaeo-Christian values (Narrain, 2001), the law remained unchallenged in India until the mid-1990s, nearly 50 years after independence and almost 40 years after its counterpart was abolished in Britain (Ramasubban, 2008). The first public protest against the law and the police harassment that was a result of the law was led by *AIDS Bhedbhav Virodhi Andolan* (campaign against discrimination related to AIDS) in 1993. From this time in 1993 until 2009, when the Delhi High Court read down section 377, decriminalising adult consensual same-sex, several LGBTQ activists and civil society stakeholders worked together not merely in a legal battle but in a political and human rights campaign for the recognition of LGBTQ people as legitimate citizens of the Indian state. However, the Delhi High Court judgment was challenged in the Supreme Court (primarily by right-wing groups). After over four years, on 11 December 2013, the Supreme Court of India set aside the Delhi High Court judgment and reinstated section 377.[3] This is a significant blow to the LGBTQ human rights campaign in the country.

Before the 2009 judgment, the threat of section 377 was used to carry out several human rights violations in the form of blackmail, extortion, threats, beating and the sexual assault of MSM, gay men, *hijras*, *kothis* and other trans people by the police (PUCL-K, 2001; Singh et al, 2012). Case records of the harassment of LGBTQ people using section 377 reveal a sorry picture. In 1994, when a group of doctors recommended that condoms be distributed in a Delhi prison, where there were reports of high homosexual activity, the prison authorities refused since homosexual sex was a crime under section 377. In 2001, some HIV and AIDS outreach workers from the Bharosa Trust and Naz Foundation International, who were carrying out HIV prevention work through the provision of sexual health information and the distribution of condoms, were arrested for running a gay 'racket' in Lucknow and charged with offences under the obscenity and indecency provisions of the IPC. The workers were beaten, kept hungry, forced to drink sewer water and refused treatment when they got sick. Despite changes in law after the 2009 judgment on section 377, the harassment of LGBT individuals has continued. For instance, in 2010, Professor Siras R, an academic in the Aligarh Muslim University in India, was suspended after having been surreptitiously photographed in a compromising position with another man within the privacy of his home (Singh et al, 2012). He was made to vacate his university quarters and moved to a rented apartment in the city. While Professor Siras's lawyers succeeded in getting his suspension cancelled, he was found dead (alleged suicide) in his apartment within weeks of this incident.

Some studies on violence among MSM, *kothis* and *hijras* in the Indian context bring out the complex relationship between marginalised sexualities and gender identities and domestic as well as state-perpetrated violence, poverty and HIV/AIDS. Research conducted by Magar and Dua (2007) with HIV-affected people who are marginalised on the basis of gender and sexuality in India revealed that poverty, harassment, physical abuse and violence due to social stigma were among the major stressors in the lives of MSM, *hijras* and *kothis*. Perpetrators of this violence ranged from intimate partners, clients and local goons to the police. Another study with 200 MSM in Chennai aimed at studying correlates of paid sex among MSM revealed that more than one third (35.0%) reported daily/weekly harassment; 40.5% reported forced sex in the previous year (Newman et al, 2008).

The limited human rights literature that exists in the context of lesbian women in India is full of testimonies of forced (heterosexual) marriages, harassment by family and the loss of jobs and residence. The most publicised example of institutional violence is the marriage of Urmila and Leela, two women from a rural background who were serving in the Madhya Pradesh police department. They got married in a temple in front of 40 witnesses and eventually with the media picking up the story, these women were labelled as 'lesbian', were asked to discontinue service and were also later separated (PUCL-K, 2001).

A study conducted in seven cities of India with 50 queer **persons assigned gender female at birth** (PAGFB)[4] found that public spaces such as schools and colleges could be a source of stigma and discrimination in the lives of queer PAGFB. PAGFB people could may face a range of violations, including attempts to correct their gender and being humiliated for their same-sex preference among their peer group and school system. Similarly for respondents who were **gender-transgressive**, spaces that were strictly gender segregated such as public toilets and women's compartments on trains were cited as spaces where they faced discrimination and violence (LABIA, 2013).

India does not yet have any non-discrimination laws that prevent discrimination on the grounds of gender or sexual orientation at work or in other public spaces. Similarly, there is no recognition of same-sex domestic partnership or same-sex marriage and thus rights related to inheritance, property, adoption and end of life decisions among same-sex partners are not available. Furthermore, there is ambiguity on the legal status of trans people and sex reassignment surgery (SRS). India has a law – section 320 – under which emasculation is an offence (Singh et al, 2012). However, whether this law could be applied in the case of SRS (where consent of the person receiving the surgery is possible) is unclear. Similarly, there is no clarity on change of documents for post-operative trans people. Currently, different states follow different practices.

Violations within the domestic/family sphere

While violations in public spheres are most visible against MSM, gay men or *hijras* and *kothis*, the domestic or family space is one of the main sources of violation in the lives of lesbian and bisexual women and trans men. The People's Union for Civil Liberties – Karnataka, which documented instances of rights violations against sexual minorities in personal as well as public spheres in Bangalore, India, acknowledges that lesbians in particular are further marginalised among sexual minorities (PUCL-K, 2001). Other studies highlight the family as a primary source of stress, and sometimes physical or psychological violence (Fernandez and Gomathy, 2001; PUCL-K, 2001; Joseph, 2005; Ghosh et al, 2011; LABIA, 2013). A book entitled *Loving women: Being lesbian in underprivileged India* (Sharma, 2006) has documented over 10 stories of women from small-town India, who wanted to live together and get married but were forced by families to separate. One study with lesbian women in India documented cases of beating and imprisonment by family members, and seeking 'remedial' treatments such as shock therapy for their lesbian daughters (Fernandez and Gomathy, 2001). Another study, which focused on disabled, lesbian and sex-working women in India, Nepal and Bangladesh, found that family violence was often heightened when the woman came out to the family or was 'outed'. Forms of violence included being beaten up, being separated from the same-sex partner, restrictions on mobility, restrictions on telephone conversations, forcible marriage and threats to life by family members. This study also reported intimate partner violence, from both gay and heterosexual partners (Dutta et al, 2012).

Research with gay men in India has emphasised the heightened stress that they face as a consequence of the family pressure for marriage, which sometimes results in forced marriages (Joseph, 2005). Research with 50 queer PAGFB people stated that depression, self-harm, cutting, staying away from home for long periods and running away from home were common responses to family violence among the respondents (LABIA, 2013).

LGBTQ health and mental health inequalities

LGBTQ health and mental health inequalities in India can be understood in the context of larger structural oppression, human rights abuses and lack of state responsiveness towards acknowledging LGBTQ people as a vulnerable group. This subsection discusses LGBTQ health and mental health inequalities in terms of the lack of adequate research on LGBTQ health, HIV and sexually transmitted infection related inequalities, barriers to accessing quality healthcare and prejudice impacting the quality of healthcare services.

In the context of LGBTQ health, much research has focused on HIV/AIDS. There is very little research on aspects of LGBTQ general healthcare and access to treatment for the same. Since lesbian and bisexual women are not considered to be part of high-risk groups for HIV infection, research focusing on their health is almost absent in India currently.

HIV Sentinel Surveillance was established in India in 1998, which monitors the HIV epidemic in the country. The 2010–11 HIV Sentinel Surveillance data show that the number of surveillance sites for MSM were increased from 40 in 2007 to 96 across 23 states in 2010–11. Among MSM, the highest HIV prevalence was recorded in the state of Chhattisgarh (15%), followed by Nagaland (13.6%), Manipur (10.5%), Andhra Pradesh (10.1%) and Maharashtra (9.9%). In total, nine states showed greater than 5% HIV prevalence (NACO, 2012), which is rather high when compared with overall adult HIV prevalence estimates (0.32% and 0.22% among adult – aged 15–49 years – males and females respectively in 2010/11). Among trans people, HIV prevalence at the three surveillance sites three (one in Maharashtra and two in Tamil Nadu) ranged from 0.8% to 18.8% (NACO, 2012). A study conducted on sexual behaviours among rural Indian men (aged 18–40 years, n = 2,910) in five districts in five states showed that 9.5% of single and 3.1% of married respondents had had anal intercourse with a man in the previous year (Verma and Collumbien, 2004). The same study also showed that only 70% of respondents had ever heard about HIV/AIDS and only 41% were aware that condom use prevented HIV infection. Only 5% of the respondents were aware about the possibility of getting HIV/sexually transmitted infection from their male partners. These studies indicate that despite over two decades of HIV/AIDS work in the country, there is still a poor reach of these services to invisible and marginalised groups such as MSM and trans people, leading to low awareness and high rates of unsafe sex among these groups.

A qualitative study among HIV-positive and high-risk *kothis* in Chennai, Tamil Nadu, about their experiences of stigma and discrimination revealed that structural violence from multiple intersecting social and institutional contexts of police, community, family and healthcare providers, placed them at a high risk of HIV infection and increased barriers to help seeking (Chakrapani, 2007).

A study conducted in Rajasthan (the largest state in India with poor human development indicators) revealed that a majority of MSM, *hijras* and other trans people in the state, both rural and urban, relied on self-medication or *hakims/dais* (traditional medical practitioners) for the treatment of sexually transmitted infections, for general health problems as well as for castration/emasculation (RSACS et al, 2007). They were reluctant to access sexual health services from government and private hospitals because of fear of harassment and lack of sensitivity among healthcare staff and counsellors. Similar findings were indicated in a study conducted with aravanis (a local term for *hijras* in Tamil Nadu) in Chennai (Chakrapani et al, 2004, 2011). Some of the problems with healthcare services were a lack of knowledge about aravanis among healthcare providers, use of abusive language by doctors as well as nurses, being forced to stay in male wards (in the case of inpatient treatment) and being mocked by other patients.

A similar trend of heterosexism and homophobia is seen among mental health professionals in India. Studies with mental health professionals in India indicate that some continue to use different methods to cure homosexuality such as masturbatory reconditioning, aversion treatments including mild shock and hormonal treatments (Narrain and Chandran, 2005; Ranade, 2009; Kalra, 2012). These methods have been internationally criticised on the grounds of both scientific efficacy and ethics (Serovich et al, 2008). In fact, the **Yogyakarta Principles** (principles on the application of international human rights law in relation to sexual orientation and gender identity; International Commission of Jurists, 2007) describe any form of treatment aimed at curing/changing sexual orientation as medical abuse. In 2001, responding to a complaint by a gay rights activist on behalf of a boy who had been administered aversion therapy and non-prescription drugs to cure his homosexuality, the National Human Rights Commission (NHRC) of India had cited section 377 of the IPC and refused to address the violation (Joseph, 2005; Khaitan, 2009). Despite this history, even today, there is no concerted dialogue or a national position regarding 'homosexuality' or use of 'conversion/reparative' treatments among professional bodies of psychiatrists, psychologists or social workers/counsellors in the country.

Similar to studies in high–income countries, a few studies that have focused on the mental health concerns of LGBTQ people in India indicate the emotional and interpersonal impact of living in a deeply homophobic environment. A qualitative exploratory study focusing on the experiences of 40 lesbian and gay individuals highlights a sense of alienation and isolation while growing up in a culture that devalues and silences same-sex desires (Ranade, 2008). Feeling guilty, living in constant fear of being found out and losing valuable relationships with peers and family are common gay-related stressors (Chakrapani et al, 2002). There have been a few reports that have documented suicides among lesbian, bisexual and trans people. A study of 50 queer PAGFB people indicated that 13 respondents had attempted suicide while still living with their family in young age due to stigma, control and violence at home (LABIA, 2013). *Humjinsi* (Fernandez, 1999), a resource book on queer rights, documented over 30 cases of lesbian couples committing suicide in a period of five years. According to Deepa V, a lesbian rights activist documenting the cases of lesbian suicides in Kerala, most women committing suicide are from *dalit, adivasi*,[5] working-class communities and have therefore been subjected to multiple discriminations (cited in Khaitan, 2004). A study conducted with 150 MSM in Mumbai city (Sivasubramanian et al, 2011) indicated that 45% reported current suicidal ideation, while 29% screened in for current major depression and 24% for any anxiety disorder. All the above studies reveal the role of social inequalities in causing mental health inequalities.

With regard to SRS in India, there is ambiguity regarding its legal status. In some states, SRS is allowed through the government-run medical facilities and in some it is not. No standard norms are followed in India regarding pre-change counselling or certification of fitness for SRS. The costs of SRS also vary widely across states (Singh et al, 2012). As a result, most trans people desirous of SRS are forced to do so in unregulated private settings. There have been instances of severe post-surgical complications, especially urological problems for male-to-female surgery (Chakrapani et al, 2004).

Conclusion

The wide range of human rights abuse of LGBTQ people, the violence they face and its impact on their health and social wellbeing call for social action at multiple levels. It is necessary to work at the socio-legal level to advocate for legislation for the protection of LGBTQ people as well as to work at the level of developing affirmative social service paradigms for LGBTQ people. The LGBTQ movement in India presently is dynamic and spreading fast throughout the country. It is raising questions related to rights, inclusion and social justice for LGBTQ people. In doing so, it is posing challenges to normative ideas of gender, sexuality and ways of relating and thereby problematising institutions of marriage and family. The movement is a good example of marginalised communities mobilising themselves to fight for their rights.

Social work education and field practice, with their grounding in values of inclusion, diversity and challenging oppression, are in a key position to align with the LGBTQ movement for change. The HIV/AIDS epidemic and social work response to the same is only the beginning. The participation of academics (social work as well as social science academics at least in major cities such as Mumbai and Delhi) and students alike in the mass protests after the Supreme Court verdict, (re)criminalising LGBTQ in India; writing protest letters to the Chief Justice of India; screening films; holding discussions on campuses – these are indications that social work education is beginning to be responsive to the concerns of LGBTQ people. A few academics and activists within social work are engaging with advocacy, research and writing that highlight the concerns of LGBTQ people and suggest more inclusive and affirmative social services for this marginalised group. While this is the beginning, there is a long way to go in terms of creating safe and inclusive services for LGBTQ people, developing inclusive policies as well as generating a sound research and knowledge base on issues that affect LGBTQ people's lives.

What we know about this already
- LGBTQ individuals in India face stigma, discrimination and violence in public and private spheres, which have an impact on their health and social wellbeing.
- A law criminalising homosexuality – section 377 of the Indian Penal Code – existed in India until it was read down to decriminalise homosexuality in 2009. The 2009 verdict was challenged in the Supreme Court, which set aside the 2009 verdict and (re)criminalised gay sex in India in December 2013.

What this chapter adds
- It provides evidence through research studies and reports of several human rights violations against LGBTQ people within families and in public spheres and the impact of these on LGBTQ people's health and mental health. It advocates for sociopolitical and legal interventions for stopping these violations.
- It documents the impact of the LGBTQ movement/s in India in addressing rights violations as well as the assertion of human rights for LGBTQ people in India.
- It highlights the need for social work curriculum and practice in India to integrate LGBTQ issues.

How this is relevant for social work and LGBT health inequalities
- The chapter states that social work education in India has neglected issues of sexual and gender minorities and underscores the need to address these in curriculum and practice.

- It argues for the need to develop LGBTQ-friendly social services and advocacy campaigns by social workers in India.
- It also argues for the need to develop LGBTQ-affirmative health and mental health services that are free of prejudice and bias.

Notes

[1] *Hijras* are usually persons assigned gender male at birth (PAGMB) and rarely persons with intersex variations but identify with the characteristics, roles and behaviours conventionally associated with the female gender. They cross-dress and live their life as a woman or may identify as belonging to a 'third gender'. They may or may not undergo castration and often live in a group with their *guru*, the head of the *hijra* household who initiates a new entrant (*chela* or disciple) into the *hijra* community through different rituals. The *guru–chela* [mentor-disciple] relationship is an important aspect of the social organisation of the *hijra* community. Most *hijras* earn a living through sex work, begging or dancing during festivals and auspicious occasions.

[2] *Kothi*: A local language term used in South East Asia to PAGMBs who identify with characteristics, roles and behaviours conventionally associated with the feminine. Kothis have also been defined as effeminate PAGMBs, who like to cross-dress and see themselves as women and use the female pronoun to describe themselves. They may take on this identity only while among their peers, but may continue to dress and act like men otherwise.

[3] This re-criminalisation of homosexuality has been met with protest and resistance not only from the LGBTQ movement but also from several progressive civil society groups, the media, politicians, business houses and academics.

[4] 'Persons assigned gender female at birth' (PAGFB) is a term used in trans feminist literature to reflect the understanding that none of us is born with a ready-made gender; gender is assigned to us at birth based on the traditional conflation of sex, in particular external genitalia. This assigned gender may or may not match our own sense of our gender.

[5] Caste hierarchies play a significant role in Indian society and determine social status, access to resources and life opportunities. In this context, being a *dalit* (belonging to one of the oppressed castes) or an *adivasi* (belonging to a tribe) implies structural oppression at multiple levels and being queer adds to the marginalisation.

References

Alphonse, M, George, P and Moffatt, K, 2008, 'Redefining social work standards in the context of globalization: lessons from India', *International Social Work*, 51, 2, 145–58

Bodhi, SR, 2011, 'Professional social work education in India – a critical view from the periphery', *Indian Journal of Social Work*, 72, 2, 289–300

CALERI (Campaign for Lesbian Rights), 1999, *A citizen's report: Khamosh! Emergency Jari Hai: Lesbian emergence*, New Delhi: CALERI

Chakrapani, V, 2007, 'Structural violence against Kothi-identified men who have sex with men in Chennai, India – a qualitative investigation;, *AIDS Education and Prevention*, 19, 4, 346–64

Chakrapani, V, Babu, P and Ebenezer, T, 2004, 'Hijras in sex work face discrimination in the Indian health-care system', *Research for Sex Work*, 7, 12–14

Chakrapani, V, Newman, PA, Shunmugam, M and Dubrow, R, 2011, 'Barriers to free antiretroviral treatment access among kothi-identified men who have sex with men and aravanis (transgender women) in Chennai, India', *AIDS Care*, first published 14 June 2011

Chakrapani, V, Row Kavi, A, Ramakrishnan, LR, Gupta, R, Rappoport, C and Raghavan, SS, 2002, 'HIV prevention among men who have sex with men (MSM) in India: review of current scenario and recommendations', www.indianlgbthealth.info/Authors/Downloads/MSM_HIV_IndiaFin.pdf

Dutta, D, Weston, A, Bhattacharji, J, Mukherji, S and Kurien, S, 2012, *Research report on violence against disabled, lesbian, and sex-working women in Bangladesh, India, and Nepal*, Delhi: CREA

Fernandez, B, 1999, *Humjinsi: A resource book on lesbian, gay and bisexual rights in India*, Mumbai: India Centre for Human Rights and Law

Fernandez, B and Gomathy, NB, 2001, *The nature of violence faced by lesbian women in India*, Mumbai: Research Centre on Violence Against Women, Tata Institute of Social Sciences, http://download.tiss.edu/fap/RCI-VAW/RCIVAW_Publications/The_Nature_of_violence_faced_by_Lesbian_women_in_India.pdf

Ghosh, S, Bandyopadhyay, BS and Biswas, R, 2011, *Vio-map: Documenting and mapping violence and rights violation taking place in the lives of sexually marginalized women to chart out effective advocacy strategies*, Calcutta: SAPPHO for Equality

International Commission of Jurists, 2007, 'Yogyakarta Principles – principles on the application of international human rights law in relation to sexual orientation and gender identity', www.yogyakartaprinciples.org

Joseph, S, 2005, *Social work practice and men who have sex with men*, New Delhi: Sage Publications

Kalra, G, 2012, 'Pathologising alternate sexuality: shifting psychiatric practices and a need for ethical norms and reforms', *Indian Journal of Medical Ethics*, 9, 4, http://www.ijme.in/index.php/ijme/article/view/1033/2357

Khaitan, T, 2004, *Violence against lesbians in India*, www.altlawforum.org/Resources/lexlib/document.2004-12-21

Khaitan, T, 2009, *NHRC, the law and the police*, http://lawandotherthings.blogspot.in/2009/07/naz-foundation-and-nhrc.html

LABIA, 2013, *Breaking the binary: Understanding concerns and realities of queer persons assigned gender female at birth across a spectrum of lived gender identities*, Mumbai: LABIA, https://sites.google.com/site/labiacollective/

Magar, V and Dua, R, 2007, *Violence in the context of HIV/AIDS in India: Gender, sexuality and risk*, Delhi: OXFAM (India) Trust

NACO (National AIDS Control Organisation), 2007, *Targeted interventions under NACP-III: Operational guidelines: Volume I: Core high risk groups*, New Delhi: NACO, Ministry of Health and Family Welfare, Government of India

NACO, 2012, *HIV sentinel surveillance 2010-11: A technical brief*, New Delhi: Department of AIDS Control, Ministry of Health and Family Welfare, Government of India

Narrain, A, 2001, 'Human rights and sexual minorities: local and global concerns', *Law, Social Justice and Global Development (LGD)*, 2, www2.warwick.ac.uk/fac/soc/law/elj/lgd/2001_2/narrain/

Narrain, A and Chandran, V, 2005, 'It's not my job to tell you that it's okay to be gay: medicalisation of homosexuality; a queer critique', in A, Narrain and G, Bhan (eds) *Because I have a voice: Queer politics in India*, Delhi: Yoda Press

Newman, PA, Chakrapani, V, Cook, C, Shunmugam, M and Kakinami, L, 2008, 'Correlates of paid sex among men who have sex with men in Chennai, India', *Sexually Transmitted Infections*, 84, 6, 434-8

PUCL-K (People's Union for Civil Liberties – Karnataka), 2001, *Human rights violations against sexuality minorities in India: A PUCL-K fact finding report about Bangalore*, Bangalore, India: PUCL-K

Ramasubban, R, 2008, 'Political intersections between HIV/AIDS, sexuality and human rights: a history of resistance to the anti-sodomy law in India', *Global Public Health*, 3, S2, 22-38

Ranade, K, 2008, 'Process of sexual identity development for young people with same-sex desires – experiences of exclusion', *Psychological Foundations – The Journal*, X, 1, 23-8

Ranade, K, 2009, *Medical response to male same-sex sexuality in Western India: An exploration of 'conversion treatments' for homosexuality*, Health and Population Innovation Fellowship Programme Working Paper, No 8, New Delhi: Population Council

RSACS (Rajasthan State AIDS Control Society), SAATHII (Solidarity and Action Against The HIV Infection in India) and OXFAM GB, 2007, *Situational analysis and strategies to upscale an evidence-based HIV response in relation to MSM, hijra and other transgender populations in Rajasthan*, London: OXFAM

Serovich, JM, Craft, P, Toviessi, SM, Gangamma, R, McDowell, T and Grafsky, E, 2008, 'A systematic review of the research base on sexual reorientation therapies', *Journal of Marital and Family Therapy*, 34, 2, 227-38

Sharma, M, 2006, *Loving women: Being lesbian in underprivileged India*, Delhi: Yoda Press

Singh, S, Dasgupta, S, Patankar, P, Hiremath, V, Chhabra, V and Claeson, M, 2012, *Charting a programmatic road map for sexual minority groups in India*, South Asia Human Development Sector Discussion Paper Series, Report No 55, Washington, DC: World Bank

Sivasubramanian, M, Mimiaga, MJ, Mayer, KH, Anand, VR, Johnson, CV, Prabhugate, P and Safren, SA, 2011, 'Suicidality, clinical depression, and anxiety disorders are highly prevalent in men who have sex with men in Mumbai, India: findings from a community-recruited sample', *Psychology, Health and Medicine*, 16, 4, 450-62

Social Work Educators' Meet, 2011, http://ssw-network.tiss.edu/reports-1/south-zone-summit-2012

UGC (University Grants Commission), 1980, Second Review Committee for Social Work Education, www.pswa.org.in/download/2%20review%20committee-SW%20edn-UGC-tiss%20doc.pdf

Verma, RK and Collumbien, M, 2004, 'Homosexual activity among rural Indian men: implications for HIV interventions', *AIDS*, 18, 13, 1845-7

Voices Against 377, 2005, *Rights for all: Ending discrimination against queer desire under section 377*, http://www.voicesagainst377.org/?page_id=61

Life in the Pink Dragon's Den: mental health services and social inclusion for LGBT people in Wales

Tracey Maegusuku-Hewett, Michele Raithby and Paul Willis

Introduction

Public understandings of the mental health needs of lesbian, gay, bisexual and trans (LGBT) people have shifted over time, from a tendency to locate the 'problem' with individual pathology, for example, in the *International classification of diseases and related health problems* (ICD; published by the World Health Organization) until 1992, to a focus on social and health inequalities that may impact negatively on mental wellbeing.

This chapter focuses attention on the Welsh context of policy making, service provision and social inclusion of lesbian, gay and bisexual (LGB) identifying adults with mental health issues. With a population of 3.1 million, Wales has its own unique history of language, cultural identity and geography, and the chapter explores areas in which Wales is making a distinctive contribution in legislative frameworks and policy initiatives regarding equalities and mental health. How these policy and societal landscapes interact with the lives of LGB people is explored further using illustrative extracts from recent Wales-wide research into LGB adults who have experienced mental health issues, and their responses to the societal attitudes and quality of services they have encountered.

The landscape of equality and mental health social care in Wales

Since the late 1990s, Scotland, Northern Ireland and Wales have been devolved nations within the United Kingdom (UK), with powers granted by the UK Parliament at Westminster to make separate legislation in some, although not all, areas of public policy. In Scotland and Wales, referenda were held in 1997, requiring a simple majority in favour of devolution. In Wales, a narrow majority in favour led to the Government of Wales Act 1998 and the establishment of the National Assembly for Wales, the legislature with powers to determine how the budget for Wales should be spent. The Government of Wales Act 2006 followed, which created the executive body of elected members: the Welsh Assembly Government. Another referendum in 2011 was in favour of further devolved powers, now named the Welsh Government (Llywodraeth Cymru) to encompass both the legislative and executive arms.

The Welsh Assembly was the first administration in the UK to introduce legislation – the Government of Wales Act 1998 – on protecting and promoting equalities in the public sector, with the duty to have due regard for the principle of equality. This was further reinforced in the Government of Wales Act 2006 (section 77), now incorporated into the Public Sector Equality Duty in the Equality Act 2010 and subsequent Equality Act 2010 (Statutory Duties) (Wales) Regulations 2011. The Public Sector Equality Duty Wales, approved in 2011, requires public bodies to have due regard to the need to eliminate unlawful discrimination, advance equality of opportunity and foster good relations between people; all relevant to LGBT people.

Wales has been particularly influential in the history of socialised healthcare across the UK. Aneurin Bevan, the Welsh Labour Party Member of Parliament and Minister of Health in the Atlee government from 1945 to 1951, followed the blueprint of his own experiences of mutual healthcare aid in his South Wales Valleys home town of Tredegar for the foundation of the National Health Service in 1948. The current Welsh Government has expressed commitment to this spirit of mutuality and collective action in its White Paper on the future of social services in Wales – *Sustainable social services* (WG, 2011a), with the principle that people in Wales should have 'a strong voice and real control' (WG, 2011a, p 9). This policy unequivocally establishes a Welsh policy direction of community and citizen-directed support, which is distinguished from a market-driven, consumerist interpretation of personalisation in England.

The Strategy for Mental Health and Wellbeing in Wales – *Together for mental health* (WG, 2012) – states the government's commitment to a human rights-based approach, fundamental to addressing inequalities and stigma, underpinned by citizen-centred delivery of public services. Reducing the inequalities, stigma and discrimination experienced by people living with mental health issues is identified as an explicit outcome. At the heart of this strategy, the Mental Health (Wales) Measure 2010 (which has the same legal status in Wales as an Act of

Parliament) expands the role of primary care as being more accessible and less stigmatised than other mental health services, as well as providing access to an independent mental health advocate for people with mental health issues who are inpatients in hospital. Another significant feature of the strategy relates to the inclusivity of citizens across all age ranges. This is a welcome shift in policy direction given that the previous approach to addressing mental health was to focus separate action plans (known as National Service Frameworks – NSFs) on children, adults of working age and older adults. This created an inequitable rate of progress, and individuals transitioning the boundaries of age often experienced patchy services and gaps in provision.

The study

Stonewall Cymru is the all-Wales LGB charity for lobbying, consultation and research, established in 2003 with support from the Welsh Assembly Government and Stonewall Great Britain. Stonewall Cymru and three partner mental health organisations identified the need to undertake research on the experiences, inclusion and access to services of LGB people in Wales living with 'mental health issues'. They obtained grant funding from the Equality and Human Rights Commission, and commissioned the chapter authors to undertake this preliminary piece of all-Wales, mixed methods research (Maegusuku-Hewett et al, 2009). A reference group made up of LGB and mental health service users, and representatives of mental health and LGB organisations, was fundamental to the success of the research. For instance, the group were instrumental in:

- the formulation of the research focus, methodological approach and scope of the definition of mental health;
- providing guidance and advice around research questions and themes;
- legitimising, gatekeeping and promoting the research to participants and organisations.

Finally, the group's membership provided a platform to promote and disseminate the findings on a national scale and to lobby the Welsh Government with key recommendations for policy and practice.

Undertaken in 2009, the study engaged with 146 people who self-identified as LGB and as having had, or currently experiencing, mental health issues via an online survey ($n = 116$) and focus groups/semi-structured interviews ($n = 30$). In reporting on our qualitative findings herein, we have used pseudonyms to protect participants' anonymity Of the 116 people completing the survey, just over half of respondents stated that they had 'fair', 'poor' or 'very poor' mental health at the time of the survey. The remaining 48% regarded themselves as having 'good', 'very good' or 'excellent' mental health now, but as having had mental health issues in the past.

The multiple dimensions of inequality in sexual orientation and mental health

The social identities of marginalised groups of people are not homogenous. Originating in Black feminist thinking (for example, Crenshaw, 1993), the concept of **intersectionality** proposes how multiple social, political and cultural identities can interact, and thereby amplify structural oppressions. LGB people may endure stigma and prejudice based on their sexual orientation while also dealing with societal bias against mental health issues and distress. LGB individuals with other marginalised identities – such as being disabled, being from a black and minority ethnic (BME) background, being trans, older or with other social identities – may therefore experience multiple sources of oppression and stigma (Fish, 2008; Cronin and King, 2010).

From our survey respondents, 33% ($n = 38$) considered themselves to be disabled under the definition originally outlined in the Disability Discrimination Act 2005 (superseded by the Equality Act 2010), 0.9% declared as being of 'mixed' background (although under-representative of the 6.8% BME population of Wales) and 23% were aged 50 **or over**. (The Welsh Government defines older people as those aged 50 or over for policy-making purposes.)

The majority of focus group participants talked about the impact that multiple stigmatised identities have on their daily lives in terms of other people's treatment of them and their level of engagement within their local communities and LGB-specific social groups and activities (some of these insights will follow in the forthcoming discussion). Our survey findings also revealed a bleak picture of community isolation wherein one third of respondents (36%, $n = 41$) said that they did not engage in any hobbies, community, social, voluntary or political activities within their local communities on a regular basis.

It is important to recognise the heterogeneity of identity-based communities, however. The impact of diversity and social difference within communities has been discussed in terms of intersectionality, or the complex and cumulative interactions between different sources of oppression, for example, by Cronin and King (2010) in relation to older LGB adults.

Study participants' access to mental health service provision

Bearing in mind the survey targeted those identifying as having/ having had mental health issues, most respondents (82%, *n* = 95) either currently accessed or had accessed mental health services, with just under half of these (44%, *n* = 42) declaring that they had accessed mental health services more or less continuously for several years. Figure 4.1 illustrates the range of services accessed. 'Talking therapies' via private or NHS counselling were the most frequently utilised form of support, for example nearly two thirds had accessed counselling in a primary care setting via their general practitioner (GP) and this preceded the introduction of the Mental Health (Wales) Measure 2010, which subsequently expanded the role of primary care. Twenty-one per cent had accessed an acute service through crisis resolution treatment, which targets services to people undergoing a crisis of such severity that they would otherwise be hospitalised.

Perceptions of the extent and benefits of service provision

It has been acknowledged by the Welsh Government in successive strategic plans that mental health services in Wales remain under-resourced and historically have been referred to as a 'Cinderella service' in relation to its 'lack of status amongst other health and social care specialisms' (NAW, 2009, p 6). Similarly, it was the general consensus within the focus groups and interviews in the present research that there were distinctive gaps in provision and several shortcomings in professional practice with LGB people. These ranged from limited specialist input, lengthy waiting lists and high threshold criteria for services, to the skills and attitudes of practitioners: "Problems are brushed under the carpet, and Prozac smarties are just dished out. They dish them out with no help for years and years. I think I went for years without seeing anyone else other than my GP for mental health problems" (Katie). Here, Katie is suggesting that underlying issues are not addressed but 'smoothed over' with the use of medication. Others in the study felt that there was a blanket approach to dealing with mental health issues, with many respondents who could afford to, paying for private counselling.

Figure 4.1: Types of mental health service accessed

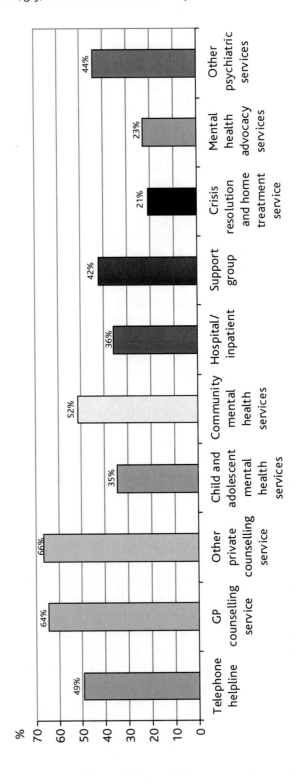

Enduring waiting lists

Several participants were dissatisfied with the length of time it took to access a range of mental health services. For example, Alun, a young gay man, stated

> 'I got put on a waiting list for anorexia in 2006 and I only just started getting treated last summer [2008]. It's just long waiting lists. When I lived in [area] I was on a psychiatric waiting list for three years and it eventually just got completely cancelled.' (Alun)

For this individual, and others with eating disorders, the longevity of being in 'limbo' without provision is not in keeping with evidence and good practice guidelines that advocate early effective treatment to be crucial in longer-term physical and emotional health (Wales NHS, 2012). That said, in 2009, the Welsh Government recognised the variability and shortcomings of eating disorder service provision across Wales and established a National Framework for Eating Disorders. The framework aims to improve funding and access to a range of eating disorder services and it reinforces that eating disorders 'can be devastating, or in a small number of cases, life-long or life-threatening' (WAG, 2009a, p 8). The framework specifically focuses on age as a risk factor, but falls short in identifying any other social characteristics that may be risk factors for developing an eating disorder. In particular, it is well established that there is a higher prevalence of eating disorders among gay and bisexual men, than among heterosexual men (Russell and Keel, 2002). Meanwhile, a national UK study by Hunt and Fish (2008, p 11), suggests that one in five lesbian and bisexual women have had an eating disorder compared with one in 20 of the general population, and 26.6% of lesbian and bisexual women who took part from Wales reported having had an eating problem.

High threshold criteria for services

> 'It sounds really bad, I was in care and I was unhappy for a long time … and I said I was unhappy and I took an overdose and they moved me. They'll start taking action when you start cutting yourself or doing things; it's almost like you have to be really bad before they'll do anything to help.' (Michael)

The prevalence of mental health problems among children in care is higher than for children in the general population (McAuley and Davis, 2009) and therefore the needs of looked-after children have been recognised in a National Service Framework for Children, Young People and Maternity Services (WAG, 2005). However, Michael's experience illustrates the gulf between policy and implementation. This experience was mirrored in a report published by the Wales Audit Office and Healthcare Inspectorate Wales (2009), which found patchy availability of early intervention, specialist, mental health services for children and young people in these circumstances.

Encounters with mental health professionals

Thirty-nine per cent of our survey respondents who were 'out' to their mental health practitioner reported heterosexist values, attitudes, knowledge and skills to have impacted on their access, experience and ultimately their treatment, with some claiming a misattribution of LGB identity as the root cause of their mental health issue: "Homosexuality to the psychiatrist was seen as a reason for greater psychological disturbances, i.e. you're gay (even when I said bi) so you must have problems. Others [psychiatrists] were good, however" (Rob).

While our findings were based on a small sample, they mirror those of King and McKeown (2003), who argue that LGB people are greater users of primary and secondary mental health services than their heterosexual counterparts. In their England and Wales survey they also found that:

> [U]p to a third of gay men, one quarter of bisexual men and over 40% of lesbians recounted negative or mixed reactions from mental health professionals when being open about their sexuality and one in five gay men and lesbians and a third of bisexual men recounted that a mental health professional made a causal link between their sexuality and their mental health problem. (King and Mckeown, 2003, p 5)

Issues of bilingualism and rurality facing LGB people in Wales

Welsh-speaking individuals may live in all areas of Wales; however, some regional and rural areas have higher numbers, for example in the local authority of Gwynedd 65% of the population are Welsh speakers. Of the respondents to our survey, 11.5% use Welsh as their first language. While this is slightly lower than the Welsh language Census statistics, which indicate that 19% of the population (or 562,000 people) can speak Welsh (ONS, 2012), the experiences reported by Welsh speakers in the survey suggest that services are not always equipped to provide a service in Welsh: "I had more trouble getting services in Welsh than from a gay-friendly practitioner" (Delyth).

The *National services model for local primary mental health support services* (WG, 2011b, p 11) recognises that '[p]oor communication can lead to misunderstanding, mistrust, misdiagnosis and subsequently inappropriate assessments, interventions and care, and potentially poorer outcomes for individuals and their carers'. It is pertinent that services take account of an individual's language, and where that language is Welsh, then public services are legislatively obliged to be proactive in providing a service in Welsh.

The Welsh Language Act 1993 was recently superseded by the Welsh Language (Wales) Measure 2011, which sought to strengthen the initial Act by way of greater obligation and accountability upon public services to facilitate the Welsh language by:

- confirming the official status of the Welsh language;
- creating duties on bodies to provide services through the medium of Welsh;
- creating a Welsh Language Commissioner with enforcement powers to protect the rights of Welsh speakers to access services through the medium of Welsh;
- providing greater accountability by establishing a Welsh Language Tribunal and right of appeal.

At the time of writing, the Welsh Language Commissioner is conducting an inquiry into primary healthcare services.

It is not known at this present time how Welsh and LGB identities may intersect and shape each other – the ways in which LGB individuals living in Wales identify and affiliate with Welsh language, identity politics and culture in parallel to LGB identity-based communities and social spaces. For Welsh speakers who identify as LGB, accessing services that are proactive in providing services in their first language of choice and that promote themselves as gay friendly and LGB inclusive presents compounded challenges. Individuals within this social bracket are more likely to have to compromise on language choice or receptiveness of helping professionals to LGB identities (or both) in order to access mental health services that meet their immediate needs. This is an important field for future enquiry and discussion with bilingual LGB adults who share close national ties with Wales, its language and its people.

Wales can be characterised by its large rural geography, farming and ex-mining communities, with just under a third of the population of Wales living in rural areas (WG, 2011c, p 2). One quarter of our sample lived in rural areas and villages. Arguably, lack of provision within rural areas impacts on all members of the community; however, given that LGB people are more likely to access mental health services, and may be isolated by their status, the proximity and availability of such services may compound their health inequalities. Study participants felt disadvantaged by transport routes and the concentration of specialist services in larger towns and cities, with some having to travel long distances to access services:

'There's self-harm support groups but I don't attend 'cos can't get to them from where I live; there should be better transport links or help to get places.' (Sian)

'There are limited mental health services in the area.' (Jodie)

Clarke et al (2010) note how rural isolation can be associated with a lack of LGBT-specific services. In addition, LGBT individuals in such areas may be reluctant to access the services that do exist, due to fear of potential victimisation should their identity become known in their community. A small-scale survey into the experiences of BME and LGB-identifying respondents living in rural North Wales, found a paradox between being highly visible minority ethnic people and invisible as LGBT individuals, thus impacting on access to services, provision of information and isolation (North Wales Race Equality Network and Stonewall Cymru, 2010).

Small, close-knit communities can embody the attributes of mutual support celebrated by the Welsh Government in its vision for social care (WG, 2011a). However, there can also be increased pressure on those perceived to be 'different' in the context of conservative social values. This is illustrated by the following experiences of two men brought up in the former coalmining communities of the South Wales Valleys:

'I had a homophobic family and growing up in the Valleys I wasn't able to accept myself let alone "come out".' (Shane)

'I had to leave the Valleys to be who I wanted to be. The first place I lived in was fine for two years until they realised I was gay; thereafter I received death threats and my property was vandalised.' (David)

Here, David's narrative can be related to the study of gay migration, which posits a unidirectional rural–urban migration. Other respondents suggested a more ambivalent relationship with the 'city', in which the city exists as a space for social practices where alternative sexualities can be experienced and explored, while at the same time for many the context in which these encounters take place remains substantially unattractive to them (Annes and Redlin, 2012):

'[T]here's no way of meeting gay men other than coming to the city … because of the depression I'm almost more hedonistic, and so I've gone out on the scene to escape, taken more risks, and drank too much to forget. It becomes a spiral of escapism.' (Mathew)

This cultural milieu is by no means exclusive to Wales. The benign image of rural life for LGBT people in England has also been critiqued by Bell and Valentine (1995) and latterly by Jones et al (2013) as part of a 'Gay and Pleasant Land?' project. Both uncover gay men and lesbians' experiences of prejudice and 'don't ask, don't tell' neighbourhood attitudes while living in rural locations.

Bell and Valentine (1995) point to the organic and self-initiated networks that may be established by LGB people residing within these contexts, and to some extent our study participants exemplified their resourcefulness in instigating and sustaining 'minority networks'. Sylvia lives rurally and depicts some rural places as 'lesbian villages'. She had lived in an area that was homophobic; however, since moving she has experienced no problems – neighbours even welcomed her and her partner with cake! Sylvia speaks of informal networks whereby friends gather at each other's houses. Even in the 1980s/1990s it was the norm to go to people's houses (researcher's notes).

'Coming out': factors that can promote resilience

The literature on LGBT communities tends to problematise in order to highlight the inequalities that exist in their health, wellbeing, human rights and quality of life. Arguably, this risks paying limited attention to resilience outcomes. An ecological approach enables a broad examination of the interplay between individual psychology and one's wider familial and social system of neighbourhood, community and service provision. These are 'social ingredients' that may mediate or add to what Mayock et al (2009) term 'minority stress' and essentially lead to poorer health outcomes and increased risk of self-harm and suicidal ideation; or, on the other hand, as Scourfield et al (2008) identify in their study of LGBT young people and self-destructive behaviour, individuals may utilise resilience strategies that mediate and strengthen LGBT identity.

Coming out is a pivotal element of LGBT identity that can be negotiated in multiple contexts across the lifecourse. Ryan et al (2009) note how young LGB adults are more likely to lose important social relationships, including those with parents, when their sexual orientation is disclosed. Furthermore, parental rejection is significantly associated with poorer health, mental ill-health and risk-behaviour outcomes. Of our survey respondents, 39% were not out to their family. One of the focus group participants reflected on the negative impact of the longevity of purporting a heterosexual identity for the sake of maintaining family relations:

> '[C]oming out meant that my homosexuality is viewed as a disease. My parents do not accept my homosexuality, and forbid me telling the rest of my family. This means I have to pretend that I am single to the rest of my family, [this] leads to low self-esteem, and used to lead to depression.' (Angharad)

Within our study we found that the level of support available to people in 'coming out' and accepting their sexual orientation (if indeed they felt the need to accept it) was crucial in bolstering their sense of identity and reducing feelings of isolation. The absence of support for some respondents served to highlight the significance of this assertion:

> 'I was in care all my life and when I came out at 16, the only people who were around me were like social workers and support workers, and I always say like that there's no support for young people who are coming out. Like there is no advisers in that service who is there specifically supporting and is there for gay people, and this is a missed area.' (Shaun)

'When I realised, at the age of 19, I was also very lonely as a result of not confiding in anyone, I felt desperate.' (Simon)

'I knew I was different but didn't know what it was. I was suicidal and reached a point and thought I either die tonight or get help.' (Paul)

We found that many participants in the study accessed online spaces to overcome isolation; however, for some, these were deemed sexualised spaces. Just under half had accessed telephone helplines and there was a call from focus group participants for LGB mental health web sources of support.

The Welsh Assembly Government's *National action plan to reduce suicide and self-harm 2009-2014* (WAG, 2009b) aims to reduce the rate of suicide and self-harm in Wales by targeting people who are at highest risk. LGBT people are acknowledged within the plan as a group of people who may experience social exclusion and stigma and fail to engage with service providers. The plan also aims to achieve wider public health goals by, for example, helping to tackle substance misuse, which is known to play an important part in suicide and self-harm, and for which, the evidence suggests, LGBT people have an elevated propensity (King and McKeown, 2003).

Where to next?

This chapter has outlined how the Welsh Government has expressed its commitment to citizen-directed services, for example in the arena of mental health, and to ensuring equal treatment for LGBT people in Wales. There are, however, some historical shortfalls in mental health provision and care across regions, specialisms and the lifespan for the population of Wales, for which recent Wales legislation and policy are aspiring to remedy. LGBT individuals are 'mainstreamed' into these; however, they have been acknowledged as a 'high risk group' within harm reduction strategies. Given the increased likelihood of mental health need among LGBT people, coupled with the evidence base around inequitable access and poor experiences of mental health providers, it is remiss that current Wales-wide provision falls short of any targeted interventions to reduce mental health inequalities for LGBT people, such as the Increased Access to Psychological Therapies pilot service in Leicester in the UK (NHS, 2013).

For social workers in Wales, the professional regulatory body provides a Code of Practice for Social Care Workers (Care Council for Wales,

2002). In common with the equivalent professional social work codes in the constituent nations of the UK, this describes the standards of conduct and practice expected of practitioners, including promoting equal opportunities for service users and carers, and respecting diversity and different cultures and values (Care Council for Wales, 2002, 1.5, 1.6). However, the qualitative evidence discussed in this chapter demonstrates that while areas of good practice exist in Wales in relation to health and social care services for LGBT people, practitioner attitudes can still lag behind policy intentions, reflecting homophobia and **transphobia** in the wider communities.

The research findings bear a number of implications for mental health service providers and social workers alike. For service providers, additional challenges remain in ensuring that services are promoted to mental health consumers as LGB inclusive and safe spaces in which service users can discuss aspects of their sexual biographies that intertwine with and sit alongside their experiences of mental distress. Preventative measures cannot be achieved without providing healthcare staff who are skilled and receptive to actively providing bilingual and LGB-inclusive services that remove initial barriers for individuals experiencing social and mental vulnerability.

For social workers, the findings highlight the importance of being mindful *and* responsive to the double stigma attached to accessing mental health services for LGB-identifying adults. The findings give examples of how prior encounters with homophobic and heterosexist attitudes conveyed by mental health professionals can foreshadow consumers' expectations of future access to vital services. For mental health practice to be truly citizen centred and human rights based, social workers need an acute understanding of how multiple social factors – including rurality, sexual identity, gender and language – intersect and shape consumers' experiences of professional services. Each of these social dimensions can operate as a source of social oppression and can compound inequities and inequalities in accessing healthcare provision.

In parallel, social workers have an advocacy role in bringing other helping professionals' attention to wider social factors that can compromise the quality of LGB consumers' everyday lives and resiliency to mental distress, such as community isolation and lack of LGB social connections. LGB consumers' former experiences of discrimination and homophobia across the lifecourse can breach their capacity to place trust in new helping professionals, including social workers.

What we know about this already

• Wales-based literature identifies strengths and limitations of mental health provision in Wales for the general population and there is evidence of the compounding factors of limitations in services for LGBT people.

• We are not aware of any research that specifically focuses on Welsh bilingualism and rurality in the context of sexuality and health inequalities; although one study reported on in this chapter explored BME LGB people living in one part of rural Wales.

• There is a plethora of research evidence outlining elevated levels of self-harm and suicidal ideation among LGBT people; little research provides a balanced perspective on resiliency strategies.

What this chapter adds

• It exemplifies Wales' ethos towards equality.

• It provides an overview of Welsh context and divergence in devolved policies and to some extent practices.

• It provides social workers and health practitioners in Wales and beyond with key messages about LGBT health inequalities and promotes good practice.

• It discusses bilingualism and rurality and provides some case examples but also identifies this as a research gap.

• It outlines a case example of strategic initiatives to promote resilience and reduce self-harm in Wales.

How this is relevant for social work and LGBT health inequalities

• Social workers need to be aware of the divergent policy and practice approaches to health and social care and equality.

• Social workers need to dissect the intersectionality of stigmatised identities.

• Social workers need to be knowledgeable of the increased risks of mental health inequalities for LGBT people and understand the social and political contributory factors.

• Social workers need to take an ecological approach to assessing and providing for the needs of LGBT service users in order to mediate stressors and improve health and wellbeing outcomes.

References

Annes, A and Redlin, M, 2012, Coming out and coming back: rural gay migration and the city, *Journal of Rural Studies*, 28, 1, 56–68

Bell, D and Valentine, G, 1995, 'Queer country: rural lesbian and gay lives', *Journal of Rural Studies*, 11, 2, 113-122.

Care Council for Wales, 2002, *Code of Practice for social care workers*, Cardiff: Care Council for Wales

Clarke, V, Ellis, SJ, Peel, E and Riggs, D, 2010, *Lesbian, gay, bisexual, trans and queer psychology: An introduction*, Cambridge: Cambridge University Press

Crenshaw, K, 1993, Mapping the margins: intersectionality, identity politics, and violence against women of color, *Stanford Law Review*, 43, 1241-99

Cronin, A and King, A, 2010, Power, inequality and identification: exploring diversity and intersectionality amongst older LGB adults, *Sociology*, 44, 5, 876-92

Fish, J, 2008, Navigating Queer Street: researching the intersections of lesbian, gay, bisexual and trans (LGBT) identities in health research, *Sociological Research Online*, 13, 1, www.socresonline.org.uk/13/1/12.html

Hunt, R and Fish, J, 2008, *Prescription for change: Lesbian and bisexual women's health check 2008*, London: Stonewall

Jones, K, Fenge, L-A, Read, R and Cash, M, 2013, Collecting older lesbians' and gay men's stories of rural life in South West England and Wales: 'We were obviously gay girls ... (so) he removed his cow from our field', *Forum: Qualitative Social Research*, 14, 2, www.qualitative-research.net/index.php/fqs/article/view/1919/3514

King, M and McKeown, E, 2003, *Mental health and wellbeing of gay men, lesbians and bisexuals in England and Wales*, London: Mind

Maegusuku-Hewett, T, Raithby, M, Huxley, P, Evans, S, Winter, B, Philpin, S and White, J, 2009, *Double stigma: The needs and experiences of lesbian, gay & bisexual people with mental health issues living in Wales*, Cardiff: Stonewall

Mayock, P, Bryan, A, Carr, N and Kitching, K, 2009, *Supporting LGBT lives: A study of the mental health and wellbeing of lesbian, gay, bisexual and transgender people*, Dublin: Gay and Lesbian Equality Network and BeLonG To Youth Service

McAuley, C and Davis, T, 2009, Emotional well-being and mental health of looked after children in England, *Child & Family Social Work*, 14, 2, 147-55

NAW (National Assembly for Wales), 2009, *Health, Wellbeing and Local Government Committee Inquiry into Community Mental Health Services*, Cardiff: NAW

NAW, 2012, Petition Committee: Child and Adolescent Eating Disorder Service P04-408, Cardiff: NAW

NHS (National Health Service), 2013, *Equality objective update, March 2013*, Leicester, Leicestershire and Rutland Integrated Equality Service, www.leicspart.nhs.uk/Library/EqualityObjectiveUpdateSheetLGBTIAPTCLINIC.pdf

North Wales Race Equality Network and Stonewall Cymru, 2010, *Dipping your toe in the water: The double jeopardy of race and sexual orientation in North Wales*, Cardiff: Stonewall Cymru

ONS (Office for National Statistics), 2012, *2011 Census: Welsh language profile unitary authorities in Wales*, table KS208WA, ONS, www.ons.gov.uk/ons/rel/census/2011-census/key-statistics-for-local-authorities-in-england-and-wales/rft-table-ks208wa.xls

Russell, J and Keel, P, 2002, Homosexuality as a specific risk factor for eating disorders in men, *International Journal of Eating Disorders*, 31, 3, 300-6

Ryan, C, Huebner, D, Diza, RM and Sanchez, J, 2009, Family rejection as a predictor of negative health outcomes in white and Latino lesbian, gay, and bisexual young adults, *Pediatrics*, 123, 1, 346-52

Scourfield, J, Roen, K and McDermott, L, 2008, Lesbian, gay, bisexual and transgender young people's experiences of distress: resilience, ambivalence and self-destructive behaviour, *Health & Social Care in the Community*, 16, 3, 329-36

WAG, 2005, *National Service Framework for Children, Young People and Maternity Services*, Cardiff: WAG

WAG, 2009a, *Eating disorders: A framework for Wales*, Cardiff: WAG, http://wales.gov.uk/docs/dhss/publications/090703eatingdisorderframeworken.pdf

WAG, 2009b *Talk to me: A national action plan to reduce suicide and self-harm 2009-2014*, Cardiff: WAG

Wales Audit Office and Healthcare Inspectorate Wales, 2009, *Services for children and young people with emotional and mental health needs*, Cardiff: Auditor General for Wales

Wales NHS (National Health Service), 2012, *Improving treatment for eating disorders*, Cardiff: NHS

WG (Welsh Government), 2011a, *Sustainable social services: A framework for action*, Cardiff: WG

WG, 2011b, *National services model for local primary mental health support services*, Cardiff: WG

WG, 2011c, *Delivering rural healthcare services*, Cardiff: WG

WG, 2012, *Together for mental health: A strategy for mental health and wellbeing in Wales*, Cardiff: WG

PART TWO

Service design and practice development

Coming into view? The experiences of LGBT young people in the care system in Northern Ireland

Nicola Carr and John Pinkerton

VIGNETTE

Simon is 16 years old and has been living with his foster parents for the past four years. He generally gets on well with his foster parents, an older couple, and his time with them has been the most settled of his life. He hasn't told his foster parents or his friends that he is gay. He recently heard his foster carers discussing a news item on gay marriage following a motion in the local parliament calling for the introduction of same-sex marriage in Northern Ireland. The proposal was rejected by politicians, and Simon's foster parents expressed their support for this position. In their discussion about the debate they sounded negative about gay people. He is starting to feel a bit down about this, particularly because some young people at school have been calling him names. His new social worker has been encouraging him to start thinking about what he wants to do when he leaves school and where he wants to live when he leaves foster care. He just wants to be himself. He hasn't told her he is gay. He thinks the best thing to do is to say nothing about that to anyone yet and wait for the day when he can leave school and leave care. It can't come too soon.

Introduction

The challenges that can go with being a care-experienced lesbian, gay, bisexual or trans (LGBT) young person, whether in out-of-home care, leaving care or after care, is an area that has received limited attention to date in terms of practice, services, policy and research. That, however, is beginning to change, encouraged by a growing international understanding regarding the importance of all facets of identity for young people in care and in their transition from the care system and their subsequent life experiences. The holistic and rights-based perspective on health and wellbeing underpinning this book is in keeping with the messages on what makes for best professional practice coming both from research and directly from young people themselves and those who care for and about them. It is that 'whole person/whole system' perspective that is needed to ensure that a care-experienced young person like Simon (see practice vignette) is positively supported.

This chapter aims to contribute to the growing awareness of the needs of LGBT young people in care, leaving care and after care through highlighting some of the key challenges that face 'sexual minority' young people in these arenas. As for all young people, this requires thinking about the sexuality of young people as a key dimension to all aspects of their needs, rights and expectations. While young people themselves must be central to this focus, attention must also be given to how their needs, rights and expectations are enabled or frustrated by the informal and formal systems of which they are a part – their 'social ecology of support'.

In this chapter, some of the key findings from the limited amount of empirical research in this area are reviewed and links are made with wider literature on LGBT young people and young people in care. These are considered in relation to the illustrative case vignette of Simon and the societal context of Northern Ireland – a post-conflict society still heavily influenced by traditional religious, community and family structures but committed to advancing human rights throughout its political structures and civil society. In this way, the chapter aims to bring into view what is available as general and contextualised knowledge, underpinning values and core skills, for anti-oppressive social work practice with LGBT care-experienced young people.

Needs, rights and expectations

In asking Simon to think about what he wants to do on leaving school and when he moves on from his foster home, his social worker is concerned to ensure that he is an active participant in planning his time in care – his 'care career'. She wants him to be able to make his voice heard at his next six-monthly formal review. As VOYPIC (Voice of Young People in Care) simply puts it in its guide for young people going into care: 'the review is about you and it is important that you have a say' (VOYPIC, no date). VOYPIC, a Northern Ireland-based non-governmental organisation set up by a group of young people in care and practitioners to improve the lives of children and young people cared for away from home, insists that all children and young people who are cared for away from home should have:

- a voice at the heart of all decision making;
- a meaningful say in their lives;
- their rights fully respected;
- the opportunity to realise their full potential in whatever they choose to do.

To help achieve that for Simon, his social worker needs to take a holistic and rights-based perspective on health and wellbeing – a 'whole person/whole system' approach towards his needs, rights and expectations, including his sexual orientation. To do that it is necessary to move beyond thinking about being in care as a discrete period in a young person's life to be managed by social services staff with the aim of achieving a set of predetermined normative outcomes appropriate to the transitional youth phase of the life cycle. A young person's in-care experience needs to be thought of as part of an individually 'lived life' in a way that connects it to pre-care and after-care experiences and to a range of emotions and relationships, past, present and future.

Care-experienced young people are involved in an ongoing developmental process of 'coping' with constantly changing physical, psychological and social circumstances. The characteristics of coping at any particular time are linked with chronological age and associated development but it is more dependent on personal agency within the 'structures of opportunity' provided by the types and qualities of formal and informal support available and availed of (Coleman and Hagell, 2007; Henderson et al, 2007; Pinkerton and Dolan, 2007). The concepts of 'resilience' and '**social capital**' are helpful in thinking about how coping is linked with existing structures of opportunity. While both terms are contested and open to different interpretations, even among those who find them helpful (Leonard, 2005; Mohaupt, 2008), they usefully capture a sense of present 'wellbeing' and future 'well becoming', which are very important dimensions to the lived experience of youth transitions.

Resilience has been defined as 'the quality that enables some young people to find fulfilment in their lives despite their disadvantaged backgrounds, the problems of adversity they may have undergone or the pressure they may experience' (Stein, 2008, p 36). Social capital can be defined as 'the sum of the resources, actual or virtual, that accrue to an individual or a group by virtue of possessing a durable network of more or less institutionalised relationships of mutual acquaintance and recognition' (Bourdieu and Wacquant, quoted in Henderson et al, 2007, p 12). These personal assets of resilience and social capital need to be situated within a social ecology of support (Pinkerton, 2011). This can be captured figuratively in a very schematic logic model linking service interventions with coping through impact on the social ecology in which formal and informal, enriching or impoverishing, networks of support resource a young person's social capital and resilience (see Figure 5.1).

Figure 5.1: A globalised social ecology of care leaving

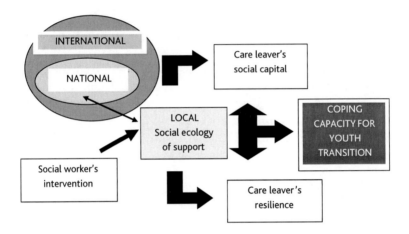

Simon knows he is gay now but is developing a coping strategy based on repressing the open expression of his sexuality until a future date. While this enables him to navigate his current living situation, the fact that he has to do this speaks to the rejection that he fears facing if he was to 'come out' (that is, disclose his sexuality) in his current care placement and raises questions regarding the type of issues that young people who are LGBT may encounter in care and how this care experience is framed by the wider social context.

Unfortunately to date, the structure of opportunity – the social ecology of support at global, national and local levels – available to care-experienced young people has tended to be very restricted. A recent literature review notes that for some young people, the outcomes based on a range of indicators (for example, housing stability, education and employment) as they transition from care are poor (Mendes et al, 2011). The review also drew attention to how specific groups of care leavers faced additional disadvantages:

- indigenous young people;
- rural and regional young people;

- young disabled people;
- unaccompanied asylum-seeking young people.

To that list can be added LGBT young people (Stein, 2012).

The poor outcomes that research to date has identified as characteristic of care leaving in a range of countries can be considered to be the outworking of low resilience and limited social capital within an impoverished social ecology of support, that is, the accumulated disadvantage of pre-care and in-care experience (Mills and Frost, 2007). Perhaps more importantly the different levels of coping between young people within care-leaving populations, which are now gaining research attention (Stein, 2008), can be seen as reflecting differences in the extent to which social capital and resilience have been garnered as developmental assets by care leavers from past and present engagement with their social ecology of support. This has particular implications for those young people facing additional challenges such as those who are LGBT (Smith, 2011).

LGBT young people in care and leaving care

There is a limited amount of empirical literature on LGBT young people in the care system, a fact we argue speaks to the relative invisibility of this group of young people and a consequent failure to adequately address their needs. There is, however, an emergent body of research that points to some of the specific issues facing lesbian, gay and bisexual (LGB) young people in care (although it is important to note that within this the specific issues facing trans young people are rarely addressed). Wider research on LGBT young people is of course relevant, and in this section we also draw on this literature.

A small number of studies (largely based in the United States) have explored specific issues for LGB young people such as differential experiences of entry into care, treatment within care and particular challenges faced when transitioning from the care system (Mallon, 1998; Dworsky, 2013). In an exploration of some of the factors that may lead to a higher representation of gay and lesbian young people in the child welfare and juvenile justice systems, Sullivan (1996) suggests parental rejection and/or abuse of a young person because of their sexuality as a possible entry route into care. Experiences of harassment in school contexts leading to absence from education can also bring young people under the ambit of child welfare or juvenile justice systems (Sullivan, 1996).

For many young people, their sexuality and/or gender identity may not have been a factor in their entry into care, but become(s) an issue in care. For some young people, this may involve having to navigate environments of heteronormativity (that is, presumed heterosexuality and gender binaries), or the absence of a safe environment in which to discuss their thoughts, feelings and desires for fear of rejection and ridicule. This is a point highlighted in the vignette at the start of this chapter, where Simon does not want to discuss his sexuality with his foster carers because he fears their potentially negative response. This raises the question of the capacity of care placements to meet the needs of LGBT young people. The experience of care may present particular challenges, for example the manner in which substitute caregivers respond to and facilitate a young person 'coming out'. In a study conducted in New York, Freundlich and Avery (2005) highlighted specific concerns of gay, lesbian, bisexual, trans and queer (LGBTQ) young people in group care settings, including concerns regarding privacy and personal safety. Sullivan et al's (2001) study of LGBT young people in foster care highlights the need to match young people with suitable foster parents. Indeed, we would further argue that there is a need for all foster carers to be aware of and sensitive to issues of sexuality and gender identity.

One of the most extensive longitudinal studies focusing on young people's transition from foster care – the American Midwest Study – found differences between LGB young people and their heterosexual peers in terms of economic wellbeing following their transition from care (Dworsky, 2013). Data from the study shows that when in care, LGB young people were more likely to have experienced more placements on average than their heterosexual peers. They were also more likely to score less well on a range of economic wellbeing indicators following their transition from care. For example, when employed, LGB young people reported less hourly earnings than their heterosexual peers and 61% of the LGB respondents experienced at least one of five economic hardships (for example, not enough money to pay rent) compared with 47% of their heterosexual peers – a statistically significant result.

Attending to the wider context

A systemic perspective (Figure 5.1) encourages attention to the very immediate social ecology of support determining the resilience and social capital of care-experienced young people. It also draws attention to the nested nature of the social ecology of care at national and international levels. Understanding and support for Simon must not only be concerned with his immediate situation, himself and his relationship with his foster family, friends and social worker but also take account of organisational and policy systems that will in turn be part of interlocking national and international systems (Pinkerton, 2008).

Care systems are situated within and are reflective of societal and structural norms and in many societies there has been a historic lack of recognition of and discrimination towards LGBT people. It is important to recall for instance that in Northern Ireland consensual sexual activity between adult males was only decriminalised in 1982 (Sanders, 1996). Social attitude surveys point towards continued high levels of discrimination against LGB people (for the Northern Ireland context see, for example, Schubotz and O'Hara, 2011; Equality Commission for Northern Ireland, 2012). Notably, the UK jurisdictions of England, Wales and Scotland have introduced legislation allowing for same-sex marriage in recent years. However, within Northern Ireland some political parties have rejected motions calling for the legislation of same-sex marriage, and this issue remains at a standstill (McAlister et al, 2014). While there have undoubtedly been advances in terms of acknowledging the social and legal rights of LGBT people in recent years, this has been by no means universal. As McDermott (2011) notes, even where rights have been advanced, the experiences of these are likely to be mediated by other factors such as class, race, gender, disability and ethnicity – and being care experienced can be added to that list.

Studies of the sexual health and educational needs of looked-after children and young people highlight traditionally poor service provision and a general reluctance on the part of care providers to engage meaningfully with issues of sex and sexuality (Broad, 2005; Dale et al, 2010). In this context, there has been a particular *lack of recognition* of the needs of LGBT young people. That said, in recent years there is evidence of attention turning towards this area. This has been informed by a number of factors, including the recognition of the relevance of identity for young people in care (Thomas and Holland, 2010; McMurray et al, 2011) and the importance of a positive sense of identity for young people leaving care in terms of longer-term outcomes (Stein, 2008). Findings from a broader and growing body of research on LGBT young people are also raising awareness of the need for more tailored and responsive social work and social care services for LGBT young people (Fish, 2012).

Wider literature on LGBT young people has explored some differential experiences and areas of increased vulnerability. For example, research on the experiences of sexual and gender minority young people in schools reveals concerns regarding negative school experiences, including homophobic and transphobic bullying and associated effects on educational attainment and school drop-out (for example, Bontempo and D'Augelli, 2002; Mishna et al, 2009). Other work has focused on mental health vulnerabilities, including risks of suicidality and self-harm among LGBT young people (for example, Fergusson et al, 1999; Van Heeringen and Vincke, 2000), while other negative social outcomes have been noted in research on LGBT young people and homelessness and alcohol and substance misuse (for example, Savin-Williams, 1994).

The picture painted here, however, is one that risks a broader pathologising of LGBT young people and this is an important critique of some of the research to date and the manner in which it has been translated into practice. Savin-Williams (2001, 2005) and Elze (2007) have pointed to some of the shortcomings in the research on sexual minority young people. These include a disproportionate focus on psychosocial risks and negative development outcomes, leading in some instances to a short-hand depiction of sexual minority young people as an 'at-risk' group (Bryan and Mayock, 2012). Conversely, limited attention has been paid to strengths and resilience (Savin-Williams, 2001). Critics have also pointed towards an overly homogenised account of sexual minority young people, which fails to adequately account for diversity (McDermott, 2011). Another concern is the failure to pay adequate attention to the intersectional nature of identity and ironically presents a normative picture of 'gay youth', one in which certain landmarks such as when to 'come out' are achieved (Talburt, 2004). Indeed, similar arguments apply to the way research on care-experienced young care leavers has been both helpful and unhelpful.

Recognising minority stress

The concept of 'minority stress' has been used to describe the stressors within the social ecology of LGBT people (for example, experiences of stigma, prejudice and discrimination) that may lead to poorer health outcomes (Brooks, 1981; Meyer and Frost, 2012). The term offers a useful analytical lens and perhaps something of a corrective to individualised accounts of risk and has been used to explain research findings, which suggest higher rates of mental distress among *some* LGBT people. It is important to note, however, that sexual minority status is not just associated with stressors and vulnerabilities and LGBT people are resilient.

This is borne out by research exploring the realities of young LGBT lives. For example, in a study focusing on young LGBT people in England and Wales, Scourfield et al (2008) found that young people adopted a range of coping strategies to manage situations of distress, which were linked to experiences of homophobia and managing socially stigmatised identities. While some young people engaged in 'self-destructive behaviours' such as self-harm as coping strategies (McDermott et al, 2008), other young people adopted strategies of resilience, such as 'fighting back' and challenging negative constructions. Similarly, in a large-scale study exploring mental health and wellbeing among LGBT people in Ireland, Mayock et al (2009) found that many respondents identified important sources of social support. Recognition of these positive features of an LGBT young person's social ecology is very important when developing service responses. There are four particularly key sources of support: friends, family, the LGBT community and school/work environments. From this list, some of the compounding factors and challenges facing young LGBT people in care will be evident.

Promoting resilience

In a review of resilience and young people leaving care, Stein (2008) identifies a range of factors that are important in promoting resilience. These include the quality of the care experience and the wider supports that young people have to draw on in care. Stein (2008, p 38) also notes the importance of helping care leavers to develop a positive sense of identity:

> Helping care leavers develop a positive identity will be linked, first of all, to the quality of care and attachments experienced by looked-after young people....; second, to their knowledge and understanding of their background and personal history; third, to their experience of how other people perceive and respond to them; and, finally, to how they see themselves, and the opportunities they have to influence and shape their own biography.

From a constructionist perspective, resilience is understood not as a trait inherent in an individual, but as a dynamic that exists between the individual and their various social worlds (for example, school, community, family, peers) (Ungar, 2004; Harvey, 2012). Harvey (2012) argues that fostering resilience among LGBT young people involves *actively affirming* their identity rather than problematising it or silencing expressions of self. Here it is also important to recognise and challenge the pervasive effects of heteronormativity in constructing and constraining both the young person's and their adult caregiver's worlds, enforcing a particular view of the norms of gender, sexuality and ways of being (Harvey, 2012).

Mallon (2006) further argues that there has been a failure of child welfare and care systems to recognise the fact that they work with LGBT people on a daily basis. Therefore a first critical step is a recognition of the diversity of sexuality and gender among young people. If we consider Simon's situation, we can see that his social worker can potentially play an important role in helping him to understand his own biography and in supporting a positive sense of identity. Here too within the wider system that the social worker operates there is a need for recognition of the diversity of sexuality and gender among people who use services and indeed those who provide them.

Conclusion

As with any socially excluded group, it is the expectations, judgements and actions of young people leaving state care themselves that will ensure the process of achieving their inclusion. The challenge to policy, to service design and to practice is to find ways to provide supportive scaffolding and to challenge and dismantle disabling barriers. Rather than locating the difficulties faced by many LGBT care-experienced young people and the capacity to resolve them solely at the level of the individual, the social ecology of support must become the focus of an anti-oppressive practice. Not only does Simon's social worker need to work alongside him to promote his individual resilience but also together they need to engage the wider systems that resource or impede his coping capacity. There is a clear need for all care-experienced young people to be supported in exploring their sexuality and gender. That must include proactively tackling homophobia and transphobia and bringing into view within the child welfare system minority sexual and gender identities.

What we know about this already
- There has been limited attention paid to the specific needs of LGBT young people within the care system.
- Existing research makes it clear that LGBT young people within the care system may face differential experiences.

- Within the UK there is a sufficient legislative mandate and policy framework within which to develop the necessary support for LGBT young people in care – but it needs to be used proactively.

What this chapter adds
- It demonstrates that more research is needed on how LGBT young people are coping with being care experienced and on how best to enhance their strategies.
- It illustrates that the concepts of 'social ecology', 'minority stress' and 'resilience' are useful when exploring the differential outcomes and experiences of LGBT young people.
- It shows that services need to develop resources and expertise focused specifically on the needs, rights and expectations of care-experienced LGBT young people.

How this is relevant for social work and LGBT health inequalities
- Anti-oppressive practice involves a holistic and rights-based approach towards promoting the health and wellbeing of LGBT young people in care.
- Professional training needs to ensure confidence and competence in addressing issues of sexual orientation as a routine aspect of the care experience.
- There is a need for a policy network focused specifically on the needs of care-experienced LGBT young people.

References

Bontempo, DE and D'Augelli, AR, 2002, 'Effects of at-school victimization and sexual orientation on lesbian, gay, or bisexual youths' health risk behaviour', *Journal of Adolescent Health*, 30, 364-74

Broad, B, 2005, *Improving the health and well-being of young people in care*, Lyme Regis: Russell House Publishing

Brooks, VR, 1981, *Minority stress and lesbian women*, Lexington, MA: Lexington Books

Bryan, A and Mayock, P, 2012, 'Speaking back to dominant constructions of *LGBT lives*: complexifying 'at riskness' for self-harm and suicidality of lesbian, gay, bisexual and transgender youth', *Irish Journal of Anthropology*, 15, 2, 8-15

Coleman, J and Hagell, A, 2007, *Adolescence, risk and resilience: Against the odds*, Chichester: John Wiley

Dale, H, Watson, L, Adair, P, Moy, M and Humphris, G, 2010, 'The perceived sexual health needs of looked after young people: findings from a qualitative study led through a partnership between public health and health psychology', *Journal of Public Health*, 33, 1, 86-92

Dworsky, A, 2013, *The economic well-being of lesbian, gay and bisexual youth transitioning out of foster care*, OPRE Report No 2012-41, Washington, DC: Office of Planning, Research and Evaluation, Administration for Children and Families, US Department of Health and Human Services

Elze, JD, 2007, 'Research with sexual minority youths: where do we go from here?', *Journal of Gay and Lesbian Social Services*, 18, 2, 73-99

Equality Commission for Northern Ireland, 2012, *Equality Awareness Survey 2011*, Belfast: Equality Commission for Northern Ireland, www.equalityni.org/archive/pdf/DYMMSurveyMainReport(webB). pdf

Fergusson, DM, Horwood, J and Beautrais, AL, 1999, 'Is sexual orientation related to mental health problems and suicidality in young people?', *Archives of General Psychiatry*, 56, 10, 876-80

Fish, J, 2012, *Social work and lesbian, gay, bisexual and trans people: Making a difference*, Bristol: Policy Press

Freundlich, M and Avery, RJ, 2005, 'Gay and lesbian youth in foster care: meeting their placement and service needs', *Journal of Gay and Lesbian Social Services*, 17, 4, 39-57

Harvey, R, 2012, 'Young people, sexual orientation and resilience', in M Ungar (ed) *The social ecology of resilience: A handbook of theory and practice*, New York, NY: Springer, 325-34

Henderson, S, Holland, J, McGrellis, S, Sharpe, S and Thomson, R, 2007, *Inventing adulthoods: A biographical approach to youth transitions*, London: Sage Publications

Leonard, M, 2005, 'Children, childhood and social capital: exploring the links', *Sociology*, 39, 605-22

Mallon, GP, 1998, *We don't exactly get the welcome wagon: The experiences of gay and lesbian adolescents in child welfare systems*, New York, NY: Columbia University Press

Mallon, GP, 2006, 'Busting out of the child welfare closet: lesbian, gay, bisexual and transgender-affirming approaches to child welfare', *Child Welfare*, 85, 2, 115-22

Mayock, P, Bryan, A, Carr, N and Kitching, K, 2009, *Supporting LGBT lives: A study of the mental health and wellbeing of lesbian, gay, bisexual and transgender people*, Dublin: Gay and Lesbian Equality Network and BeLonG To Youth Services

McAlister, S, Carr, N, and Neill, G, 'Queering the family: attitudes towards lesbian and gay relationships and families in Northern Ireland', Belfast: ARK. Available at: http://www.ark.ac.uk/publications/ updates/Update89.pdf

McDermott, L, 2011, 'The world some have won: sexuality, class and inequality', *Sexualities*, 14, 1, 63-78

McDermott, L, Roen, K and Scourfield, J, 2008, 'Avoiding shame: young LGBT people, homophobia and self-destructive behaviours', *Culture, Health and Sexuality*, 10, 8, 815-29

McMurray, I, Connolly, H, Preston-Shoot, M and Wigley, V, 2011, 'Shards of the old looking glass: restoring the significance of identity in promoting positive outcomes for looked-after children', *Child and Family Social Work*, 16, 2, 210-18

Mendes, P, Johnson, G, Moslehuddin, B, 2011, *Young people leaving state out-of-home care: Australian policy and practice*, Melbourne: Australian Scholarly Publishing

Meyer, IH and Frost, DM, 2012, 'Minority stress and the health of sexual minorities', in CJ Patterson and AR D'Augelli (eds) *Handbook of psychology and sexual orientation*, New York, NY: Oxford University Press, 252-66

Mills, S and Frost, N, 2007, 'Growing up in substitute care: risk and resilience factors for looked-after young people and care leavers', in J Coleman and A Hagell (eds) *Adolescence, risk and resilience: Against the odds*, Chichester: John Wiley

Mishna, F, Newman, PA, Daley, A and Solomon, S, 2009, 'Bullying of lesbian and gay youth: a qualitative investigation', *British Journal of Social Work*, 39, 8, 1598-614

Mohaupt, S, 2008, 'Review article: resilience and social exclusion', *Social Policy and Society*, 8, 1, 63-71

Mullan, C, McAlister, S, Rollock and Fitzsimons, L, 2007, 'Care just changes your life': factors impacting upon the mental health of children and young people with experiences of care in Northern Ireland, *Child Care in Practice*, 13, 4, 417-34

Pinkerton, J, 2008, 'States of care leaving: towards international exchange as a global resource', in M Stein and ER Munro (eds) *Young people's transitions from care to adulthood: International research and practice*, London: Jessica Kingsley Publishers

Pinkerton, J, 2011, 'Constructing a global understanding of the social ecology of leaving out of home care', *Children and Youth Service Review*, 33, 2412-16

Pinkerton, J and Dolan, P, 2007, 'Family support, social capital, resilience and adolescent coping', *Child and Family Social Work*, 12, 3, 219-28

Sanders, D, 1996, 'Getting lesbian and gay issues on the international human rights agenda', *Human Rights Law Quarterly*, 18, 1, 67-106

Savin-Williams, RC, 1994, 'Verbal and physical abuse as stressors in the lives of lesbian, gay male, and bisexual youths: associations with school problems, running away, substance abuse, prostitution and suicide', *Journal of Consulting and Clinical Psychology*, 62, 2, 261-9

Savin-Williams, RC, 2001, *Mom, dad, I'm gay*, Washington, DC: American Psychological Association

Savin-Williams, RC, 2005, *The new gay teenager*, Cambridge, MA: Harvard University Press

Schubotz, D and O'Hara, M, 2011, 'A shared future? Exclusion, stigmatisation and mental health of same-sex-attracted young people in Northern Ireland', *Youth and Society*, 43, 2, 486-506

Scourfield, J, Roen, K and McDermott, L, 2008, 'Lesbian, gay, bisexual and transgender young people's experiences of distress: resilience, ambivalence and self-destructive behaviour', *Health and Social Care in the Community*, 16, 3, 329-36

Smith, WB, 2011, *Youth leaving foster care: A developmental, relationship-based approach to practice*, New York: Oxford

Stein, M, 2008, 'Resilience and young people leaving care', *Child Care in Practice*, 14, 1, 35-44

Stein, M, 2012, *Young people leaving care: Supporting pathways to adulthood*, London: Jessica Kingsley Publishers

Sullivan, C, 1996, 'Kids, courts and queers: lesbian and gay youth in the juvenile justice and foster care systems', *Law and Sexuality: A Review of Lesbian and Gay Legal Issues*, 6, 31-62

Sullivan, C, Sommer, S and Moff, J, 2001, *Youth in the margins: A report on the unmet needs of lesbian, gay, bisexual, and transgender adolescents in foster care*, New York, NY: Lambda Legal Defense and Education Fund

Talburt, S, 2004, 'Constructions of LGBT youth: opening up subject positions', *Theory into Practice*, 43, 2, 116-21

Thomas, J and Holland, S, 2010, 'Representing children's identities in core assessments', *British Journal of Social Work*, 40, 8, 2617-33

Ungar, M, 2004, 'A constructionist discourse on resilience: multiple contexts, multiple realities among at-risk children and youth', *Youth and Society*, 35, 3, 341-65

Van Heeringen, C and Vincke, J, 2000, 'Suicidal acts and ideation in homosexual and bisexual young people: a study of prevalence and risk factors', *Social Psychiatry and Psychiatric Epidemiology*, 35, 11, 494-9

VOYPIC (Voice of Young People in Care), no date, *Care… but not as we know it*, Belfast: VOYPIC, www.voypiccareguides.org/DOWNLOADS/GUIDES/VOYPIC_11-15_guide.pdf

SIX

Social services for LGBT young people in the United States: are we there yet?

Elizabeth A. Winter, Diane E. Elze, Susan Saltzburg and Mitchell Rosenwald

VIGNETTE

The bus was late again. Sari was used to this. Since 'hitting' the streets, she needed the bus to get around. Aged 16, Sari had been homeless for three months. Originally, she stayed at a young people's shelter, but ran away when slurs like "queer bitch" from other young people became too much. The staff knew and did not seem to care.

Sari preferred staying on her own, sometimes couch-surfing with her girlfriend or making enough money selling marijuana to stay in a cheap motel. Sari did not have to sleep in an alley yet. She refused to sell her body, but she knew more than anything that she did not want to return to her mother's home.

Her mother couldn't understand why Sari was 'different'. Sari referred to herself as female but disliked labels; she felt the same about 'lesbian' or 'straight'. Her very religious mother thought Sari's lifestyle was against God's will, and reacted by verbally and physically abusing Sari. On the street, Sari was determined to make it on her own. Yet quietly, she was not always sure how.

Introduction

Although Sari is fictional, her experience at the youth people's shelter, meant to be a safe haven, is common. Lesbian, gay, bisexual and trans (LGBT) young people in the United States (US), despite advances in legal protections and cultural visibility, still face barriers in accessing culturally competent care throughout service delivery systems. Trans young people, homeless LGBT young people and LGBT young people involved in child welfare and juvenile justice systems are highly vulnerable to stigmatisation, victimisation and inadequate, insensitive service delivery. The US lags behind other countries in applying a human rights framework in assessing social, cultural and economic policies (Reichert, 2007). Human rights language is absent from the Institute of Medicine's report on the health of LGBT Americans (IOM, 2011) and from *Healthy People 2020* – the federal government's 10-year national health promotion agenda (USDHHS, 2010). However, both reports draw attention to social determinants associated with physical and mental health disparities affecting LGBT citizens (that is, stigmatisation, violence, oppression and discrimination).

LGBT young people frequently experience policies and practices within US service delivery systems that violate the Convention on the Rights of the Child (UN, 1989), which the US has not ratified. Discriminatory, differential treatment of LGBT young people persists in:

- child welfare settings (Woronoff et al, 2006);
- schools (Kosciw et al, 2012);
- programmes for runaway and homeless young people (Ray, 2006);
- juvenile courts and detention facilities (Majd et al, 2009).

Victimisation includes:

- harassment (Woronoff et al, 2006);
- physical, sexual and emotional abuse by peers and professionals (Ray, 2006; Woronoff et al, 2006; Kosciw et al, 2012);
- denial of medically necessary hormone treatments to trans young people (Majd et al, 2009).

LGBT young people can be forced to undergo 'conversion therapy' aimed at changing sexual orientation (Woronoff et al, 2006), a practice denounced by major national professional associations – for example, the American Psychological Association (APA Task Force, 2009), the National Association of Social Workers (2000), the Pan American Health Organization and the World Health Organization (PAHO and WHO, 2012). California recently became the first state to prohibit reparative therapy for minors; the ban was upheld on appeal (Lovett, 2013).

Schools frequently violate LGBT young people's rights to freedom of expression and association, and freedom from harm, by prohibiting students from organising school-based gay–straight alliances (GSAs), banning same-sex couples from school dances, ignoring harassment and bullying of LGBT students (Kosciw et al, 2012) and preventing trans young people from wearing clothing and using facilities congruent with their gender identity (Sausa, 2005). Futhermore, the Affordable Care Act 2010 restored US$50 million annually for abstinence-only-until-marriage educational programmes. Such curricula violate international human rights standards guaranteeing young people access to scientifically accurate and comprehensive health and sexuality information (UN High Commissioner for Human Rights, 2011).

This chapter addresses policies and practices promoting equitable services for LGBT young people by presenting the case study of Sari, a young person involved in multiple service systems. The chapter describes the ideal, seamless cross-system service delivery using promising practices and recommended policies. Progress achieved towards providing quality services for US LGBT young people and key next steps are described.

Homeless and runaway young people

Sari was beginning to realise that street life is challenging. As a 'runaway', Sari escaped her mother's abusive behaviour for what she thought was freedom. She experienced an unwelcoming shelter, where young people harassed her and the staff did not protect her. She had left the shelter a week ago and could only stay with her girlfriend for two days at a time. This was Sari's fourth week on the streets and she was scared.

That evening, a police officer found Sari, shivering with cold; he wanted to take her to the shelter she had just left! When she told him that they did not like queer people, he suggested a local safe house for LGBT young people that provided warm meals, a shower and a bed. Staff would work with her and the child welfare system to help find permanency for her. Sari said she would try it and felt relieved once she arrived and settled in. What a difference a welcoming environment meant!

Sari is part of the larger group of young people and young adults escaping abuse, or who are ejected from their homes due to familial rejection of their sexual orientation or gender identity and become homeless. These young people lack permanent housing and are homeless under the definition of the US Department of Housing and Urban Development (2011). Lesbian, gay and bisexual (LGB) young people comprise 15% to 36% of homeless young people, while only representing 1.3% to 3.8% of young people in general (Rosario et al, 2012). Annually, approximately 80,000 lesbian, gay, bisexual, trans and queer (LGBTQ) young people are homeless for more than one week

(National Alliance to End Homelessness, 2013). On the street, young people face increased risk of sexual exploitation, violence, substance abuse and suicidality (Ray, 2006). They also struggle to find services that are respectful of variance in sexual orientation and gender identity (National Alliance to End Homelessness, 2013).

The second shelter Sari visits exemplifies ideal service delivery for LGBT homeless and runaway young people, in which staff would be proficient in LGBT diversity issues. For young people in general, the US government provides US$114 million dollars (fiscal year 2014) under The Runaway and Homeless Youth Act 1974 (as amended) to fund the provision of concrete resources (The Basic Centre Programme), up to 18 months of residential care for 16- to 21-year-olds (The Transitional Living Programme) and crisis intervention for street young people (The Street Outreach Programme) (National Alliance to End Homelessness, 2014). Yet, despite this focus on homeless and runaway young people, the US has not prioritised the needs of LGBT young people.

Quintana et al (2010), echoing recommendations in the LGBT Youth National Policy Statement (National Alliance to End Homelessness, 2012), argue that the federal government should do more to help LGBT young people, including family strengthening, safe schools, expanding housing for this population when homeless, and conducting research.

Child welfare

After dropping Sari off at the shelter, the police officer contacted the local child welfare agency. Sari's new child welfare caseworker started helping Sari to find safe housing. The caseworker contacted Sari's mother to talk about Sari returning home. Sari's mother would neither let her return, nor make other arrangements, saying: "She can live with those women she hangs around." Seeking a family placement, the caseworker arranged a placement with foster parents who had successfully fostered LGBT young people. The foster parents had attended relevant training events and Parents and Friends of Lesbians and Gays (PFLAG) meetings. PFLAG supports LGBT people and their families, provides advocacy and education, and has chapters in over a dozen countries.[1]

At the court hearing, the judge confirmed the foster placement and ordered family therapy for Sari and her mother, to support the goal of reunifying Sari and her mother. The judge ordered that the family group decision making (FGDM) process be used (American Humane Association, 2008). In FGDM, caring adults connected to a

116

young person collaborate to recommend the best placement option to the court. This group may include family members, teachers, clergy, a caseworker and, for Sari, perhaps a PFLAG member and LGBT-affirmative therapist.

Following the Fostering Connections to Success and Increasing Adoptions Act 2008, the caseworker located Sari's other relatives and told them they could be considered as placement resources. The caseworker contacted relatives who had lost touch with the family, since estranged LGBT adult family members may provide support or placement. The caseworker provided Sari with copies of *It's your life* (Desai, 2010) and *Getting down to basics* (CWLA and Lambda Legal Defense, 2012), which detail LGBTQ young people's legal rights and other important child welfare system information).

In the US, governmental agencies hold primary responsibility for administering child protective services (Child Abuse Prevention and Treatment Act 1974). These child welfare agencies investigate child maltreatment reports and are responsible for connecting children, young people and their families to resources to meet child welfare system goals of safety, wellbeing and appropriate permanent living arrangements (Adoption and Safe Families Act 1997). A key child welfare principle is helping children to achieve permanency with their family of origin or other relatives. If this is impossible, the permanency goal becomes adoption or legal guardianship with other adults. This concept of 'permanency' involves legal relationships (such as adoption), physical permanency (a physical home) and relational permanency (an ongoing connection to caring adults) (Mallon, 2011).

Sari's child welfare agency had developed LGBT-appropriate services using best practice guidelines (CWLA et al, 2012); all agency personnel were trained using nationally recognised curricula on services to LGBT young people in out-of-home care (Elze and McHaelen, 2009). The child welfare agency also held regular case consultations with an LGBT-competent agency.

In practice, the services provided to Sari may not follow best practice guidelines. Little is known about how many child welfare agencies provide appropriate services for LGBT young people. An exploratory study of private and public child-serving agencies found modest advances in changing policies and providing LGBT-appropriate services (Rosenwald, 2009). The federal government has noted the over-representation of LGBT young people in the child welfare system and the need for appropriate services (Children's Bureau, 2011). Safety and placement stability are challenging for LGBT young people placed out of home, who risk victimisation because of sexual orientation or gender identity and so are more likely to run away (Woronoff et al, 2006). In one group home study, 70% of sexual minority young people reported violence and 78% were subsequently removed or ran away (Feinstein et al, 2001). Most of these young people reported feeling 'safer' on the streets than in group or foster homes. Forums conducted with US LGBT young people and adults (Woronoff et al, 2006) have confirmed the need for systemic changes in child welfare to account for how LGBT people build community and family.

Minority ethnic young people are also over-represented in child welfare (Child Welfare Information Gateway, 2011). Although little is known about the intersection of racial and sexual minority status, black and minority ethnic (BME) young people are probably over-represented among LGBT child welfare-involved or homeless young people (Quintana et al, 2010). Promising child welfare models such as FGDM, developed for other underserved populations, could benefit LGBT young people with minimal adaptation.

The school system

At Anytown High School, Sari met Ms Andrews, the school social worker, who provides school-based services to homeless young peoples under the McKinney-Vento Homeless Assistance Act 1987. Sari noticed colourful posters on the walls advertising a GSA for LGBT students and their friends. Ms Andrews explained that she protects the educational rights of students who are homeless or in foster care, and that she and Sari's caseworker would gather immunisation and educational records and secure school transportation for Sari. Under the law, even without records, Sari can attend school.

They discussed Sari's class schedule and previous school experiences. Ms Andrews invited Sari to check in later that day, telling Sari that students see her for many reasons, everything from "stress with academics or friends, to concerns about sexual orientation or gender identity, or just to chat". Ms Andrews handed Sari the school's policies, including one 'prohibiting discrimination, harassment, and bullying for reasons like race, ethnicity, sexual orientation, gender identity, physical and mental abilities, religion, and being from another country'.

Ms Andrews walked Sari to her English class with Mr Rudnick. He greeted Sari, handing her a copy of *The picture of Dorian Gray*. Moments into the discussion, one boy called Oscar Wilde "a fag". Mr Rudnick stopped him and reminded everyone that such words hurt and devalue people; the student apologised. Mr Rudnick continued: "Oscar Wilde lived in a time when loving someone of the same sex was illegal and he was imprisoned for that reason. How do you think his sexual orientation influenced his writing?" A spirited discussion ensued.

While changing classes, Sari saw teachers everywhere in the hallways, calling students by name, asking about Saturday's game and interrupting disrespectful language before situations escalated. At lunchtime, Sari noticed the GSA's informational table; many students were buying tickets for the GSA dance. Sari thought she might talk with Ms Andrews about her struggles around gender identity and sexual orientation. She was not totally sure, but she felt hopeful for the first time in a long time.

Decades of research with LGB young people, and recently with trans young people, show that they report significantly more school-based victimisation and discrimination than their heterosexual peers (IOM, 2011) and higher rates of psychological distress and health-risk behaviours (Centers for Disease Control and Prevention, 2011). Multiple studies have shown an association between school-based victimisation and higher rates of suicidality, substance use and risky sexual behaviours among sexual minority young people (IOM, 2011), poorer educational outcomes and other school-related problems (Greytak et al, 2009), particularly for LGBT BME (Diaz and Kosciw, 2009). Evidence exists that these health disparities continue into young adulthood (Russell et al, 2011).

Policy advocates, educators, parents and students have made considerable progress in:

- securing state and school district-level policies prohibiting harassment and discrimination in US educational settings;
- winning judgments against districts that fail to protect victimised students;
- organising school-based GSAs;
- successfully challenging, under the federal Equal Access Act 1984, districts' attempts to ban such clubs;
- raising public awareness about bullying severity.

Since 2001, the Gay, Lesbian, and Straight Education Network's (GLSEN) biennial national school climate surveys have provided critical data for change efforts (Kosciw et al, 2012).

Lawsuits have upheld LGBT young people's constitutional rights to equal protection from harm and freedom of expression, including trans young people's right to express their gender identity within schools (NCLR and GLSEN, 2012). Approximately 13 states and the District of Columbia prohibit discrimination against students based on sexual orientation and gender identity (Human Rights Campaign, 2013a). Some additional states and the District of Columbia specifically include LGBT students in laws and/or administrative regulations that address harassment and bullying, but most do not (Human Rights Campaign, 2013b). State bullying laws vary widely in content and scope, including definitions of bullying and mandates placed on state education departments and school districts (US Department of Education, 2011).

Nearly 4,000 school-based GSAs or LGBT-positive diversity clubs are registered with GLSEN (Kosciw et al, 2010) and are the primary vehicles through which LGBT students and their allies create LGBT-affirming school climates (Russell et al, 2009). GSA presence in schools is also associated with the following among sexual minority young people:

- greater psychological wellbeing and educational attainment (Toomey et al, 2011);
- school belonging (Heck et al, 2011);
- feeling safe;
- academic achievement;
- less truancy (Walls et al, 2010);
- less suicidality (Goodenow et al, 2006).

Findings are mixed as to whether GSA presence is associated with less school-based victimisation (Walls et al, 2010).

BME students may feel excluded from GSAs due to racially defined social boundaries limiting participation in extracurricular activities, privileging of white students' experiences, and adult advisers' shortcomings in effectively addressing the needs of BME students (McCready, 2004). Promising practices for creating safer, more affirming school climates include teacher training on LGBT issues and bullying prevention, LGBT resources and the integration of LGBT issues into curricula (Russell et al, 2010). The Obama Administration has issued statements reminding educational authorities of their legal obligations to stop discrimination, bullying and harassment, including gender-based discrimination (Ali, 2010), and to support LGBT students in establishing GSAs under the Equal Access Act 1984 (Duncan, 2011).

Mental health

Aware of the increased risks facing homeless LGBT young people, including personal assault, prostitution or drug trafficking as means to survive, and exposure to health disorders (Cochran et al, 2002), the arms of the 'systems of care' model (Stroul and Friedman, 1996) unfold when responding to Sari's mental health needs. Establishing mental health services for Sari quickly is critical; the child welfare caseworker refers Sari to a clinical social worker with expertise in LGBT young people.

Approaching the first session, Sari worries that the therapist may think she needs 'fixing' or will expect Sari to teach her about trans identities. Surprised when she enters the agency, Sari notices culturally diverse posters, including some with LGBT young people, plus stickers designating 'safe and accepting' space for LGBT young people.

The therapist's ways of engaging Sari reflect training in cultural competence (Van Den Bergh and Crisp, 2004) and affirmative counselling (Matthews, 2006). Not assuming heterosexuality or cisgender identity, affirmative practitioners possess self-awareness of biases, communicate affirmation (Matthews, 2006) and understand the effects of 'minority stress' (Meyer, 2003). Following mental health and substance abuse assessments, the therapist evaluates for the intersectionality of cultural influences. Validating Sari's experiences of family rejection, community prejudice and hardship on the streets, the therapist employs affirming practices, such as narrative therapy (Saltzburg, 2007), to externalise the effects of heterosexism. Cognisant of the victimisation suffered by homeless LGBT young people, trauma-informed care (Huckshorn and Lebel, 2013) also informs therapeutic interventions.

Identifying family support as crucial in protecting young people from depression, substance abuse and suicide (Ryan et al, 2009) and recalling positive adjustments observed with other families, the therapist views 'family-focused' interventions as key for reunification. While some parents experience the coming out of adolescents as an adaptive transition to a new way of knowing their children, the therapist recognises the role of religious culture in mothers' adverse reaction, suggesting the importance of cultural awareness in supporting adjustment. Despite increased LGBT young people visibility, parental experiences of adolescent children coming out may precipitate crisis, leading to periods of emotional detachment (Saltzburg, 2004), and conflict, abuse and rejection (Ryan et al, 2009). The more children present as gender non-conforming, the greater likelihood of family crisis (Saltzburg, 2004). Using strength-based approaches, like narrative therapy (Saltzburg, 2007), as Sari relates events preceding leaving home, the therapist listens for storylines suggesting more hopeful times.

Angst may set in for young people, as parents grapple with the significance of children coming out, eroding hope for restoration of the relationship (Saltzburg, 2005). Because young people are vulnerable to depression and suicide under such duress (D'Augelli et al, 2005), there is greater urgency to provide interventions. Working with the foster family while family therapy gets under way, will further promote Sari's wellbeing. The foster family's training with LGBT young people (Mallon et al, 2002) may help to establish a mentoring relationship with Sari's mother. Therapy will employ family systems approaches that have shown promise in working with LGBT young people (LaSala, 2010), such as narrative therapy (Saltzburg, 2007).

As the therapist empathically validates both mother's and daughter's journey, she plans to connect Sari and her mother with community supports to facilitate family healing. Community-based organisations for LGBT young people provide safe havens for young people whose parents are not accepting, offering emotional support, socialisation opportunities and linkage with community resources. They also may serve as bridges between young people and parents, as LGBT adults mentor parents about what it means to grow up gay (Saltzburg, 2005). With Sari's agreement, the therapist introduces her to the local LGBT youth centre; Sari begins attending a 'gender-queer' group. Since parents are not always emotionally ready to attend PFLAG meetings (Saltzburg, 2004), the therapist provides resources from the Family Acceptance Project (Ryan et al, 2009) to introduce the mother to other parents struggling to accept LGBT adolescents and to ways that will increase affirming behaviours on her part. Highlighting the importance of keeping young people in their homes, the project's booklets, website resources and videos provide information to assuage parents' apprehension and confusion. Videos reflect families from diverse ethnic backgrounds relating healing stories of family reunification.

As trust is established, the therapist will refer Sari's mother to the local PFLAG chapter, first introducing her to a parent who understands her struggles first hand, and later encouraging her to attend meetings. As the mother finds comfort from other parents, therapy will help her to be open to examining the effects of heterosexist discourse on making meaning of Sari's identity (Saltzburg, 2007). By entering into conversations that deconstruct heterosexist and cisgender assumptions, the mother will have the opportunity to understand Sari's life from a new perspective, becoming re-engaged with the whole person that constitutes her daughter. The therapist feels optimistic as family work gets under way, seeing the promise and possibilities ahead for Sari and her mother. Together they are re-authoring the mother's emotional investment in her daughter, Sari's renewed trust in her mother and Sari's emotional wellbeing.

Conclusion

Although progress in serving US LGBT young people has been achieved, serious gaps exist between available knowledge and provider behaviour within and across service delivery systems. Despite availability of recommended best practices and policies, LGBT young people still experience human rights violations and disparate treatment associated with health inequalities. LGBT-affirmative organisational transformation is needed that sets the following in motion:

- clear expectations for competent service delivery;
- institutionalised LGBT-affirmative policies and practices;
- LGBT-competent supervision;
- system-wide accountability.

What we know about this already
- LGBT young people have higher risk profiles, more negative outcomes and unique service needs.
- Best practices exist for delivering effective care across systems.
- Appropriate services are not yet widely available.

What this chapter adds
- It gives a view of one young person's trajectory through systems employing best practices.
- It highlights the importance of the integration of an intersectionality and human rights approach to service provision.
- It provides a case study illustrating the gap between best practice and possible young people's and family experience.

How this is relevant for social work and LGBT health inequalities
- The chapter highlights the urgency for organisational development, policy making, capacity building and institutionalised accountability using a systems-of-care approach.
- It reiterates the need for education, training and LGBT-affirmative supervision to ensure the implementation of best practices.
- Continued dissemination and utilisation of best practices can reduce health disparities for LGBT young people.

Note

[1] See http://community.pflag.org/Page.aspx?pid=194&srcid=-2

References

Ali, R, 2010, *Dear colleague letter: Harassment and bullying*, Washington, DC: US Department of Civil Rights, www2.ed.gov/about/offices/list/ocr/letters/colleague-201010.pdf

American Humane Association, 2008, *Family group decision making in child welfare: Purpose, values and processes*, www.americanhumane.org/assets/pdfs/children/fgdm/purpose.pdf

APA Task Force on Appropriate Therapeutic Responses to Sexual Orientation, 2009, *Report of the Task Force on Appropriate Therapeutic Responses to Sexual Orientation*, Washington, DC: American Psychological Association, www.apa.org/pi/lgbt/resources/therapeutic-response.pdf

Centers for Disease Control and Prevention, 2011, 'Sexual identity, sex of sexual contacts, and health-risk behaviors among students in grades 9-12 – Youth Risk Behavior Surveillance, selected sites, United States, 2001-2009', *Morbidity and Mortality Weekly Report Early Release*, 60, 1-133, www.cdc.gov/mmwr/pdf/ss/ss60e0606.pdf

Child Welfare Information Gateway, 2011, *Addressing racial disproportionality in child welfare*, Washington, DC: Children's Bureau, US Department of Health and Human Services

Children's Bureau, US Department of Health and Human Services, 2011, *Information memorandum, ACYF-CB-IM-11-03*, Washington, DC: US Department of Health and Human Services.

Cochran, B, Stewart, A, Ginzler, J and Cauce, AM, 2002, 'Challenges faced by homeless sexual minorities: comparison of gay, lesbian, bisexual, and transgender homeless adolescents with their heterosexual counterparts', *American Journal of Public Health*, 92, 5, 773-77

CWLA (Child Welfare League of America), American Bar Association Center on Children and the Law, Elze, D, Family Acceptance Project, Lambda Legal Defense, Legal Defense Services for Children et al, 2012, *Recommended practices to promote the safety and well-being of lesbian, gay, bisexual, transgender and questioning youth and youth at risk of or living with HIV in child welfare settings*, Washington, DC: CWLA.

CWLA and Lambda Legal Defense, 2012, *Getting down to basics: Tools to support LGBTQ youth in care*, New York, NY and Arlington, VA: CWLA and Lambda Legal Defense, www.lambdalegal.org/take-action/tool-kits/getting-down-to-basics/

D'Augelli, AR, Grossman, AH, Salter, NP, Vasey, JJ, Starks, MT and Sinclair, KO, 2005, 'Predicting the suicide attempts of lesbian, gay, and bisexual youth', *Suicide and Life-Threatening Behavior*, 35, 6, 646-60

Desai, K, 2010, *It's your life*, Chicago, IL: American Bar Association

Diaz, EM and Kosciw, JG, 2009, *Shared differences: The experiences of lesbian, gay, bisexual and transgender students of color in our nation's schools*, New York, NY: Gay, Lesbian and Straight Education Network.

Duncan, A, 2011, *Key policy letters from the Education Secretary and Deputy Secretary*, Washington, DC: US Department of Education, www2. ed.gov/policy/elsec/guid/secletter/110607.html

Elze, D and McHaelen, R, 2009, *Moving the margins: Training curriculum for child welfare services with LGBT youth in out-of-home care*, Washington, DC: National Association of Social Workers with Lambda Legal Defense, www.lambdalegal.org/publications/moving-the-margins

Feinstein, R, Greenblatt, A, Hass, L, Kohn, S and Rana, J, 2001, *Justice for all? A report on lesbian, gay, bisexual and transgendered youth in the New York juvenile justice system*, New York, NY: Urban Justice Center.

Goodenow, C, Szalacha, L and Westheimer, K, 2006, 'School support groups, other school factors, and the safety of sexual minority adolescents', *Psychology in the Schools*, 43, 573-89

Greytak, EA, Kosciw, JG and Diaz, EM, 2009, *Harsh realities: The experiences of transgender youth in our nation's schools*, New York, NY: Gay, Lesbian and Straight Education Network.

Heck, NC, Flentje, A and Cochran, BN, 2011, 'Offsetting risks: high school gay-straight alliances and lesbian, gay, bisexual, and transgender (LGBT) youth', *School Psychology Quarterly*, 26, 2, 161-74

Huckshorn, K and Lebel, JL, 2013, 'Trauma informed care', in K Yeager, D Carter and D Svendson (eds) *Modern community mental health*, New York, NY: Oxford Press, 62-83

Human Rights Campaign, 2013a, *Statewide school non-discrimination laws and policies*, Washington, DC: Human Rights Campaign, www.hrc. org/files/assets/resources/school_non-discrimination_laws_062013. pdf

Human Rights Campaign, 2013b, *Statewide school anti-bullying and laws and policies*, Washington, DC: Human Rights Campaign, www.hrc. org/files/assets/resources/school_anti-bullying_laws_062013.pdf

IOM (Institute of Medicine), 2011, *The health of lesbian, gay, bisexual, and transgender people: Building a foundation for better understanding*, Washington, DC: The National Academies Press

Kosciw, JG, Greytak, EA, Bartkiewicz, MJ, Boesen, MJ and Palmer, NA, 2012, *The 2011 National School Climate Survey: The experiences of lesbian, gay, bisexual and transgender youth in our nation's schools*, New York, NY: Gay, Lesbian and Straight Education Network, www.glsen. org/sites/default/files/2011%20National%20School%20Climate%20 Survey%20Full%20Report.pdf

Kosciw, JG, Greytak, EA, Diaz, EM and Bartkiewicz, MJ, 2010, *The 2009 National School Climate Survey: The experiences of lesbian, gay, bisexual and transgender youth in our nation's schools*, New York, NY: Gay, Lesbian and Straight Education Network, http://glsen.org/ sites/default/files/2009%20National%20School%20Climate%20 Survey%20Full%20Report.pdf

LaSala, M, 2010, *Coming out, coming home*, New York, NY: Columbia University Press

Lovett, I, 2013, 'Law banning "gay cure" is upheld in California', *The New York Times*, 29 August, www.nytimes.com/2013/08/30/us/ law-banning-gay-cure-is-upheld-in-california.html?_r=0

Majd, K, Marksamer, J and Reyes, C, 2009, *Hidden injustice: Lesbian, gay, bisexual, and transgender youth in juvenile courts*, San Francisco, CA: Legal Services for Children, National Juvenile Defender Center and National Center for Lesbian Rights, www.equityproject.org/pdfs/ hidden_injustice.pdf

Mallon, GP, 2011, 'Permanency for LGBTQ youth', *Protecting Children*, 26, 1, 49-57, www.americanhumane.org/assets/pdfs/children/ protecting-children-journal/pc-26-1.pdf

Mallon, GP, Aledort, N and Ferrera, M, 2002, 'There's no place like home: achieving safety, permanency, and well-being for lesbian and gay adolescents in out-of-home care settings', *Child Welfare*, 81, 2, 407-39

Matthews, CR, 2006, 'Affirmative lesbian, gay and bisexual counseling with all clients', in KJ Bieschke, RM Perez and KA DeBord (eds) *Handbook of counseling and psychotherapy with lesbian, gay, bisexual and transgender clients*, Washington, DC: American Psychological Association, 201-20

McCready, L, 2004, 'Some challenges facing queer youth programs in urban high schools: racial segregation and de-normalizing whiteness', *Journal of Gay and Lesbian Issues in Education*, 1, 37-51

Meyer, IH, 2003, 'Prejudice, social stress, and mental health in lesbian, gay, and bisexual populations: conceptual issues and research evidence', *Psychological Bulletin*, 129, 5, 674-90

National Alliance to End Homelessness, 2012, *LGBTQ youth national policy statement*, Washington, DC: National Alliance to End Homelessness, www.endhomelessness.org/library/entry/lgbtq-youth-national-policy-statement

National Alliance to End Homelessness, 2014, 'Homeless youth legislation', www.endhomelessness.org/pages/youthlegislation

National Association of Social Workers, 2000, *'Reparative' and 'conversation' therapies for lesbians and gay men: Position statement.*, Washington, DC: National Association of Social Workers, http://www.socialworkers. org/diversity/lgb/reparative.asp

NCLR (National Center for Lesbian Rights) and GLSEN (Gay, Lesbian and Straight Education Network), 2012, *Expensive reasons why safe schools laws and policies are in your district's best interest*, San Francisco, CA: NCLR, www.nclrights.org/legal-help-resources/resource/ expensive-reasons-why-safe-schools-legislation-is-in-your-states-best-interest/

PAHO (Pan American Health Organization) and WHO (World Health Organization), 2012, '"Therapies" to change sexual orientation lack medical justification and threaten health', 17 May, http://new.paho. org/hq/index.php?option=com_content&view=article&id=6803 &Itemid=1926

Quintana, NS, Rosenthal, J and Krehely, J, 2010, *On the streets: The federal response to gay and transgender homeless youth*, Washington, DC: Center for American Progress, 28, http://cdn.americanprogress.org/ wp-content/uploads/issues/2010/06/pdf/lgbtyouthhomelessness.pdf

Ray, N, 2006, *Lesbian, gay, bisexual and transgender youth: An epidemic of homelessness*, New York, NY: National Gay and Lesbian Task Force Policy Institute and the National Coalition for the Homeless, www. ngltf.org/reports_and_research/homeless_youth

Reichert, E, 2007, 'Human rights in the twenty-first century: creating a new paradigm for social work', in E Reichert (ed) *Challenges in human rights: A social work perspective*, New York, NY: Columbia University Press, 1-15

Rosario, M, Schrimshaw, EW and Hunter, J, 2012, 'Homelessness among lesbian, gay, and bisexual youth: implications for subsequent internalizing and externalizing symptoms', *Journal of Youth and Adolescence*, 41, 5, 544-60

Rosenwald, M, 2009, 'A glimpse within: an exploratory study of child welfare agencies' practices with LGBTQ youth', *Journal of Gay and Lesbian Social Services* 21, 4, 343-56

Russell, ST, Kosciw, J, Horn, S and Saewyc, E, 2010, 'Safe schools for LGBTQ students', *Social Policy Report*, 24, 4, 1-17, www.srcd.org/ sites/default/files/documents/spr_24_4_final.pdf

Russell, ST, Muraco, A, Subramaniam, A and Laub, C, 2009, 'Youth empowerment and high school gay–straight alliances', *Journal of Youth and Adolescence*, 38, 891-903

Russell, ST, Ryan, C, Toomey, RB, Diaz, RM and Sanchez, J, 2011, 'Lesbian, gay, bisexual, and transgender adolescent school victimization: implications for young adult health and adjustment', *Journal of School Health*, 81, 223-30

Ryan, C, Huebner, D, Diaz, RM and Sanchez, J, 2009, 'Family rejection as a predictor of negative health outcomes in white and Latino lesbian, gay and bisexual young adults', *Pediatrics*, 123, 1, 346-52

Saltzburg, S, 2004, 'Learning that an adolescent child is gay or lesbian: the parent experience', *Social Work*, 49, 1, 109-18

Saltzburg, S, 2005, 'Co-constructing adolescence for GLBT youth and their families', in G, Mallon and P, McCourt-Hess (eds) *Child welfare for the twenty-first century: A handbook of practices, policies, and programs*, New York, NY: Columbia University Press

Saltzburg, S, 2007, 'Narrative therapy pathways for re-authoring with parents of adolescents coming-out as lesbian and gay', *Contemporary Family Therapy: An International Journal*, 29, 57-69

Sausa, L, 2005, 'Translating research into practice: trans youth recommendations for improving school systems', *Journal of Gay and Lesbian Issues in Education*, 3, 1, 15-28

Stroul, BA and Friedman, RM, 1996, 'The system of care concept and philosophy', in BA Stroul (ed) *Children's mental health: Creating systems of care in a changing society*, Baltimore, MD: Paul H. Brookes Publishing, 3-23

Toomey, RB, Ryan, C, Diaz, RM and Russell, ST, 2011, 'High school gay–straight alliances (GSAs) and young adult well-being: an examination of GSA presence, participation, and perceived effectiveness', *Applied Developmental Science*, 15, 4, 175-85

UN (United Nations), 1989, *Convention on the Rights of the Child*, Geneva: UN, www.ohchr.org/EN/ProfessionalInterest/Pages/CRC. aspx

UN (United Nations) High Commissioner for Human Rights, 2011, *Discriminatory laws and practices and acts of violence against individuals based on their sexual orientation and gender identity: Report of the United Nations High Commissioner for Human Rights*, Geneva: UN, www2.ohchr.org/ english/bodies/hrcouncil/docs/19session/A.HRC.19.41_English.pdf

US (United States) Department of Education, 2011, *Analysis of state bullying laws and policies*, Washington, DC: US Department of Education

US Department of Housing and Development, 2011, 'Homeless emergency assistance and rapid transition to housing: defining "homeless"', *Federal Register*, 76, 233, 75994-6019, www.gpo.gov/fdsys/pkg/FR-2011-12-05/html/2011-30942.htm

USDHHS (US Department of Health and Human Services), 2010, *Healthy People 2020, Lesbian, gay, bisexual and transgender health*, Washington, DC, http://healthypeople.gov/2020/topicsobjectives2020/overview.aspx?topicid=25

Van Den Bergh, N and Crisp, C, 2004, 'Defining culturally competent practice with sexual minorities: implications for social work education and practice', *Journal of Social Work Education*, 40, 2, 221-38

Walls, NE, Kane, SB and Wisneski, H, 2010, 'Gay–straight alliances and school experiences of sexual minority youth', *Youth and Society*, 41, 3, 307-32

Woronoff, R, Estrada, R and Sommer, S, 2006, *Out of the margins: A report on regional listening forums highlighting the experiences of lesbian, gay, bisexual, transgender, and questioning youth in care*, New York, NY: Lambda Legal Defense and Education Fund

Unique experiences and needs of LGBT older people: one community in rural California responds

Elizabeth Breshears and Valerie Lester Leyva

VIGNETTE

Mike, a slight man in his mid-sixties, stood in the crowded room of healthcare professionals and told his story – life as a young trans person, undergoing counselling, living as a male, and implementing a hormone therapy regimen prior to breast removal. Mike shared that he had not pursued surgeries on his 'lower half' to turn his vagina into a penis, because of cost, complexity and questionable success. Having recently lost his partner of many years, Mike predicted that a time would come when, unable to care for himself, he would need to reside in a nursing home. In a soft-spoken voice he concluded by saying, "When that happens, I don't want to be viewed as abhorrent. I don't want to know that workers are repulsed when they touch me. I am a person." The silent audience could hear Mike's vulnerability as he shared these feelings during a training sponsored by the LGBT Roundtable of San Joaquin County, California.

Introduction

This chapter presents the efforts of one community in the United States (US) to better understand and address health and ageing needs of lesbian, gay, bisexual and trans (LGBT) older people, including Mike. The chapter introduces readers to the LGBT Roundtable of San Joaquin County, California; it describes how this collaborative advocates for equal access to services and to eliminate heteronormative bias in services to LGBT older people. The chapter reviews the societal context for Mike's lived experience of growing old and being LGBT in the US and how that experience differs from those of heterosexual older people as well as younger LGBT populations. The chapter discusses the seminar at which Mike presented his story and identifies training content that can be adapted for use by local communities. Lastly, the chapter examines the importance of social workers and other health providers taking immediate steps to make services to ageing individuals, including Mike, more LGBT-competent and friendly.

Origin and composition of the collaborative

In 2007 and 2009, California implemented two important laws to prevent discrimination based on gender identity and sexual orientation of LGBT older people such as Mike. The Older Californians Equality and Protection Act 2006 required ageing services agencies to identify and address the needs of LGBT older people through culturally competent service delivery systems. The LGBT Senior Care Training Act 2008 required licenced health providers in skilled nursing facilities, including doctors and nurses, to obtain training in LGBT elder care.

California's 58 counties were charged to develop strategies to comply with these laws. With the guidance of Donna Anderson, a licensed clinical social worker and chief of the County's Department of Aging and Community Services, San Joaquin County chose to form a collaborative using snowball recruitment. Snowball recruitment is a methodology that reaches out to known members of a hard-to-reach group, such as LGBT older people, who are hidden as a result of social stigma or personal vulnerability (Gorbach et al, 2009). Initial members identify other members. Thus, LGBT older people and consumers of services, along with partners, family members and allies, were recruited along with stakeholder representatives from religion, local business, an advocacy law firm (California Rural Legal Assistance), the American Association of Retired Persons (AARP), the Commission on Aging and several county agencies including Adult Protective Services. The local university's Social Work Department also became a partner. The collaborative named itself the LGBT Roundtable of San Joaquin County (hereafter referred to as Roundtable). By early 2009, the Roundtable was actively engaged and had sponsored a daylong training on issues unique to serving LGBT older people. It was at that daylong training that one of the authors was introduced to Mike. Two years later, the Roundtable organised its second all-day training for service providers.

California is generally viewed as accepting of differences in lifestyle, gender identity and sexual orientation. However, less than 160 kilometres east of San Francisco, named one of the 'gayest cities in America' (Breen, 2013), is one of the state's most conservative regions – the Central Valley. It is here that San Joaquin County, home of the Roundtable, is located. The farming communities that comprise the Central Valley are known for their conservative views. As one Roundtable member said: "With 300 days of sunshine, everything grows in this Valley but equal rights and social justice."

The important role of a collaborative

The previous section discussed creation of the LGBT Roundtable. This section asks: How can a collaborative, such as the Roundtable, play a pivotal role in community change? It was important to ensure that voices of LGBT older people were heard and that 'business as usual' was unacceptable. In the ongoing development of the Roundtable, Anderson's approach modelled her underlying commitment to inclusion and social justice.

Anderson pursued dialogical methods reflecting power *with* rather than power *over* LGBT older people. Breshears and Volker (2013) discuss that in power over practices, those with more power use their power to obtain what they want from those with less power; it is antithetical to social work best practice. Power *with* is a shared use of power in which all members of a group are valued for their contributions and viewed as important co-creators of knowledge. In the terms of Freire (2000, p 48), for real change to occur, it was important that the plan be 'forged *with*, not *for*, the oppressed'. Individuals who might be the subject of change thus became partners as co-investigators and change agents, a process known as community action research. Jewell et al (2009, p 311) write:

> Personal and political power for those involved has the ability to challenge the status quo that marginalizes and oppresses people.... The process of self-advocacy transforms the lives of those engaged in community organizing and leads to both individual and collective empowerment.... On the community level, organizing can dismantle the structural laws, policies and mind-sets that maintain the unjust system.

This potential for empowerment became a reality in the Roundtable. The Roundtable's initial role was to advise. However, as Roundtable members became empowered, they engaged more directly in advocacy and education and began to learn about other LGBT advocacy coalitions and activities. The Roundtable forged a bridge with *Lavender Seniors of the East Bay*[1] whose focus on service provider education resonated with Roundtable members. The Roundtable also co-sponsored with a local church a community screening of the award-winning documentary, *Gen Silent*.[2]

The Roundtable's self-empowerment and evolving role was timely. Ageing services needed to 'become more multicultural to appropriately serve diverse and disenfranchised people' (Hyde, 2004, p 7). As the Roundtable's strength and stature grew, it also provided a meaningful experience for its members. On macro and micro levels, the Roundtable offered community for LGBT older people and their allies; it provided space for dialogue and it validated their experiences. Perhaps most important, it served to buffer the dominant US culture's dismissal of the experience of being old and LGBT. To this end, the Roundtable elevated awareness of issues that historically were ignored or unknown. Some of these issues are addressed in the next section.

The intersection of being old and LGBT

Is Mike's story unique? Unfortunately, Mike is only one of many LGBT older people deeply concerned about future wellbeing. The post-Second World War baby boom, better diets and more accessible healthcare have led to rising growth in the number and lifespan of older people. United Nations estimates are that by 2050, two billion people will be aged 60 or older and four of every 10 older adults will need some form of long-term care (Reyna et al, 2007). Current US population estimates project that by 2030, fully one fourth of the nation's population will be aged 65 or older and by 2020, 12 million US older people will be in need of long-term care (Jimenez, 2010, p 373).

Projecting future numbers of LGBT older people is complicated as no statistical method for an accurate count is currently available. Little consensus exists on what percentage of the total population is gay (or lesbian, bisexual or trans) and even less is known about how many LGBT individuals are aged 65 or older. One widely accepted estimate is that the number of LGBT older people over the age of 65 will total about six million in the US by 2030 (Fredricksen-Goldsen and Muraco, 2010). Whatever the actual number of LGBT older people, there is consensus that older LGBT adults comprise a significant minority that will continue to increase proportionately as the ageing population grows.

Within the expanding ageing population, the context of growing old and being LGBT in the US creates a multiplicity of significant issues. The following two subsections describe the powerful and often negative nexus of ageism and heterosexism and the deep distrust that many LGBT older people feel about health and social welfare service systems.

Ageism

Ageism involves 'stereotyping and discrimination against people simply because they are old' (Butler, 2010, p 557). Derogatory nicknames (for example, old goat, old hag, fossil) and myths about functioning (for example, doddering, cranky, forgetful, rigid) are examples of ageist stereotypes within the dominant construct of being old (Butler, 2010). In many cultures, myriad products promise to stop ageing, reflecting a youth-centric ideal and society's negative view of becoming or even appearing to look old.

Within dominant ageist stereotypes is 'perhaps the ultimate insult in our society': being depicted as 'sexless' (Butler, 2010, p 558). Rarely are older people asked about their sexual orientation, because a heterosexual history is presumed (Thompson, 2008). Mallon (2009, p 5) described the desire to avoid thinking about older people as sexual beings as the 'ick' factor. Barusch (2009) states that social workers need to advocate for older people who want to express love and intimacy. She points out that in residential care facilities, safety issues may preclude locking a door, but similar to a hotel, privacy should be available to older people with something as simple as a 'do not disturb' sign. Barusch contends that to believe infatuation and romance are solely the purview of the young is ageism and actions based on ageist stereotypes are discriminatory.

In many ways, LGBT older people's experiences of ageist comments and treatment are comparable to their heterosexual peers. However, significant differences also exist between LGBT and heterosexual older people of the same age cohort. Fewer LGBT older people have strong family connections in old age, fewer have children who are part of their lives and more have created families of choice or other diverse family structures (National Resource Centre on LGBT Aging, 2012). Studies report that more LGBT older people will live alone: twice as many gay and bisexual men and one third more lesbian and bisexual women as compared to the general population (Grant, 2010). While some studies discuss increased vulnerability in terms of safety, diet and isolation, others identify strengths of increased resilience and greater coping abilities for living alone as a result of their LGBT experience (Grant, 2010).

Heterosexism

The second 'ism' – heterosexism – alleges that sex between a man and a woman is the only right and normal sexuality (National Centre for Lesbian Rights, 2012). To competently and sensitively provide services to LGBT older people, social workers and other health providers must gain an understanding of the overwhelming influence of heteronormativity in the dominant culture.

Young LGBT adults may have difficulty relating to the experiences prevalent in the older LGBT population. Young LGBT individuals' experience of personal power and acceptability of being 'out' differs from individuals who may be the age of their parents or grandparents. The social environment of US views and laws affecting LGBT individuals are changing from judgemental and discriminatory to increasing social acceptance and equal rights. Catalano and Shlasko (2010) assert that growing acceptance of LGBT people is occurring in mainstream culture, reflected by regular portrayal of LGBT individuals in the media.

However, the historical social environment of the pre-Stonewall era resulted in fundamental differences in the lives of LGBT older people compared with younger LGBT post-Stonewall generations. David and Cernin (2008) emphasise that the imprint and residue of lived experiences of LGBT older people remain powerful influences. These authors write that those from the pre-Stonewall cohort are less likely to be forthcoming regarding their sexual orientation, have experienced more stigma and access fewer community-based LGBT services. One of the differences between Mike and a young LGBT individual is that for two thirds of Mike's life, being gay was diagnosed as a mental disorder. It was not until 1986 that 'homosexuality' was fully eliminated as a psychiatric condition (Jimenez, 2010).

As a female to male (FtM) trans person, Mike must further deal with the reality that the current American Psychiatric Association's *Diagnostic and statistical manual of mental disorders* (DSM-V) continues to include a trans diagnosis pathology, although it has been incorporated into the '**gender dysphoria**' diagnosis as opposed to the previous DSM edition's 'gender identity disorder' (Beredjick, 2012; Johnson, 2013). Trans advocates and other differently sexed persons lobbied for full removal from the DSM, but to date have been unsuccessful.

Having sex with a same-sex partner was not only considered a mental illness, it was also illegal in many states during much of Mike's life. Not until 2003, as a result of the US Supreme Court decision on *Lawrence v Texas* (539 US 558, 2003) was homosexuality decriminalised in the last 13 states. That same year, noted psychiatrist Robert Spitzer (2003) published a study concluding that reparative therapy to eliminate homosexuality was efficacious if an individual was sufficiently motivated to go through the treatment. Nine years later, Spitzer retracted his conclusions in a letter of apology reprinted in the *New York Times*, which stated in part: 'I believe I owe the gay community an apology for my study making unproven claims of the efficacy of reparative therapy' (Carey, 2012, para 9). Fundamentalist Christianity continues to preach that homosexuality is 'unnatural' and an 'abomination' (Barton, 2010).

Given the factors above, it may be understandable why many LGBT older people adopted heterosexual lifestyles in their youth to avoid being outed and continue to 'struggle with the vestiges of stigma and shame' attached to homosexuality (Thompson, 2008, p 132). Many have chosen to 'come out of the closet' at some point during their lives. However, research suggests that a number of LGBT older people are going back into the closet over concerns about vulnerability and abuse at the hands of caregivers and in nursing facilities. Rea Carey, executive director of the US National Gay and Lesbian Task Force contends: 'The scenario of LGBT adults being forced back into the closet for safety in hostile elder environments is alarming and disgraceful' (as quoted in Grant, 2010, p 5).

Although LGBT older people in the US are witnessing many changes in societal attitudes regarding sexual orientation, the intersectionality of age, gender identity and sexual orientation still creates barriers to receiving adequate services. Trans individuals, in particular, are still at significant risk of discrimination and exposure to abuse. These factors motivated the Roundtable to develop and implement training for ageing services providers.

Provider training to improve services to LGBT older people

This section describes the daylong training – *The Special Needs of LGBT Seniors: Developing Understanding, Empathy, and Respect* – designed by the Roundtable. The section discusses the training's philosophical underpinnings and content. It reviews the seven modules and offers considerations to groups who hope to initiate community training on the needs of LGBT older people residing in their locale.

One of the tenets of good social work practice is to 'begin where the client is' (Miley et al, 2013, p 134). Targeted attendees for the Roundtable's training included educated and licensed health providers, many with decades of experience working with ageing clients. However, for most, this training was their first introduction to experiences and needs of LGBT older people. The Roundtable sought to create connections between attendees and the LGBT older population and explicitly incorporated the terms 'understanding', 'empathy' and 'respect' in the workshop title.

Three modules were designed to facilitate empathy and understanding of LGBT older people as unique and complex individuals:

- The morning 'Welcome' incorporated a reading of 'Letter to Mama' – a young man's poignant coming-out letter (Maupin, 1978).
- During lunch, participants selected, from handouts of documented discrimination and rights violations of LGBT older people and/or their partners, one story that was particularly meaningful to them. Participants discussed their selection with a partner and identified actions needed to change outcomes.
- During the final module, six LGBT older people shared life stories and answered written questions that participants were hesitant to ask verbally. Participant evaluations described the panel's contribution as profoundly moving and effective.

Four modules included panels of *subject experts* from health and legal sectors. A critical part of the training design was that each panel also included LGBT older people who spoke as *experts of their lived experiences* in that topic area.

- One module reviewed acceptable and derogatory terms and definitions.[3]
- Another module discussed how to make services/agencies more LGBT-friendly particularly when working with trans clients and co-workers, how to improve intake forms and how to conduct organisational self-evaluation.
- One module examined concerns and vulnerabilities identified by LGBT older people regarding long-term care and dependence on skilled out-of-home care. Patients' rights and recourse when violations occur were outlined.
- The fourth module addressed legal advocacy in multiple life areas, including: shared property; wills and survivor benefits; health-related decisions and communication; and same-sex partner/spouse visitation. Attorney panellists cautioned the necessity of accessing local legal and healthcare expertise responsive to LGBT concerns because of complexity and geographic differences in law and policy.[4]

In summary, the Roundtable goals for the training were to:

- facilitate empathy and understanding of LGBT older people's experiences and needs;
- increase awareness that individual occurrences of discrimination often reflect systemic oppression;
- challenge participants to examine the adequacy of and discriminatory assumptions embedded in their agencies and services to this population;
- leave with a sense of urgency to act.

Participants were challenged to identify changes that could be made immediately to better serve those who receive or need services from their programmes but may not be known as members of the LGBT community.

The Roundtable, with the help of their university social work partners, conducted a pre- and post-test evaluation of the training. Of the 129 attendees, 115 completed the pre-test and 112 completed the post-test. Results of the evaluation are not the focus of this chapter; however, post-test scores reflected increased knowledge, skills and positive attitude for all participants. Gay attendees reflected greater knowledge, skills and positive attitude than their straight counterparts; however, unlike the results at pre-test, the difference between the gay and straight training participants was not significant at post-test (Leyva et al, 2014).

Conclusion and the importance of immediate action

Why is it imperative that social workers act to improve services to LGBT older people? It certainly can be argued that a sea change is occurring in the cultural acceptance of LGBT people and relationships. LGBT roles occur in movies and television with some regularity. However, research reveals that within LGBT media roles, almost all trans (and other differently sexed) people are depicted 'either as victims or as medical anomalies, and not as complex people with lives and interests beyond their gender' (Catalano and Shlasko, 2010, p 423).

Blumenfeld (2010, p 378) asserts that in the US, LGBT people remain 'among the most despised groups'. Older LGBT individuals and couples continue to experience discrimination and stigma in many areas, ranging from discriminatory tax laws to policies regarding marriage and relationships. For example, same-sex lovers and partners are often denied access to loved ones with serious health problems when hospital policy allows 'only blood relatives or a legal spouse visitation rights' (Blumenfeld, 2010, p 379). Should a hospital social worker or a social work practicum student let such a policy go unchallenged?

As a values-driven profession guided by a Code of Ethics, social work *practice* must grow its capacity and competence in serving the older LGBT population. A major US social work initiative – the Council on Social Work Education Gero-Ed Center (2010, p 6) – has adopted principles to inform education and practice with ageing clients. Two are particularly germane to serving LGBT older people:

- Racism, sexism, classism, heterosexism and other forms of discrimination influence the opportunities of individuals over the lifecourse, and systems of care for older people must address the needs of those who have been marginalized or disadvantaged during their lives.
- The growing diversity of the older population in ethnicity, language, culture, and immigration status must be reflected in culturally competent staff and program design.

The closing thoughts in this chapter address the role of an individual social worker who might ask, 'What can I do? I am a mere student' or 'caseworker', 'supervisor', etc. Breshears and Volker (2013, p 10) maintain that leadership 'can occur from any chair around the table'. These authors make a case that one does not need to be 'appointed' nor does one need 'authority' to be a leader. Heifetz (1994, p 183) argued: 'The scarcity of leadership from people in authority makes it all the more critical ... that leadership be exercised by people without authority'. Each of us has the opportunity to lead. Sometimes the answer is about asking the right questions, then facilitating small and practical changes.

No one appointed Christine Jorgensen, who fought in the Second World War as Private George Jorgensen, to become an internationally known advocate for trans people. Jorgensen's celebrity resulted from sex reassignment surgery and a 1952 *New York Daily News* headline 'Ex-GI becomes blond beauty' that catapulted her into the public eye (Walsh, 2012). Rather than shrink from exposure, Jorgensen used her notoriety to educate and advocate for trans people. Jorgensen believed the public's interest in her sexual reassignment surgery was an early step in the sexual revolution of the 1960s, and said 'she never regretted her decision' (Walsh, 2012).

Similarly, when Harvey Milk was told no gay man could be elected to public office, he ran anyway and, after three attempts, was the first openly gay person elected to the San Francisco Board of Supervisors. Milk, called one of *Time*'s most influential people of the 20th century (Cloud, 1999) used his social capital to advocate for all civil rights and once declared: 'Rights are won only by those who make their voices heard' (Milk, 2012). Not all of us can be a Jorgensen or a Milk, but all have before us the issue of social justice for LGBT older people – an issue that should no longer be ignored. What can you do? You can be a person that speaks out for social justice. You can be a change agent in everyday situations to improve the health and lives of LGBT older people.

What we know about this already
- Older people are living longer and are projected to become a larger percent of the world's population; however, no accurate population statistics regarding numbers of LGBT older people are available.
- LGBT older people experience greater health and social inequalities than their heterosexual counterparts.
- Marginalised populations, including LGBT older people, have the right to receive culturally competent and sensitive services.

What this chapter adds
- It shows why LGBT older people may be less willing to 'come out' to service providers than younger LGBT populations and why some may go back into 'the closet'.
- It describes how one community is working to raise awareness, increase sensitivity and competence, and make ageing services more LGBT-friendly.
- It explores how societal stigma around ageism and heterosexism place LGBT older people at increased risk of social and health inequalities.

How this is relevant for social work and LGBT health inequalities
- As the ageing population continues to increase, more social workers will be needed with expertise in gerontology *and* competence in serving LGBT older people.
- This chapter offers social workers a context for a strengths-based, participatory approach to work collaboratively with LGBT older people as co-investigators and co-creators of the knowledge, action and system change necessary to reduce social and health inequalities.
- Social workers can advocate to ensure that their agencies are LGBT-friendly and that all marginalised populations, including LGBT older people, receive culturally competent and sensitive services.

Notes

[1] For more information about Lavender Seniors of the East Bay, see www. lavenderseniors.org/

[2] For information about *Gen Silent*, see http://stumaddux.com/gen_silent_about.html; excerpts are available on YouTube.

[3] For a helpful glossary, see National Resource Center on LGBT Aging (2012, pp 26-7).

[4] Social workers may benefit from in-country legal advocacy organisations and publications similar to National Center for Lesbian Rights (2009).

References

Barton, BJ, 2010, '"Abomination": life as a Bible belt gay', *Journal of Homosexuality*, 57, 4, 465-84

Barusch, AM, 2009, 'Love and ageism: a social work perspective', *Social Work Today*, 9, 1, 12-17

Beredjick, C, 2012, 'DSM-V to rename gender identity disorder "gender dysphoria"', Advocate.com, 23 July, www.advocate.com/politics/transgender/2012/07/23/dsm-replaces-gender-identity-disorder-gender-dysphoria

Blumenfeld, WJ, 2010, 'How homophobia hurts everyone', in M Adams, WJ Blumenfeld, R Castañeda, HW Hackman, ML Peters and X Zúñiga (eds) *Readings for diversity and social justice* (2nd edn), New York, NY: Routledge, 376-85

Breen, M, 2013, 'Gayest cities in America, 2013', Advocate.com, 9 January, www.advocate.com/print-issue/current-issue/2013/01/09/gayest-cities-america-2013?page=full

Breshears, E and Volker, R, 2013, *Facilitative leadership in social work practice*, New York, NY: Springer

Butler, RN, 2010, 'Ageism: another form of bigotry', in M Adams, WJ Blumenfeld, R Castañeda, HW Hackman, ML Peters and X Zúñiga (eds) *Readings for diversity and social justice* (2nd edn), New York, NY: Routledge, 557-62

Carey, B, 2012, 'Psychiatry giant sorry for backing gay "cure"', *New York Times*, 18 May, www.nytimes.com/2012/05/19/health/dr-robert-l-spitzer-noted-psychiatrist-apologizes-for-study-on-gay-cure.html?pagewanted=all

Catalano, C and Shlasko, D, 2010, 'Transgender oppression: introduction', in M Adams, WJ Blumenfeld, R Castañeda, HW Hackman, ML Peters and X Zúñiga (eds) *Readings for diversity and social justice* (2nd edn), New York, NY: Routledge, 423-9

Cloud, J, 1999, 'Time 100 persons of the century', *Time Magazine*, 153, 23, http://content.time.com/time/magazine/article/0,9171,991227,00.html

CSWE (Council on Social Work Education) Gero-Ed Center (2010) *Advanced gero social work practice*, Alexandria, VA; CSWE Gero-Ed Center

David, S and Cernin, P, 2008, 'Psychotherapy with lesbian, gay, bisexual, and transgender older adults', *Journal of Gay & Lesbian Social Services*, 20, 1, 31-49

Fredriksen-Goldsen, K and Muraco, A, 2010, 'Aging and sexual orientation: a 25-year review of the literature', *Research on Aging*, 32, 3, 372-13

Freire, P, 2000, *Pedagogy of the oppressed*, New York, NY: Continuum

Gorbach, PM, Murphy, R, Weiss, RE, Hucks-Ortiz, C and Shoptaw, S, 2009, 'Sex with men and women in a street-based sample in Los Angeles', *Journal of Urban Health*, 86, 1, doi: 10.1007/s11524-009-9370-7

Grant, JM, 2010, *Outing age 2010: Public policy issues affecting lesbian, gay, bisexual and transgender elders*, New York, NY: National Gay and Lesbian Task Force

Heifetz, RA, 1994, *Leadership without easy answers*, Cambridge, MA: Belknap Press

Hyde, CA, 2004, 'Multicultural development in human services agencies: challenges and solutions', *Social Work*, 49, 1, 7-16

Jewell, JR, Collins, KV, Gargotto, L and Dishon, AM, 2009, 'Building the unsettling force: social workers and the struggle for human rights', *Journal of Community Practice*, 17, 3, 309-22

Jimenez, J, 2010, *Social policy and social change: Toward the creation of social and economic justice*, Thousand Oaks, CA: Sage Publications

Johnson, L, 2013, 'From disorder to dysphoria: transgender identity and the DSM-V', *429 Magazine*, 9 May, http://dot429.com/articles/2125-from-disorder-to-dysphoria-transgender-identity-and-the-dsm-v

Lawrence v Texas (02-102) 539 US 558 (2003) 41 S. W. 3d 349, reversed and remanded.

Leyva, V, Breshears, E and Ringstad, R, 2014, 'Assessing the efficacy of LGBT cultural competency training for aging services providers in California's Central Valley', *Journal of Gerontological Social Work*, 57, 2-4, 335-348

Mallon, M, 2009, 'The ick factor', *Social Work Today*, 9, 1, 5

Maupin, A, 1978, *Tales of the city*, New York, NY: Harper & Row

Miley, KK, O'Meliea, MW and DuBois, BL, 2013, *Generalist social work practice: An empowering approach* (7th edn), New York, NY: Pearson

Milk, H, 2012, 'The city weeps', in V Emory (ed) *The Harvey Milk interviews: In his own words*, San Francisco, CA: Vince Emery Productions

National Center for Lesbian Rights (2009) *Planning with purpose: Legal basics for LGBT elders*, www.nclrights.org/legal-help-resources/resource/planning-with-purpose-legal-basics-for-lgbt-elders/

National Resource Center on LGBT 'Aging' (2012) *Inclusive services for LGBT older adults: A practical guide to creating welcoming agencies*, New York, NY: National Resource Center on LGBT Aging, www.n4a.org/files/programs/resources-lgbt-elders/InclusiveServicesGuide2012.pdf

Reyna, C, Goodwin, EJ and Ferrari, JR, 2007, 'Older adult stereotypes among care providers in residential care facilities', *Journal of Gerontological Nursing*, 33, 2, 50-5

Spitzer, RL, 2003, 'Can some gay men and lesbians change their sexual orientation? 200 participants reporting a change from homosexual to heterosexual orientation', *Archives of Sexual Behavior*, 32, 5, 403-17

Thompson, EH, 2008, 'Do we intend to keep this closeted?', *The Gerontologist*, 48, 1, 130-2

Walsh, M, 2012, 'It's been 60 years since the first he turned she: Bronx-born Christine Jorgensen's historic sexual reassignment surgery in Denmark', *New York Daily News*, 30 November, www.nydailynews.com/news/world/60-years-christine-jorgensen-born-article-1.1211068

Good practice in health and social care provision for LGBT older people in the UK

Sue Westwood, Andrew King, Kathryn Almack, Yiu-Tung Suen and Louis Bailey

VIGNETTE

Laura, Gary, Bridget, Chris and Theresa have been referred to social services. Laura is an 83-year-old White British lesbian. Her civil partner died last year and she now lives alone in their large multi-storey house in a rural area. She has several private pensions. Her eyesight is deteriorating and she can no longer drive. She is lonely and depressed. Gary is a single 70-year-old gay man of African Caribbean decent, living in an inner-city local authority flat and reliant on state pensions and other forms of welfare support. He is showing signs of memory loss and confusion. Bridget is a 65-year-old bi-identifying woman of White Irish Catholic origin. She lives in the suburbs with her partner, Chris, aged 69, a White British bisexual man who has multiple sclerosis, needing increasing care and support. Their daughter is supportive, but lives a long distance away. Theresa is a 61-year-old heterosexual trans woman with an Asian/White British heritage, who **transitioned** three years ago. She has a son, but they are estranged. She lives in a sheltered housing scheme for people with mental health issues. Theresa has complained that staff are discriminating against her.

What would good practice look like for each of these people?

Introduction

Lesbian, gay, bisexual and trans (LGBT) ageing occurs in wide-ranging socio-legal contexts. In countries where there is a lack of legal recognition and social protections, the health of LGBT people is impacted not only by the accumulated effects of discrimination but also by the fact that their older age care needs are served by health and social care systems that offer little or no recognition of their minority identities (AGE Platform Europe and ILGA-Europe, 2012). Even in more liberal countries offering some forms of legal rights, older LGBT people experience a range of health inequalities (Fish, 2007). These disadvantages (Fredriksen-Goldsen et al, 2013a, 2013b) can be clustered into four main areas:

- the cumulative physical and psychological effects of discrimination, stigma and marginalisation across the lifecourse;
- a relative lack of social capital, particularly informal social support, compared with heterosexual and cisgender older people;
- health and social care provision that is ill-equipped to recognise and meet the needs of older LGBT people (Fish, 2007; 2009);
- the intersection between increased need for formal support and a reluctance on the part of older LGBT people to access health and social care provision because of concerns about how they will be treated (Ward et al, 2011).

This chapter will first locate older LGBT health inequalities in a theoretical context before outlining core areas of good practice for older LGBT people across health and social care contexts. It will then explore specific areas of good practice linked to vignettes, which are composites, drawn from our respective pieces of empirical research.

Context

Older LGBT health inequalities can be understood through the lens of both health determinants and resilience. From a health determinants perspective (Williams et al, 2013), the impact of 'minority stress' (that is, the cumulative effects of having a marginalised identity) is now recognised as having a major effect on older LGBT people's health and wellbeing (Fredriksen-Goldsen et al, 2013a, 2013b) and can result in depression, self-harm and lifestyle issues such as drug and alcohol use and obesity (Witten and Eyler, 2012). Moreover, many older LGBT people are ageing with reduced social capital (Cronin and King, 2013), which in turn has an impact on health. Older LGBT people are more likely than their heterosexual peers to be single and living alone, to be childless and to have less contact with biological family (Stonewall, 2011; Fredriksen-Goldsen et al, 2013a). While older LGBT people have 'families of choice' (Weeks et al, 2001) networks, they are often of the same generation, so that as friends die there is no younger cohort available for ongoing informal care and support. It is now generally recognised that older LGBT people are in need of formal health and social care provision sooner than their heterosexual peers, because of relatively diminished social support networks, and because of health needs linked to minority stress.

Yet at the same time, the quality of health and social care provision for older LGBT people is extremely variable. Some European countries lack policies that are responsive to and reflective of older LGBT people's needs, while in other countries those policies are in place but are not appropriately implemented (AGE Platform Europe and ILGA-Europe, 2012). Even where policies are effectively in place, **cisnormativity**, **heteronormativity**, **homophobia**, **biphobia** and **transphobia** can mean that older LGBT people go unrecognised at best and experience discrimination at worst (Ward et al, 2011).

Social work has a major role to play in addressing and redressing these health inequalities (Coren et al, 2010), through both tackling LGBT stigma and marginalisation, and thereby reducing/mitigating their effects on health. Additionally, taking a resilience approach (understanding the complex interplay of risk and protective factors) to the lives of older LGBT adults can involve both risk reduction and also protection enhancement (Fredriksen-Goldsen et al, 2013a, 2013b). In particular, improved social support has a key role to play in both reducing risk associated with social isolation and enhancing resilience in terms of social support (Knocker et al, 2012). Health and social care providers should not only become more inclusive in the services they offer, but should also work on preventative issues, particularly the need for more, better-resourced, older LGBT people support networks.

While older LGBT people continue to be marginalised in both services for older people and generic services for LGBT people, there is a growing number of publications that identify good health and social care practice guidelines in working with older LGBT people (Knocker, 2006; Concannon, 2009; GRAI and CHIRI, 2010; Opening Doors London, 2010; Age UK, 2011; LGBT MAP and SAGE, 2012; National Resource Center on LGBT Aging, 2012; Stonewall, 2012). These highlight seven main areas of good practice:

- inclusive consultation in service design and delivery;
- appropriate equality and diversity *and* LGBT-specific policies;
- creating a safe working and living environment for staff and service users;
- a robust staff training strategy;
- appropriate language and cultural representation;
- person-centred assessment and care planning;
- setting and auditing standards.

Each of these will now be addressed.

Inclusive consultation

Older LGBT people should be included in the design, implementation and monitoring of service provision, through:

- community group liaison;
- confidential monitoring of sexual orientation and gender identity among staff and service users;
- service user feedback, including via safe and supportive LGBT staff and service user networks (for example, Anchor Housing; see Stonewall, 2012).

Appropriate policies

Services should employ staff and service user equality policies that explicitly address sexual orientation, gender identity and gender expression. Anti-discrimination policies should be clearly displayed in publications and on public display. Managers should make clear to staff and service users that discrimination is not tolerated, staff should be confident that they will be supported in challenging discrimination and there should be a safe, confidential and robust complaints procedure.

A safe working and living environment

LGBT staff need to be made to feel confident and comfortable in the workplace, by creating a culture of inclusion. If LGBT staff are comfortable at work it is much more likely that LGBT service users will be as well.

A robust staff training strategy

There should be comprehensive training about older LGBT people on all social work training courses, as well as for managers, practitioners, educators and healthcare staff. Practitioners and policy makers need to appreciate how LGBT histories inform their fears about engaging with health and social care provision (River and Ward, 2012). 'Homosexuality' was classified as a psychiatric disorder under the *Diagnostic and statistical manual of mental disorders* (DSM-II) until it was removed by the American Psychiatric Association from its seventh printing in 1973 (McCommon, 2009) and many older LGB people will have experienced enforced psychiatric 'cures'. Many trans people continue to be pathologised under the DSM-V diagnosis of 'gender dysphoria' (APA, 2013), making them particularly wary of engaging with mental health services (McNeil et al, 2012).

Appropriate language and cultural representation

All staff should be careful not to use language that makes assumptions about someone's sexual orientation or gender identity. Promotional materials (brochures, leaflets, websites and so on) for older people should include visual representations of older LGBT people and should make explicit a service's commitment to working with older LGBT people. Healthcare, day care and residential establishments should have pictures and photographs representing older LGBT people, display LGBT publications and advice sheets, and hold LGBT social events and celebrations.

Person-centred assessment and care planning

LGBT people do not want to have the added hassle of explaining or defending their sexualities and/or gender identities when they may already be stressed and/or in crisis. They want personalised care plans that take all intersecting aspects of their identity into account, tying in with the United Kingdom (UK) government's personalisation agenda, which emphasises individualised care packages rather than 'one size fits all' (DH, 2007). Examples of good care planning include:

> George would like to have his subscription to *Gay Times* continued. He enjoys having some of the articles read out to him. He likes going through the 'personal ads' column thinking about who he might like to contact.

> Rosaria would like to go out to a local gay pub with three of her closest female friends on a monthly basis. (Knocker, 2006, p 28)

Age UK highlights areas of good practice with older trans people. Sometimes small choices can make a big difference. For example, if a trans man in a nursing home has feet that are too small for men's slippers, rather than buying women's slippers, service providers should purchase boy's slippers instead (Age UK, 2011, p 24).

Setting and auditing standards

A number of ways have been suggested to raise the bar for LGBT health and social care provision, including:

- kite-marking;
- commissioners requiring service providers tendering for contracts to evidence how their service meets the needs of older LGBT people;
- mobilisation of equality and human rights legislation to challenge inadequate provision.

The next section considers these good practice guidelines in the contexts of the vignettes.

Implications for social work practice

Laura

Laura is an 83-year-old White British lesbian ...

Some older lesbians have identified and lived as lesbians all their lives. The oldest are most likely to have led hidden lives and not to have children. They may belong to a rich informal network of other women/lesbians, but are all of a similar age, meaning that they may develop extra care needs at around the same time. Some women have lived a significant part of their lives as heterosexuals, but in later life form same-sex relationships, some identifying as bisexual, some as lesbian and others mobilising a sexual fluidity discourse. These women are more likely to enjoy informal support from children and grandchildren but have greater difficulty meeting and socialising with other lesbians (Cronin and King, 2013).

LGBT people living in rural areas, who may have geographically dispersed communities, may find it more difficult to access those communities in later life, leading to loneliness and isolation, which in turn can lead to depression (Jones et al, 2013). LGBT bereavement is less likely to be recognised, supported and socially validated, which in turn leads to 'disenfranchised grief' and an increased risk of depression (see Chapter Ten, this volume).

An assessment of Laura's needs should take into account her recent bereavement, and her low mood. In terms of her loneliness, referring Laura to a local day centre, where there may be no other 'out' lesbians, may only add to her sense of isolation (Langley, 2001). Local and national support networks for older lesbians should be considered, as well as how she can be supported to maintain/restore pre-existing social networks.

If Laura decides that she wishes to live in sheltered housing, she should be supported in identifying suitable provision. There should be a menu of housing choices available to older lesbians and all older LGBT people. For example, a significant number of older lesbians want LGBT-specific housing, and many want it to be women-only or lesbian-only (Stonewall, 2011; Averett and Jenkins, 2012). Others want 'LGBT-friendly' mainstream provision, fearing ghettoisation in specialist services. Emergent projects in Australia, Spain and the United States suggest that some specialist housing projects and/or collective co-commissioning of services might be a possibility (Carr and Ross, 2013). Addressing Laura's housing and social support needs will both reduce the risk of loneliness and depression (and consequent effects on her physical health), and promote her resilience to physical and mental health issues.

Gary

Gary is a single 70-year-old gay man of African Caribbean descent ...

Older gay and bisexual men experience elevated health risks compared with both the general population and older lesbian/bisexual women, including in relation to drug and alcohol use, increased internalised stigma and associated mental health problems and less social support, again impacting on physical and mental health (Fredriksen-Goldsen et al, 2013b). Older gay men ageing with HIV are especially vulnerable to deficiencies in informal social support (Rosenfeld et al, 2012) and this in turn impacts their resilience in coping with their health needs. Black older gay men also report significantly higher levels of perceived ageism and social exclusion than white older gay men (David and Knight, 2008).

Gary has very limited material and social resources, which impact his ability to maintain social networks in later life, in turn affecting overall wellbeing (Heaphy, 2009). He is also showing the early signs of dementia. While dementia among black and minority ethnic (BME) populations is receiving increasing attention (APPG, 2013), there is very little awareness so far about dementia among LGBT individuals. Much of dementia care is geared towards people with heterosexual and gender-congruent identities (Price, 2008). So while Gary, if assessed and given a diagnosis, may be recognised as a black man with dementia, he is less likely to be recognised as a gay man with dementia, and even less likely to be recognised as a black, gay man with dementia. Dementia care spaces are dominated by women, as both care providers (because of the gendering of care work) and service users (because women live longer than men). This means that Gary, going into any form of dementia provision, be it day care or residential care, may experience a triple inequality because he is black, gay and a man.

As with Laura, Gary's social isolation will affect his overall health. Interventions that provide social support to and community links for older LGBT people, including outreach projects such as Opening Doors in London (Knocker, 2012) and SAGE in New York (Kling and Kimmel, 2006), are vital as a means of mitigating the negative health effects of social isolation and enhancing wellbeing. Had such support been in place before Gary became confused, others may have picked up on his deteriorating mental state sooner and advocated on his behalf. Given Gary's present circumstances, the social worker working with him should be aware of older LGBT issues and/or seek guidance and support from older LGBT networks, which should also be responsive to issues of ethnicity (Price, 2008). Current provision offers limited options to Gary and this needs to be improved (Fish, 2012). Providing him with services that appreciate the importance of his identity as a gay man will be essential to promoting his wellbeing.

Bridget and Chris

Bridget is a 65-year-old bi-identifying woman of White Irish Catholic origin and her partner Chris, aged 69, is a White British bisexual man …

Much of 'LGBT' ageing research omits bisexuality or conflates bisexual women's experiences with those of lesbians, and bisexual men's experiences with those of gay men (Dworkin, 2006). Health and social care staff often think of service users in binary terms (that is, either heterosexual or lesbian/gay) rather than being open to the possibility that someone might be bisexual. Very often a bisexual man or woman in an opposite-sex relationship will be assumed to be heterosexual while those in a same-sex relationship will be assumed to be lesbian or gay. This means that services often fail to recognise, and appreciate, the issues for (older) bisexual service users (Jones, 2010). At the same time, lack of visibility and relatively lower levels of social support can mean heightened risks to the physical and mental health of older bisexual people (Fredriksen-Goldsen et al, 2013b). On a more general point, LGBT carers of older people (often older people themselves) may go unrecognised, because of heteronormative models of care and carers (Willis et al, 2011). This means that they often do not receive the services and support to which they are entitled as carers.

For Bridget and Chris, the first issue is to recognise Bridget as a carer and ensure that she knows what her rights are and what support is available to her. Assumptions should not be made about Bridget's or Chris' sexual orientation and this should be made clear via open-ended questioning. The extent to which Bridget and Chris wish their respective sexual orientations to be recognised and/or how they apply to their current situation should be explored with them sensitively. Whether and how religion is important to Bridget should also be explored. If she has experienced rejection from mainstream religious support, she might find LGBT faith groups spiritually sustaining. If Bridget and Chris wish to take up respite care, then they should be supported in selecting day and/or residential provision that they feel comfortable with. If such provision is not available, then a more individualised care package may need to be considered. Much more research is needed about bisexual lives in general and about bisexual ageing in particular, and only then will it be clearer what good practice would look like to a broad range of older bisexual individuals.

Theresa

Theresa is a 61-year-old heterosexual trans woman with an Asian/White British heritage …

Despite the significant growth of the trans population in recent years (Reed et al, 2009), there is a lack of research on trans ageing and, consequently, a lack of understanding about the specific needs and experiences of older trans people. Those who transitioned 30 or 40 years ago will have different needs from those who transition in later life (Bailey, 2012). There may be possible health risks associated with long-term exposure to hormone therapy (Age UK, 2011) and the experimental nature of some surgeries (Cook-Daniels, 2006).

In the UK, medical and/or legal gender reassignment (under the Gender Recognition Act 2004) is contingent upon a psychiatric diagnosis of gender dysphoria, and so trans people are inevitably caught up in the psychiatric system if they want gender reassignment. Many trans campaigners wish to see trans identities conceptualised away from a psychiatric model (GRAI and CHIRI, 2010). Many trans people have experienced major mental health problems prior to transitioning (particularly BME trans people; NGLTF, 2011), which often improve post-transitioning, providing that sufficient support is made available. However, many have experienced a lack of understanding in psychiatric contexts and so avoid accessing mental health services if their mental health subsequently deteriorates (McNeil et al, 2012).

This may be what has happened in Theresa's situation, where there may be a complex interplay between her recent transitioning and her mental state, together with a possible reluctance to seek psychiatric help. The quality of post-transitioning support will have been crucial for Theresa, both formal provision, that is, her housing arrangement, and informal social support. The estrangement from her son will be a profound loss, which will inevitably impact on her mental and physical health (Fredriksen-Goldsen et al, 2013a). Her concerns about the staff in the sheltered housing that she lives in may be based in reality, may be a reflection of her mental state or may be interconnected.

Theresa should be provided with a trans-friendly mental health assessment and be supported by an independent and trans-aware mental health advocate. Her concerns should be addressed via the organisation's complaints procedure. Consideration should be given to what trans awareness training the staff team have had, staff attitudes, the overall ethos of the sheltered housing and whether it is supportive of diversity, particularly around trans and BME issues (National Resource Center on LGBT Aging, 2012). Joined-up working between teams needs to be in place Theresa's post-transitioning support should be reviewed and, if necessary, strengthened. She should be provided with a safe space to explore what her transitioning means to her, and to address the issues with her son. Once the situation is resolved to Theresa's satisfaction, there should be ongoing monitoring and support to sustain Theresa in her housing situation, and wider social context.

Conclusion

Much more needs to be done to achieve greater health equity for older LGBT people, particularly in terms of health and social care provision (Fish, 2010). Standards of care for older LGBT people have the potential to become a litmus test for person-centred and anti-discriminatory health and social care (Ward et al, 2011). Improved recognition and respect for individuality and diversity have the potential to promote health equity among all older people, not only those who identify as LGBT.

What we know about this already
- Older LGBT people are very worried about relying on formal health and social care provision in older age.
- Older LGBT people are more likely to be earlier and disproportionate users of social care than their heterosexual counterparts.

- Current health and social care provision is ill-equipped to meet the needs of older LGBT people.

What this chapter adds
- It identifies core good practice guidelines for all older LGBT people.
- It explores specific areas of good practice for LGBT people.
- It highlights the importance of appreciating diversity and intersectionality among older (and all) LGBT people.

How this is relevant for social work and LGBT health inequalities
- The chapter offers clear strategies for improving services for older LGBT people.
- It emphasises the importance of respecting each individual's identity, life story and personal needs.
- It indicates how addressing social exclusion and reducing social isolation can promote wellbeing among older LGBT people.

References

AGE Platform Europe and ILGA-Europe, 2012, *Equality for older lesbian, gay, bisexual, trans and intersex people in Europe*, Brussels: Age Platform Europe and ILGA-Europe

Age UK, 2011, *Trans issues in later life*, London: Age UK

APA (American Psychiatric Association),1973, *Diagnostic and statistical manual of mental disorders* (2nd edn) (DSM-II), Arlington, VA: APA

APA (American Psychiatric Association), 2013, *Diagnostic and statistical manual of mental disorders* (5th edn) (DSM-V), Arlington, VA: APA

APPG (All Party Parliamentary Group), 2013, *Dementia does not discriminate: The experiences of black, Asian and minority ethnic communities*, London: The Stationery Office

Averett, P and Jenkins, C, 2012, 'Review of the literature on older lesbians: implications for education, practice, and research', *Journal of Applied Gerontology*, 31, 4, 537-61

Bailey, L, 2012, 'Trans ageing: thoughts on a life course approach in order to better understand trans lives', in R, Ward, I, Rivers and M, Sutherland (eds) *Lesbian, gay, bisexual and transgender ageing: Biographical approaches for inclusive care and support*, London and Philadelphia, PA: Jessica Kingsley Publishers, 51-66

Carr, S and Ross, P, 2013, *Assessing current and future housing and support options for older LGB people*, York: Joseph Rowntree Foundation

Concannon, L, 2009, 'Developing inclusive health and social care policies for older LGB citizens', *British Journal of Social Work*, 39, 403-17

Cook-Daniels, L, 2006, 'Trans ageing', in D Kimmel, T Rose and S David (eds) *Lesbian, gay, bisexual and transgender ageing*, New York, NY: Columbia University Press, 20-35

Coren, E, Iredale, W, Bywaters, P, Rutter, D and Robinson, J, 2010, *The contribution of social work and social care to the reduction of health inequalities: Four case studies*, Research Briefing 33, London: Social Care Institute for Excellence

Cronin, A and King, A, 2013, 'Only connect? Older lesbian, gay and bisexual (LGB) adults and social capital', *Ageing and Society*, First View Article, January, 1-22

David, S and Knight, BG, 2008, 'Stress and coping among gay men: age and ethnic differences', *Psychology and Aging*, 23, 1, 62-9

DH (Department of Health), 2007, *Putting people first: A shared vision and commitment to the transformation of adult social care*, London: DH

Dworkin, SH, 2006, 'The ageing bisexual: the invisible of the invisible minority', in D, Kimmel, T, Rose and S, David (eds) *Lesbian, gay, bisexual and transgender aging*, New York, NY: Columbia University Press, 36-52

Fish, J, 2007, *Reducing health inequalities for lesbian, gay, bisexual and trans people: A series of briefings for health and social care staff*, London: Department of Health.

Fish, J, 2010, Promoting equality and valuing diversity for lesbian, gay, bisexual and trans patients, *InnovAiT*, 3, 6, 333-8.

Fish, J, 2012, Older people, in J, Fish, *Social work and lesbian, gay, bisexual and trans people: Making a difference*, Bristol: Policy Press

Fredriksen-Goldsen, KI, Cook-Daniels, L, Kim, H-J, Erosheva, EA, Emlet, CA, Hoy-Ellis, CP, Goldsen, J and Muraco, A, 2013a, Physical and mental health of transgender older adults: an at-risk and underserved population, *The Gerontologist*, first published online 27 March 2013, doi: 10.1093/geront/gnt021

Fredriksen-Goldsen, KI, Emlet, CA, Kim, HJ, Muraco, A, Erosheva, EA, Goldsen, J and Hoy-Ellis, CP, 2013b, The physical and mental health of lesbian, gay male, and bisexual (LGB) older adults: the role of key health indicators and risk and protective factors, *The Gerontologist*, 53, 4, 664-75

GRAI and CHIRI (GLBTI Retirement Association Inc and Curtin Health Innovation Research Institute), 2010, *Best practice guidelines: Accommodating older gay, lesbian, bisexual, trans and intersex (GLBTI) people*, Perth: GRAI and CHIRI

Heaphy, B, 2009, Choice and its limits in older lesbian and gay narratives of relational life, *Journal of GLBT Family Studies*, 5, 1/2, 119-38

Jones, K, Fenge, LA, Read, R and Cash, M, 2013, Collecting older lesbians' and gay men's stories of rural life in South West England and Wales: 'we were obviously gay girls ... (so) he removed his cow from our field', *Forum: Qualitative Social Research*, 14, 12, www.qualitative-research.net/index.php/fqs/article/view/1919/3515

Jones, R, 2010, Troubles with bisexuality in health and social care, in RL, Jones and R, Ward (eds) *LGBT issues: Looking beyond categories: Policy and practice in health and social care (10)*, Edinburgh: Dunedin Academic Press, 42–55

Kling, E and Kimmel, D, 2006, SAGE: New York City's pioneer organization for LGBT elders, in D, Kimmel, T, Rose and S, David (eds) *Lesbian, gay, bisexual and transgender aging*, New York, NY: Columbia University Press, 265–76

Knocker, S, 2006, *The whole of me: Meeting the needs of older lesbians, gay men and bisexuals living in care homes and extra care housing*, London: Age Concern England

Knocker, S, 2012, *Perspectives on ageing lesbians, gay men and bisexuals*, London: Joseph Rowntree Foundation

Knocker, S, Maxwell, N, Phillips, M and Halls, S, 2012, Opening doors and opening minds: sharing one project's experience of successful community engagement, in R, Ward, I, Rivers and M, Sutherland (eds) *Lesbian, gay, bisexual and transgender ageing: Biographical approaches for inclusive care and support*, London and Philadelphia, PA: Jessica Kingsley Publishers, 150–64

Langley, J, 2001, Developing anti-oppressive empowering social work practice with older lesbian women and gay men, *British Journal of Social Work*, 31, 917–32

LGBT MAP (Movement Advancement Project) and SAGE (Services and Advocacy for Gay, Lesbian, Bisexual and Transgender Elders), 2012, *Improving the lives of transgender older adults: Recommendations for policy and practice*, New York, NY: SAGE and National Center for Transgender Equality

McCommon, B, 2009, Sexual orientation and psychiatric diagnosis: issues to consider for DSM-V and beyond, *Journal of Gay & Lesbian Mental Health*, 13, 94–99

McNeil, J, Bailey, L, Ellis, S, Morton, J and Regan, M, 2012, *Trans Mental Health and Emotional Wellbeing Study 2012*, Edinburgh: The Scottish Transgender Alliance

National Resource Center on LGBT Aging, 2012, *Inclusive services for LGBT older adults: A practical guide to creating welcoming agencies*, New York, NY: Services and Advocacy for Gay, Lesbian, Bisexual and Transgender Elders

NGLTF (National Gay and Lesbian Task Force), 2011, *Injustice at every turn: A look at black respondents in the national transgender discrimination survey*, New York, NY: National Center for Transgender Equality and National Black Justice Coalition, www.thetaskforce.org/reports_and_research/ntds_black_respondents

Opening Doors London, 2010, *Supporting older lesbian, gay, bisexual and transgender people: A checklist for social care* providers, London: Age Concern

Price, E, 2008, Pride or prejudice? Gay men, lesbians and dementia, *British Journal of Social Work*, 38, 1337-52

Reed, B, Rhodes, S, Schofield, P and Wylie, P, 2009, *Gender variance in the UK: Prevalence, incidence, growth and geographic distribution*, Ashtead, UK: Gender Identity Research and Education Society

River, L and Ward, R, 2012, Polari's life story: learning from work with older LGBT people, in R, Ward, I, Rivers and M, Sutherland (eds) *Lesbian, gay, bisexual and transgender ageing: Biographical approaches for inclusive care and support*, London and Philadelphia, PA: Jessica Kingsley Publishers, 135-49

Rosenfeld, D, Bartlam, B and Smith, R, 2012, Out of the closet and into the trenches: gay male baby boomers, aging, and HIV/AIDS, *The Gerontologist*, 52, 2, 255-64

Stonewall, 2011, *Lesbian, gay bisexual people in later life*, London: Stonewall

Stonewall, 2012, *Working with older lesbian, gay and bisexual people: A guide for care and support services*, London: Stonewall

Ward, R, Pugh, S and Price, E, 2011, *Don't look back? Improving health and social care service delivery for older LGB users*, London: Equality and Human Rights Commission

Weeks, J, Heaphy, B and Donovan, C, 2001, *Same sex intimacies: Families of choice and other life experiments*, London: Routledge

Williams, H, Varney, J, Taylor, J, Fish, J, Durr, P and Elan-Cane, C, 2013, *The lesbian, gay, bisexual and trans public health outcomes framework companion document*, London: National LGB&T Partnership, Public Health England and Department of Health

Willis, P, Ward, N and Fish, J, 2011, Searching for LGBT carers: mapping a research agenda in social work and social care, *British Journal of Social Work*, 41, 1304-20

Witten, T and Eyler, AE (eds), 2012, *Gay, lesbian, bisexual and transgender aging: Challenges in research, practice and policy*, Baltimore, MA: Johns Hopkins University Press

A theoretical model for intervening in complex sexual behaviours: sexual desires, pleasures and passion – *La Pasión* – of Spanish-speaking gay men in Canada

Gerardo Betancourt

VIGNETTE

Carlos, a Latino Colombian gay man, came to the first session of Chicos Net, an HIV prevention behavioural intervention. He has lived in Canada for the past four years. During the process, he told the group that he had unprotected sex the week before. His reasoning was based on how much he was attracted to the guy he had sex with, and that he was so 'into' the moment that he 'let things happen'. He was worried about the event. The group provided support and feedback. A discussion about similar situations in which other participants had been involved made Carlos feel a little bit better. "We have all been there," a participant said. Then the group moved the focus of the night's discussion to sexual desires, pleasures and passions.

Introduction

In order to understand HIV infection and its relation to social determinants of health, it is relevant to touch on the conditions in which sexualities and gender relations are socially enacted and constructed. Logie (2012, p 1243) invites us to think about gender and sexual orientation as an intervening factor that affects an individual's wellbeing: 'sexual minorities experience significant and pervasive health disparities'.

Different disciplines in social science have centred their attention on the social environments in which the HIV epidemic has evolved, particularly among homosexual communities. Moreover, scholars have long promoted the understanding and analysis of the role of social work in the field of sexualities and HIV prevention when working with gay populations.

According to Hicks (2008, p 66), social work is a discipline that should examine various forms of thinking of what sexuality is, and disentangle it from 'dominant versions of "sexuality"'. This analysis is relevant because dominant forms of understanding sexuality have historically marginalised certain practices or individuals according to the particular historical moment and geographic locations. In consequence, those individuals practising 'that' kind of sex are often repressed, and forced to hide or live in fear. The social inequality comes from the idea that some forms of sexual expression or sexual practices are more acceptable than others, and in some extreme cases, some forms are banned or even illegal.

Health inequalities

Krieger (2001) invites us to think about 'social epidemiology' and how many health constructs that have been considered and analysed from a biological perspective are truly socially constructed. Factors such as discrimination and stress lead to job-related illnesses, infections and diseases, which are unequally socially distributed.

The purpose of this chapter is to propose an analysis of a particular group that is at higher risk of getting infected with HIV due to the epidemiology of the infection – unprotected anal intercourse (UAI) – but also due to the particular social characteristics and cultural dynamics that posit men who have sex with other men as having a higher risk of infection, particularly for ethnoracial groups. Other approaches have focused on localising client needs, cultures and contexts, particularly in the area of sexuality with a strong recognition of the role of pleasure and sexual desires (Boyce et al, 2007). In the context of HIV prevention, social workers can lead participants to a fuller understanding of the interplay between these various life factors, social contexts and the decision-making process.

Latino gay men and HIV

Spanish-speaking men are at higher risk of contracting HIV in Canada. In 2005, a survey conducted during PRIDE, Toronto (The Ontario HIV Treatment Network, 2007) showed that Latino men are more than twice as likely to engage in UAI. In addition, Remis and Lui (2007) published epidemiological data on the number of HIV infections among Spanish-speaking populations from 1981 to 2005 in Canada.

More recently in 2010, the *Cuentame* (Adam et al, 2011) study analysed Latino gay men's qualitative narratives of man-on-man sexual activities, depicting the difficult sexual health dilemmas that this particular group faces in Canada in relation to being sexually active and dealing with HIV prevention practices.

Canadian research and reports about Latino gay men and HIV are in tune with those from the United States (US) (Carballo-Diéguez et al, 2005; Bianchi et al, 2007; Organista, 2012) where HIV prevention research in Spanish-speaking gay communities consistently points out the following factors that are associated with UAI events:

- sexual migration: according to Diaz (1998) and Muñoz-Laboy (2004), sexual migration is a common experience among Spanish-speaking gay men, who use migration as a strategy to deal with highly gendered contextualised environments, rejection and violence. Men migrate to other locations or cross borders (North America for instance) as a strategy to deal with repressive, homophobic environments in Latin America (personal shame, family loyalty).
- difficulties in dealing with new environments: this search for new geographies where there is more sexual freedom – particularly, big North American cities that function as 'gay epicentres' (Carrillo, 2004; Bianchi et al, 2007; Vasquez del Aguila, 2012) or in Latin America countries, by moving from rural to urban settings – leads to a new environment that Spanish-speaking men are not prepared to deal with due to factors such as isolation, a lack of social networks, race (Latino), culture (Spanish-speaking social norms), economics (poverty, unemployment, underemployment), migration status, access to services, language barriers and so on (Halkitis and Perez Figueroa, 2013);
- lack of personal control, self-awareness, self-esteem, self-efficacy and safe sex strategies (Diaz, 1998; Adam, 2006; Diaz et al, 2012);
- lack of current knowledge about HIV and its transmission, and poor understanding of HIV infection low viral load (Diaz, 1998; Vega et al, 2011; Gay Men's Sexual Health Alliance and AIDS Committee of Toronto, 2013);
- sexual urges, passion, desires, pleasures, the need for sexual intimacy and physical sensations, emotional commitment and romance – the need for Spanish-speaking gay men to connect with other men, both sexually and romantically, presents challenges related to safe and unsafe sexual behaviours (Adam et al, 2000; Fontdevila, 2009).

Research in the HIV field has analysed empirical and theoretical approaches to intervene and the factors associated with *UAI* events. Those efforts have focused on developing behavioural interventions that aim to decrease the number of infections by promoting condom use and the choosing of lower-risk sexual behaviours. Some interventions have aimed to provide more HIV information, such as *Hermanos de Luna y Sol* (Diaz, 1998) and *SOMOS* (Vega et al, 2011). Others have concentrated on increasing empowerment and the individual's resilience (Zea et al, 2003; Carballo-Diéguez et al, 2005; Ramirez-Valles, 2007). Others still have focused on how knowledge, skills, self-awareness and judgement can be better predisposed to more effectively deal with different sexual situations with inherent HIV infection risks (Martin et al, 2005; Sandfort et al, 2007; Kissinger, 2012).

Approaching the study of sexualities; theoretical frameworks

In order to intervene in unsafe sexual behaviours, one must understand the way sexualities are experienced by Spanish-speaking gay men. The ways sexualities are realised are closely connected and contextualised with social constructions of gender and are deeply grounded in cultural understandings: 'Gender is a multidimensional social construct that is culturally based and historically specific, and thus constantly changing' (Johnson et al, 2009, p 3). Furthermore, Krieger (2003, p 653) refers to gender as 'a social construct regarding culture-bound conventions, roles, and behaviors'. Thus, gender is a central focus in examining sexual behaviours, particularly in the study of sexualities, where race, masculinity, class and sexual orientation define an individual's experiences. This approach has been termed 'intersectionality':

> Intersectionality is concerned with simultaneous intersections between aspects of social difference and identity (as related to meanings of race/ethnicity, indigeneity, gender, class, sexuality, geography, age, disability/ability, migration status, religion) and forms of systematic oppression…. (Dhamoon and Hankivsky, 2011, p 16)

In short, 'intersectionality' provides us with a more refined lens through which to examine the contemporary construction of masculinities and therefore the sexual practices and behaviours in which those male individuals engage.

As such, those masculine social expectations might promote risky behaviours: 'social practices that undermine men's health are often signifiers of masculinity and instruments that men use in the negotiation of social power and status' (Courtenay, 2000, p 1385), especially when those are framed in such complex domains where sexuality is intertwined with emotional, physical and social frameworks.

Moreover, those sexual expressions play a role in the realisation of sexual behaviours and how they are connected to sexual encounters. They are individually experienced and are located in a particular geographic, historical, economic and social contexts. Sometimes those contexts have been supportive of those particular behaviours and practices (homosexuality), and sometimes they have not.

For instance, in analysing Latino gay men, Vasquez del Aguila (2012) examines the Latino construction of sexualities, masculinities and identities. In his article, '"God forgives the sin but not the scandal": coming out in a transnational context – between sexual freedom and cultural isolation' (2012), he analyses sociological factors in the migration of Latino men to North America with the intention to live their sexual lives away from the social scrutiny of family and communities of origin, demonstrating that sexuality is a strong drive that socially organises individuals' lives.

This drive that structures and organises sexual lives also dictates and provides meaning to the sexual practices and behaviours realised by individuals. This is the connection with efforts and challenges in relation to HIV infection. As such, I propose an approach for the understanding of an intervention in behaviours and practices based on sexuality: sexual desires, pleasures and passions for Spanish-speaking gay men.

Sexual health dilemmas and *La Pasión*

For more than 30 years since the HIV/AIDS epidemic started, the dominant discourse for prevention has concerned the use of a physical barrier: the condom. The downside of condom use is that some people experience a reduction in pleasure, and for many gay men, it also means a lessening in the sense of connection and deep intimacy between sexual partners. This situation has created a jeopardised equation, in which sexual desires, pleasures and passions are in conflict with safe-sex prevention efforts. This equation is embodied by individuals who have different approaches and rationales – some gay men may prioritise pleasure over risk and health-related consequences (Adam, 1992, 2006, 2011).

Health dilemmas (Fontdevila, 2009) need to be discussed in HIV behavioural interventions. Spanish-speaking gay men who have sex with men have to make sense of safe-sex health strategies and make decisions in regards to how (safely or unsafely) and to what degree they deal with their sexual experiences (in intercourse activities), and their needs for intimacy and pleasure; *La Pasión* must be understood as playing a central role in their lives.

La Pasión is the experience of sexual desires, pleasures and passions of Spanish-speaking gay men who want to better understand both their sexual behaviours and how to enact their sexual intimacy and need for romance with other men in the context of HIV prevention (Adam et al, 2000; Boyce et al, 2007). It helps to develop better frameworks for engaging in meaningful conversations, social actions and behavioural interventions that recognise the role of sexualities in the lives of Spanish-speaking men. This framework recognises that some men find it challenging to incorporate safe-sex practices in their daily lives, or are not able to change their unsafe sexual practices unless sexual behavioural interventions provide better and more encouraging approaches that truly address gay men's sexuality needs.

Understanding that the sexual decision-making process is interconnected with multiple aspects of Spanish-speaking gay men's lives, other approaches that analyse complex decision-making behaviours may be adapted and applied in HIV intervention models.

Intervening in sexual behaviours and practices

Different disciplines in the social and health sciences are concerned with explaining and understanding complex sexual behaviours. Some theoretical approaches have tried to shed light on the relationship between thinking, doing and the reflection of behavioural patterns, with the intention of proposing models and maps that could be useful in health promotion efforts.

Knowledge/skills extend beyond a pure understanding of a particular factual scenario, but include other factors that at the time do not seem to be relevant to the decision at hand (such as marginalisation, racialisation or other social barriers). In other words, HIV skills knowledge includes knowing more about one's self than simply asking whether one knows how the virus is transmitted or how to use a condom. By applying a social work approach towards understanding how various life factors and social contexts play into their sexual health, participants are better prepared to apply the new knowledge/skills in their decision making.

The new model: intervening in safe-sex practices

There is need for a model that assists in the integration of more complex approaches for intervening in sexual practices, behaviours and knowledge. If adapted for the HIV prevention field, it will help to address a set of complex sexual behaviours and the theoretical areas involved in safe-sex practices. These areas include HIV prevention *knowledge*, *self-regulation* and *decision making*, among other internal and personal processes that are, according to empirical research (Carballo-Diéguez et al, 2005; Ramirez-Valles, 2007; Adam et al, 2011a, 2011b; Vega et al, 2011), involved in sexual intercourse events and influence whether safe-sex behaviours are present or absent.

The *knowledge* relates to knowing how HIV is transmitted (factual information), as well as to attitudes towards and awareness of HIV, condom use and safe-sex practices (Diaz 1998; Vega et al, 2011). Research has shown that the area of *knowledge* – negotiating condom use with partners, along with bringing condoms to dates and using them in sexual intercourse – is relevant for informed safe-sex practices (Diaz, 1998; Bianchi et al, 2007) and is intimately related to and associated with levels of HIV knowledge.

At the same time, there is evidence of the internal, personal factors that intermingle in sexual intercourse events, which according to HIV literature (Diaz, 1998; Carillo, 2004) are represented by *self-regulation*. According to Diaz (1998, p 142), self-regulation is 'the human capacity to plan, guide and monitor one's behavior flexibly in the face of difficult and challenging circumstances'. Thus, the importance of self-regulation lies in the ability to plan one's sexual activities while recognising:

- highly risky HIV sexual activities;
- one's sexual desires, pleasures and passions/romance needs;
- *decision making* in regards to safe sex needs to be promoted and realised.

This final point, the *decision-making* aspect, is where behaviours are realised into effective/ineffective safe-sexual practices. *Decision-making* actions are the final choice where individuals do or do not incorporate HIV prevention and sexual health discourses. The 'Rational Man' (Adam, 1992, 2006) notion of being able to prevent risky activities that could have health consequences is confronted with the sexual discourses of desires, pleasures and passions – *La Pasión* – of Latino gay men.

Chicos Net: an HIV intervention

Chicos Net is an HIV prevention programme – facilitated at the Centre for the Spanish-Speaking Peoples in Toronto, Canada – that aims to intervene in sexual behaviour among Latino men in the city. The intervention was born in 2008, when it was called *Mano en Mano*. In 2012, the intervention changed its name to *Chicos Net* and adapted a model of incorporating art-based outputs and modern internet activities such as the production of videos, a podcast on sexual health, a radio-novella (radio dramatisation) and a photo-voice model (photos and narratives taken by participants). Although it is a very brief intervention consisting of four sessions of three hours each, it aims to allow participating Latino men to interact in Spanish and get to know more peers who speak Spanish as a first language and who may be dealing with similar experiences as immigrants to Canada.

The most important aspect of this project – having a group of friends and becoming socially integrated and reducing the individual's isolation – is operationalised in the *Chicos Net* intervention by the creation of groups of eight to 12 Spanish-speaking gay men who will '*hang out*' during the sessions. These groups get together to talk about sexual experiences, challenges in dating, homophobia, life experiences and work/careers among other topics – always within the context of discussion of sexual desires, pleasures and passions, and factors that enable or prevent safe-sex behaviours and practices.

Objectives of Chicos Net

The first objective of *Chicos Net* is to reduce the individual's isolation, since it is a social determinant of health (Dennis, 2009), and a factor that is related to HIV risk. As Diaz (1998) states, many Latino men come from social contexts of rejection, shame, violence and painful experiences. The practical perspective of this objective is achieved by providing social opportunities for Latino gay men to meet other peers. This is done by placing recruitment posters in places and locations that Latino gay men attend such as bars, social services and medical services.

The second objective of *Chicos Net* is to increase knowledge of HIV and safe-sex practices. In the intervention, we have approached the concept of 'safe-sex practices' from the broader perspective of sexual health (Boyce et al, 2007). 'Sexual health' is understood in a holistic way as a complex concept integrating physical health in general, mental health and a sex-positive approach. Empirical research has shown that there is a direct correlation between safe-sex knowledge and the reduction of UAI events (Vega et al, 2011). Thus, participants learn more than just medical facts and the correct way to use a condom. They learn about measuring and appraising infection risks with certain sexual activities and practices. In consequence, knowledge becomes more than just information; it also can be translated into skills (how to navigate the sexual field) and judgement (when, how, why, how, etc). In this way, condoms are incorporated into the individual's sexual repertoire as part of having intercourse in the context of HIV prevention, allowing better decision making in regards to condom use, or other safe-sex practices.

The third objective of *Chicos Net* is to develop participants' critical awareness and empowerment. This objective is achieved throughout the intervention's activities by implementing three major theoretical approaches found in Freire's (2000) *Pedagogy of the oppressed*, Foucault's *History of sexuality I* (1978), *II* (1984) and Butler's (1990) *Gender trouble*:

- Freire proposes that oppressed people could become empowered and free if they could gather together and talk about the factors and structures that oppress them. Thus, in *Chicos Net*, participants share their experiences and how they solve problems related to homophobia, racialised experiences, dating, online cruising, body image and migration issues, among others, particularly surrounding sexual desires, pleasures and passions.
- Foucault analyses the role of historical discourses (historical ways in which sexuality has been understood or approached) in relation to sexuality and how sexual practices have historically defined identities. Understanding this is important in order to promote change and wellness with this particular group due to the feelings of social shame, rejection and isolation that Latino gay men have experienced because of their sexual desires, pleasures and passions towards other men.
- Butler helps us to understand and to develop critical awareness of the societal conceptualisation of gender, in this case in regard to Latino masculinities. Her theoretical framework questions and dissects the attributed gender expectations and how they are socially constructed from the biological sex, and how sexual desires and pleasures are also predetermined by society. This aspect is important for understanding the heavy burden with which Latino men are raised in their home communities in Latin America, whereby Spanish-speaking men are expected to comply with the masculine role imposed by Latin cultures, in which men are expected to get married, raise families

and be productive in society. Any attempt to defy this role is deemed as a failure and produces family and social shame.

Finally, the fourth objective of *Chicos Net* is to increase the individual's resilience, personal agency and *self-regulation*. Literature in HIV studies (Diaz, 1998; Carballo-Diéguez, 2005; Ramirez-Valles, 2007) stresses the role of these factors in enabling behaviours that support condom use.

In consequence, *self-regulation* becomes a personal strength that could help to operationalise self-awareness, self-reflection and self-assessment. These are all important aspects for HIV prevention, particularly working with gay men in Spanish-speaking populations, where the lack of understanding of self-emotions and the role of sexualities in one's life represent an everyday life challenge. The absence of role models for showing ways to enact love and romantic relationships among men may limit thinking and consideration in connection with behaviours, particularly in the realm of sexualities.

Conclusions and social work implications

According to Carballo-Diéguez et al (2005), HIV interventions have traditionally focused on intervening in individuals' sexual behaviours by focusing on self-empowering approaches, providing HIV and safe-sex information, developing resilience attitudes and reducing the individual's social isolation. Studies in social human sexuality are central to understanding the motivations, actions, decision making and judgement involved in safe-sex practices. The community/group discussion by *Chicos Net* participants allows one to hear the rationales surrounding how they place, make sense of and organise their sexual lives around sexual desires, pleasures and passions. However, there remains the inherent challenge of making an impact on individualistic dimensions of personality such as sexualities. This model shows promising theoretical and empirical features for future implementation of interventions that are community-accessible and that need to be properly evaluated quantitatively and qualitatively (Lipsey and Cordray, 2000; Boydell et al, 2012). *Chicos Net* incorporates a theoretical model in order to evaluate and standardise this intervention.

La Pasión is a model that helps social workers to understand and intervene in sets of complex sexual behaviours when working with groups of Latino gay men in relation to *knowledge*, *self-regulation* and *decision making*, with a strong accent in recognising sexual desires, pleasures and passion, and the role that those emotions and factors play in HIV prevention intentions and efforts.

As for Carlos, he is now able to apply the skills and knowledge learned about himself, *la pasión* and HIV sexual health decisions. He reported back to the group that he now understands better the interplay between the seemingly unrelated aspects of his life and his sexual health. Carlos' story is but one, but he speaks for many.

What we know about this already

- Health inequalities affect disproportionately individuals belonging to particular groups or categories such as women, black and minority ethnic women, immigrants, refugees, members of the working class and LGBT communities. The intersection of one or more of those categories increases the inequality of individuals in the overlapping groups.
- Gender, sexual orientation and ethnoracial minorities have traditionally been affected by health inequalities and poorer levels of access to health.
- Traditional approaches to HIV prevention in the US have included safe-sex prevention initiatives. In Canada, efforts with Latino gay men are very new.

What this chapter adds

- It shows that marginalised ethnoracial men are at higher risk of contracting HIV due to their vulnerable situation as immigrants, who belong to minority groups. They also may not have training or the acquired skills to deal with their sexual desires, pleasures and passions, in the context of HIV prevention.
- It provides new knowledge to intervene in sexual HIV risk behaviours among Latino gay men, particularly those living in Canada.

How this is relevant to social work and LGBT health inequalities

- A theoretical approach that recognises the role of sexual desire, pleasure and passion – *La Pasión* – promotes open discussion and a constructive approach to intervening in HIV risk sexual behaviours among Latino gay men.

References

Adam, B, 1992, 'Sociology and people living with AIDS', in J Huber and BE Schneider, eds, *The social context of AIDS,* Newbury Park, California: Sage Publications, ch 1

Adam, B, Sears, A, and Schellenberg, G.E, 2000, 'Accounting for unsafe sex: interviews with men who have sex with men', *The Journal of Sex Research,* 37, 24-36

Adam, B, 2006, 'Infectious behaviour: imputing subjectivity to HIV transmission', *Social Theory and Health,* 4, 168-179

Adam, B., 2011, 'Epistemic fault lines in biomedical and social approaches to HIV prevention', *Journey of the International AIDS Society*, 14(2), 1-9

Adam, B, Betancourt, G, and Serrano-Sanchéz, A, 2011a, 'Development of an HIV prevention and life skills program for Spanish-speaking gay and bisexual newcomers to Canada', *The Canadian Journal of Human Sexuality*, 20, I, 11-17

Adam, B, Rangel, C, Serrano, A, and Betancourt, G, 2011b, 'An analysis of sexual decision making for Spanish-speaking gay, bisexual and men who have sex with men', in The Ontario HIV Treatment Network, *OHTN 2011 Research at the front lines: Influencing policy, practice and programs*, Toronto, Ontario, Canada 14-15 November 2011, Toronto: Canada, www.ohtnweb.ca/OHTNRCProgram2011/frmPrintAbstracts.aspx?ID=954852983

Bianchi, FT, Reisen, CA, Zea, MC, Poppen, PJ, Shedlin, MG, and Penha, M, 2007, 'The sexual experiences of Latino men who have sex with men who migrated to a gay epicentre in the USA', *Culture Health and Sexuality*, 9, 5, 505-18

Boyce, P, Huang Soo Lee, M, Jenkins, C, Mohamed, S, Overs, C, Paiva, V, Reid, E, Tan, M, and Aggleton, P, 2007, 'Putting sexuality (back) into HIV/AIDS: Issues, theory and practice', *Global Public Health*, 2, 1, 1-34

Boydell, KM, Gladstone, BM, Volpe, T, Allemang, B, and Stasiulis, E, 2012, 'The production and dissemination of knowledge: A scoping review of Arts-based health research', *Forum: Qualitative social research*, 13, 1-12

Butler, J, 1990, *Gender trouble*, New York: Routledge

Carballo-Diéguez, A, Dolezal, C, Leu, C-S, Nieves, L, Díaz, F, Decena, C, and Balan, I, 2005, 'A randomized controlled trial to test an HIV-prevention intervention for Latino gay and bisexual men: Lessons learned', *AIDS Care*, 17, 3, 314-328

Carillo, H, 2004, 'Sexual migration, cross-cultural sexual encounters, and sexual health', *Sexuality Research and Social Policy*, 1, 3, 58-70

Courtenay, WH, 2000, 'Constructions of masculinity and their influence on men's well-being: a theory of gender and health', *Social Science and Medicine*, 50, pp. 1385-1401

Dennis, R, 2009, *Social determinants of health*, Toronto, Canada: Canadian Scholar's Press Inc

Dhamoon, RH and Hankivsky, O, 2011, 'Why the theory and practice of intersectionality matter to health research and policy', in O Hankivsky, S de Leeuw, J Lee, B Vissandjée and N Khanlou, eds, *Health inequities in Canada: Intersectional frameworks and practice.* Vancouver, Canada: UBC Press

Diaz, RM,1998, *Latino gay men and HIV*, New York: Routledge

Diaz, RM, Sanchez, J, and Schroeder, K, 2012, 'Inequality, discrimination, and HIV risk: a review of research on Latino gay men', in KC Organista, ed, *HIV prevention with Latinos: Theory, research and practice*, New York: Oxford University Press, ch 7

Fontdevila, J, 2009, 'Framing dilemmas during sex: A micro-social approach to HIV', *Social Theory and Health*, 7, 241-263

Foucault, M, 1978, *The history of sexuality: An introduction, volume 1*, New York: Vintage Books

Foucault, M, 1984, *The history of sexuality, volume 2*, New York: Vintage Books

Freire, P, 2000, *Pedagogy of the oppressed*, New York: Continuum

Gay Men's Sexual Health Alliance and AIDS Committee of Toronto., 2013, *Undetectable viral loads and HIV transmission: What we know*, Toronto, Canada

Halkitis, PN, and Perez Figueroa R, 2013, 'Sociodemographic characteristics explain differences in unprotected sexual behavior among young HIV-negative gay, bisexual, and other YMSM in New York City', *AIDS Patient Care and STDs*, 27, 3, 181-190

Hicks, S, 2008, 'Thinking through sexuality', *Journal of Social Work*, 8, 1, 65-82

Johnson, JL, Greaves, L, and Repta, R, 2009, 'Better science with sex and gender: facilitating the use of a sex and gender-based analysis in health research', *International Journal for Equity in Health*, 8, 14, 1-11

Kissinger, P, Kovacs, S, Anderson-Smits, C, Schmidt, N, Salinas, O, Hembling, J, Beaulieu, A, Longfellow, L, Liddon, N, Shedlin, M, 2012, 'Patterns and predictors of HIV/STI risk among Latino migrant men in a new receiving community', *AIDS and Behavior*, 16, 1, 199-213

Krieger, N, 2001, 'A glossary for social epidemiology', *Journal Epidemiol Community Health*, 55, 693-700

Krieger, N., 2003, 'Genders, sexes, and health: what are the connections — and why does it matter?', *International Journal of Epidemiology*, 32, 652-7

Lipsey, MW and Cordray, DS, 2000, 'Evaluation methods for social intervention', *Annual Review of Psychology*, 51, 1, 345-75

Logie, C, 2012, 'The case for the World Health Organization's Commission on the Social Determinants of Health to Address Sexual Orientation', *American Journal of Public Health*, 102, 1243–6

Martin, M, Camargo, M, Ramos, L, Lauderdale, D, Krueger, K, and Lantos, J, 2005, 'The evaluation of a Latino community health worker HIV prevention program', *Hispanic Journal of Behavioral Sciences*, 27, 3, 371–84

Muñoz-Laboy, MA, 2004, 'Beyond "MSM": sexual desire among bisexually-active Latino men in New York City', *Sexualities*, 7, 1, 55–80

Organista, KC (ed), 2012, *HIV prevention with Latinos: Theory, research, and practice*, New York: Oxford University Press

Ramirez-Valles, JJ, 2007, 'The quest for effective HIV-prevention interventions for Latino gay men', *American Journal of Preventive Medicine*, 32, 4, 34–5

Remis, RS and Liu, J, 2007, *Epidemiologic trends in HIV infection among men who have sex with men in Ontario: The situation in 2007*, Toronto: Ontario Ministry of Health and Long-Term Care, AIDS Bureau, Gay Men's HIV Prevention Working Group. Pdf available at: www.ohemu.utoronto.ca/doc/MSM_Sept_2007.pdf

Sandfort, TM, Melendez, RM and Díaz, R, 2007, 'Gender noncomformity, homophobia, and mental health in Latino gay men', *Journal of Sex Research*, 44, 2, 181–9

The Ontario HIV Treatment Network, 2007, *Risk management in circuits of gay and bisexual men: Results from the Toronto pride survey*, Ontario HIV Treatment Network, www.actoronto.org/research.nsf/pages/riskmanagement/$file/Risk%20Management%20in%20Circuits%20of%20Gay%20and%20Bisexual%20Men.pdf

Vasquez del Aguila, E, 2012, '"God forgives the sin but not the scandal": Coming out in a transnational context –between sexual freedom and cultural isolation', *Sexualities*, 15, 2, 207–24

Vega, MY, Spieldenner, AR, DeLeon, D, Nieto, BX, and Stroman, CA, 2011, 'SOMOS: Evaluation of an HIV prevention intervention for Latino gay men', *Health Education Research*, 26, 3, 407–18

Zea, MC, Reisen, CA, and Díaz, RM, 2003, 'Methodological issues in research on sexual behavior with Latino gay and bisexual men', *American Journal of Community Psychology*, 31, 3-4, 281–91

TEN

Research and policy about end of life care for LGBT people in the UK

Kathryn Almack, Tes Smith and Bridget Moss

VIGNETTE

Joan has end-stage heart failure. She hopes to be cared for at home as long as she can but is unsure how she will cope as she lives alone. Joan has a partner, Richard. They live separately; Richard lives in a flat adapted for his disabilities. Joan is also supported by an ex-partner, Margaret and Margaret's daughter Tracey. They lived together for 15 years from when Tracey was four years old. Tracey thinks of Joan as her second mother; she is now married with small children and they see Joan and Richard as another set of grandparents. However, Richard and Margaret have not always got on together. Both Richard and Margaret want to move in with Joan to support her. This would be difficult for Richard due to his disabilities; he has contacted his social worker to see what could be done to assist them to support Joan.

How might social workers support Joan and the people closest to her?

Introduction

Social workers support vulnerable people at critical times in their lives. This can include supporting people at the end of life, which could be said to be one of the most critical times in someone's life. There is just the one chance to get things right for both the individual who is dying and those close to them. In the United Kingdom (UK), the importance of end of life care (EoLC) for social work practice is now included in the Professional Capabilities Framework (Social Work Reform Board, 2012). EoLC should be an everyday part of social work and social care practice rather than being an exclusive domain allocated to palliative care social workers (NEoLCP, 2010, 2012a). Social workers, for example, have the expertise to support the people surrounding the individual at the end of life, that is, anyone the individual regards as being important to them, which is central to any EoLC support provision. At times when there are divergent or conflicting perspectives on the needs of the dying person, social workers can exercise their skills in mediation and negotiation.

There is scant research that addresses EoLC experiences of lesbian, gay, bisexual and trans (LGBT) individuals (Harding et al, 2012) to develop evidence-based social work interventions for this client group. Nevertheless, sexual orientation and gender identity are identified as issues of social difference in relation to EoLC (DH, 2007; Cox, 2011). The next section of this chapter will outline existing (albeit limited) research addressing LGBT end of life concerns and experiences. It should be noted that where publications state lesbian, gay and bisexual (LGB) rather than LGBT as the focus of their study, this acronym is used. Overall, however, the chapter aims to be inclusive of LGBT people. There is also a body of research specifically concerned with palliative care for gay men with HIV. This chapter does not deal with this in detail (for an overview, see Stall et al, 1988). It largely stems from a period when an HIV/AIDS diagnosis was accompanied by a short prognosis; it carried a particular social stigma and involved experiences for the bereaved of multiple losses and 'survivor guilt' (Wright and Coyle, 1996). More recently, as a result of improvements in life-extending treatments, HIV is now considered a long-term condition, albeit potentially life-limiting and not without complications (Rosenfield et al, 2012). This research may have some relevance to the broader experiences of LGBT people in learning from evidenced good practice (although this has seldom permeated into the more general service delivery of palliative care and EoLC) but there are also substantive differences. There is also a significant body of literature from broader health and social care perspectives regarding LGBT communities. Again, there may be some overlaps here with EoLC (for an overview relating to older LGBT people, see Chapter Eight, this volume).

The international context

This chapter is written from a United Kingdom (UK) perspective. The International Gay and Lesbian Human Rights Commission[1] and Amnesty International[2] provide useful information regarding the cultural, legal and political position for lesbian and gay people internationally. Many LGBT citizens throughout the world are still criminalised rather than protected by laws such as those that now exist in Australia, Canada, the United States (US), the UK and other parts of Europe. In such contexts, LGBT individuals facing life-threatening illness have to hide their sexual orientation, their partner, aspects of their lifestyle and culture. Where same-sex relationships are not legally recognised, this may mean that one's partner is not involved in one's care or that dying wishes may not be recognised by families of origin, who may override decisions. Differing legislation provides a complex backdrop in which to practise EoLC and surrogate decision making.

Research background

While LGBT and heterosexual individuals may share EoLC experiences and concerns, there are additional issues that need to be addressed among LGBT people. Evidence suggests that the mental and physical health of LGBT people is poorer than that of their heterosexual counterparts, with associated consequences for people's lifespan (examples include King et al, 2003; King and Nazareth, 2006; Mayer et al, 2008; McNeil et al, 2012). In a large part, these issues are attributed to behaviours seen as health risks, which in turn are linked to minority stress. This may include experiences of stigma, marginalisation or discrimination, which have been acknowledged as social determinants of health and which may have a significant impact on the health and wellbeing of LGBT people (GLMA, 2001; Mulé et al, 2009).

Consultation for the English End of Life Care Strategy Equality Impact Assessment (DH, 2008) noted that in terms of quality of EoLC, LGBT people were most likely to be at risk of discrimination; it also noted that there was scant evidence available about LGBT people's concerns and needs at the end of life. A recent systematic review of the literature (Harding et al, 2012) of research into palliative care and EoLC in LGBT populations (published between 1990 and 2010) confirms this. The authors identified only 12 relevant papers (the criteria excluded papers not published in English). Most came from studies in the US and the primary focus of the research was the cancer experiences of lesbian women and gay men. There was little evidence pertaining to bisexual experience and no papers reporting on trans people's experiences. The review noted the educational needs of healthcare professionals to develop a greater understanding of LGBT patients; this could perhaps equally apply to a wider group of services including social care and social work working with LGBT people and those close to them, to avoid discrimination and to facilitate safe environments for disclosure.

EoLC is increasingly associated with the experience of being old (Seale, 2004, p 37). One critical review explored a wider literature about the health and social care needs of older LGB people, EoLC and bereavement (Almack, 2007). The evidence suggests that older LGB people may receive suboptimal care at the end of life due to assumed heterosexuality, lack of awareness and/or homophobia, and gaps in knowledge (Röndahl, et al, 2006; Green and Grant, 2008; Hunt and Fish, 2008; Higgins and Glacken, 2009). More recently, the concerns and needs of older LGB people have become clearer through UK research and reflection on practice in social care and housing with regard to the EoLC needs of older LGB people (Almack et al, 2010) and older LGBT people (NCPC, 2011; Stein and Almack, 2012). This adds to the evidence base about the challenges for current generations of older LGB people but there are many gaps, not least relating to trans and bisexual people. The reasons why older LGBT people may be particularly reluctant to disclose their sexual orientation or hesitant to approach services are well rehearsed (Almack et al, 2010; Cox, 2011) but these are important to understand and to address in relation to EoLC.

It is often assumed that issues raised relating to EoLC will be exclusive to our oldest generations of LGBT people and that younger LGBT generations will feel more able to request services addressing their specific needs. However, we know little about points of transition in older age or ill-health and the consequences of these. For example, levels of confidence and assertiveness may be affected in transitions from active and independent lives through to frailty or dealing with conditions that require care and support (Jones, 2011, and Carr and Ross, 2013, offer rare insights into anticipated futures of LGB younger generations getting older).

To be living with a life-limiting condition, to be dying or bereaved, can be a socially excluding experience and there are additional layers of exclusion that LGBT people may face at these times. This may include feeling unable to disclose their sexual orientation or their gender identity or other aspects of their lifestyle and culture due to previous experiences or concerns about discrimination from wider society (and sometimes for bisexual and trans people, discrimination from within lesbian and gay communities). Other issues include a potential lack of support networks, loss and grief not being fully acknowledged. Evidence specific to EoLC experiences is currently limited but the following section draws on qualitative data from three sources (see Table 10.1) to explore some of these issues further.

Table 10.1: Details of data sources

Source	Description	Reference
1	Data from a series of stakeholder discussion groups held around the UK for older LGBT people and those who work with them. Some older LGBT people's experiences were followed up to develop case stories.	NEoLCP (2012b)
2	Data from a series of focus groups to discover views, concerns and experiences about EoLC and to gather opinions about information and education needs.	Seymour et al (2009), Almack et al (2010)
3	Personal correspondence reproduced with permission, from discussions that informed the development of a research project: 'The Last Outing: exploring end of life experiences and care needs in the lives of older LGBT people' (Almack et al, University of Nottingham).	www. nottingham. ac.uk/ nmpresearch/ lastouting/home. aspx

LGBT experiences and concerns towards end of life

Many people express a preference to die at home, which can necessitate the need to have a range of health and social care professionals coming into their home. For LGBT people who are likely to be adept at managing their social networks to minimise exposure to discriminatory behaviour or attitudes, this can be daunting:

> 'We had to have carers coming into our home to help me look after Dorothy.... I sometimes felt like a stranger in my own home. We were prayed over once – and not in a good way; I used to hide photographs of me and Dorothy and just pretend I was her friend, not her partner of 50 odd years.' (Marjorie, source 1)

LGBT people may be faced with decisions about hiding items associated with their sexual orientation or gender identity, disclosing information or outing themselves to every visiting professional, with associated further loss of privacy. Or it can mean being exposed to discriminatory attitudes, which individuals may feel too vulnerable or dependent on care services to be able to challenge. In the instance Marjorie referred to, she interpreted this as religious intolerance. Another aspect of religious intolerance or evangelism is that people from LGBT communities may find themselves excluded or on the fringes of their particular religious communities and may not be able to draw on the very source of support they need at the end of life.

Trans people can face further dilemmas between privacy and disclosure. Service providers often have even less knowledge about the issues relating to trans people than LGB individuals. This can mean that an 'educative burden' is placed on the trans individual and/or others supporting them, which can be particularly onerous when someone is ill or dying and exacerbated if the same explanations are required numerous times in encounters with different staff. Trans people can face particular challenges if they have to negotiate intimate care with carers who may not be aware of their particular needs. It is important to be aware of the diversity among trans people; some will have spent most of their lives with a gender identity and body other than the one assigned at birth, while for others this may be a relatively recent transition. Others might not have undergone any form of gender reassignment surgery at all. Some who fall under the definition of trans may not necessarily see themselves as trans. They may instead refer to 'trans' as an aspect of their status or history, but not current identity.

- *What can social workers do to address these aspects of discrimination outlined here and to support LGBT people who may be encountering forms of discrimination at the end of life?*

In the case study outlined at the start of this chapter, we did not state Joan's sexual orientation but it is illustrative of an individual whose past and current relationships have been with both sexes – it is possible she may at various times have identified as heterosexual, bisexual, lesbian or other. We have not specified whether she identifies as trans or has a trans history.

- *What assumptions (if any) did you make about Joan? How might a social worker explore and identify the important aspects of Joan's identity with her?*

LGBT people are not only managing actual and feared homophobic/biphobic/transphobic prejudice but in also may be called upon to deal with a 'far more pervasive experience of heterosexism' (Cox, 2011, p 194), that is, the assumption that they are heterosexual, which can render a central aspect of their identity as invisible.

Access to other service provision

Existing evidence suggests that older LGBT people are often more isolated than their counterparts (Stonewall, 2011). As a result, they may be more dependent on formal services to support them at the end of life. Often service providers do not consider that some service recipients may be LGBT (see, for example, GRAI, 2010). Further issues for trans people, reported in several studies, include concerns about being placed in inappropriate hospital wards or having inadequate access to services (Whittle et al, 2007).

- *How can social workers contribute to helping improve access to services to support LGBT people who may feel isolated?*

It can be difficult to be open or assertive in the face of deteriorating health and increasing dependency on others. Feelings of exclusion may be exacerbated for LGBT people in a range of settings, such as nursing or care homes or communal areas of supported living, due either to prejudicial attitudes expressed by other residents or more subtle forms of exclusion such as feeling that they do not have common experiences to talk about with their peer group:

> 'The conversations are all about husbands, wives, grandchildren. If there was another gay person who I could have a little chat with and then we could both chat to the others it would be different. But on my own, I just don't feel I can join in, what can we talk about, would I be accepted?' (Barbara, source 1)

- *How might a social worker support care home staff to facilitate Barbara feeling more included in the home?*

Supportive networks

On the other hand, LGBT people may have strong supportive networks – these may 'look' different from those of heterosexual individuals, as illustrated by our case study. Some may include family of origin. Others who have lost touch with their family of origin may rely on and prefer alternative networks of support and people who are important to them. These networks may be fragile in the sense of a lack of recognition and legal protection (Knauer, 2010). Members of a 'chosen' family are often of the same generation; ageing without an intergenerational support system may lead to further social isolation for older LGBT people. However, there are also other more positive stories emerging that suggest access to networks that may serve people well when in need of support. Colin spoke of being part of the chosen family of a friend who died of a brain tumour:

> 'His family as far as he was concerned were his friends and we were his next of kin. His parents were dead and he was estranged from some of his relatives. We were the ones making decisions about his care … staff never challenged the fact that we were next of kin.' (Colin, source 2)

The term 'next of kin' is used widely in health and social care but there is a common misunderstanding that it refers to and needs to be a person related by blood or marriage (for further discussion, see NEoLCP, 2012b, p 7). It can be a concern for LGBT people that someone close to them will be denied visiting rights and information because they are not seen as the 'next of kin'.

- *How can social workers identify an individual's key sources of support and those who are important to the person? What approaches might facilitate doing so in a sensitive manner?*

Bereavement and loss

LGBT people may have particular support needs following loss of a partner. The full extent of their grief and loss may not be acknowledged. Doka (1989) refers to this as 'disenfranchised grief'. When a heterosexual spouse dies, the surviving partner has a recognised social role of widow/er, which carries a certain social status and a permissible range of emotional expression. These kinds of 'privileges' may be denied a same-sex partner.

Michael recalled a friend who received very little recognition of his loss when his partner died, other than from close friends:

> 'I went to his funeral and the family were none too happy with the situation, I don't think they wanted people knowing their son, brother was gay and my friend who was grieving, he's been with his partner for years, he never got a mention from the vicar, not one.' (Michael, source 2)

As noted by Cox (2011), funerals are significant spaces/occasions within which the deceased person's sexual orientation or gender identity should be recognised – and bereaved partner/friends can be publicly validated. Trans people may have particular concerns that the gender they have lived in is respected after death.

LGBT people as staff and as family members or people caring for a friend/partner at the end of life

Inevitably, staff bring their own experiences, feelings and views into their work. However, this necessitates the need to develop a level of self-awareness. Being aware of their own feelings enables staff to be better able to attune to other people's feelings and able to provide the best care and support for people needing their services. Some staff will be LGBT; it is important that they are supported and they are not left to be the sole champions of LGBT issues.

LGBT people will also be friends and partners of people who are dying (Price, 2012). Carol and Sarah are a lesbian parent couple who cared for their son, Stuart, at home in the last few months before he died. Carol spoke about carers coming into their home who made all kinds of assumptions:

> 'One carer asked me who was Stuart's real mum so I said what do you mean? I knew what she meant but I didn't have the strength at that point in time to deal with it ... someone else asked our friend Tom if he was Stuart's Dad.' (Source 3)

Carol and Sarah's family was – in a normative framework – quite complex to follow; Stuart's father for example, was viewed by them to be a family friend rather than a 'Dad'; Carol's eldest daughter's father had more of a 'fatherly role' with Carol and Sarah's three children.

- *How might a social worker explore who was important in Stuart's life, without asking inappropriate questions or falling back on/making heterosexist assumptions?*

> 'I visited my elderly aunt in her care home and I decided to tell her I was going to go through transition. What I didn't expect was that she would be on the receiving end of ridicule and micky-taking about me. This was happening after each visit and it made things really tough and upsetting.' (Anna, source 1)

These kinds of assumptions and behaviours exacerbate situations that can already be very difficult and stressful times in people's lives. Fortunately in the cases outlined here, there were positive experiences too. Carol was very moved by one particular general practitioner who, upon coming into their home, said: 'Before I do anything, I just want to thank you for the privilege of letting me come into your home' (Carol, source 3). This was in contrast to some others who Carol and Sarah felt 'came in as if they owned the place'; it just requires a degree of sensitivity, which should be accorded to anyone in similar circumstances, but it was particularly meaningful to them given the assumptions and misunderstandings they had to deal with at a time when they were facing a terrible loss.

Anna reported how the situation she outlined was resolved by her aunt's carers and social worker once they became aware of what was happening; Anna now feels she would be happy to choose this same care home should she ever need to be cared for in a nursing home at the end of her life.

Conclusion

In the last year of life, individuals and those important to them may need access to a complex array of services across different settings. *It is important not to make assumptions about someone's sexual orientation or gender identity but, instead, to take cues from the individual as to how they describe themselves and those important to them. As we noted earlier with reference to our case study, Joan may,* across her lifecourse, have identified as heterosexual, bisexual, lesbian or other. Her current identity may be bisexual but if she chooses not to disclose that, it may be 'hidden' due to her relationship with Richard and people making assumptions of heterosexuality. *If there is any doubt or someone is not wanting or not able to engage in conversations, staff should stay open to all possibilities. At the same time, it is important to note that sexual orientation and gender identity are about so much more than who a person has sex with; it is about a person's whole identity and whole way of life for that individual.* LGBT people and those close to them need to feel safe in approaching services for assistance; if they are not confident about services or staff, they may not seek support.

How we care for the dying is an indicator of how we care for all sick and vulnerable people. It is a vital time to get things right; how someone dies remains a lasting memory for the individual's friends, family and staff involved. All people who live within our communities should be afforded the same care, compassion and dignity through life and at the end of life. The fact is that inequalities in terms of access to services, lack of confidence to access services and discriminatory attitudes sadly remain. The challenge for those who are in a position to do so is to advocate/influence and facilitate better inclusive services for all. Addressing the distinct complex multiple needs of LGBT people holds the potential to develop non-discriminatory services that will benefit everyone.

What we know about this already
- LGBT people may be reluctant to disclose aspects of who they are at a vulnerable time in their life.
- LGBT people may have had previous negative experiences with health and care services, which could also impact on seeking support at the end of life.
- There is currently little research as to actual experiences of EoLC for those within the LGBT descriptors.

What this chapter adds
- It gives explanations as to why it is important to look at the whole person without heterosexist assumptions and emphasises the importance of respecting each individual's life story.
- It identifies key research and commentators in this area.
- It highlights particular concerns relating to EoLC and bereavement.

How this is relevant for social work and LGBT health inequalities
- The chapter poses questions that social workers must consider to ensure that they advocate for LGBT people.
- It identifies that there is a clear role for challenge and negotiation for social workers to ensure inclusion for all members of the community.
- It reminds social workers as to the need for honest, reflexive practice to ensure self-awareness.

Notes

[1] www.iglhrc.org

[2] www.amnestyusa.org/our-work/issues/lgbt-rights/decriminalizing-homosexuality

References

Almack, K, Seymour, J and Bellamy, G, 2010, 'Exploring the impact of sexual orientation on experiences and concerns about end of life care and on bereavement for lesbian, gay and bisexual elders', *Sociology*, 44, 5, 908-24

Almack, K, 2007, 'Palliative and end of life care for the non-heterosexual community', *End of Life Care for Nurses*, 1, 2, 27-32

Carr, S and Ross, P, 2013, *Assessing current and future housing and support options for older LGB People*, York: Joseph Rowntree Foundation

Cox, K, 2011, 'Sexual orientation', in D Oliviere, B Monroe and S Payne (eds) *Death, dying and social difference* (2nd edn), Oxford: Oxford University Press, 191-9

DH (Department of Health), 2007, *Bereavement: A guide for transsexual, transgender people and their loved ones*, London: DH

DH, 2008, *The End of Life Care Strategy: Equality impact assessment*, London: DH

Doka, K (ed), 1989, *Disenfranchised grief*, Boston, MA: Lexington Books

GLMA (Gay and Lesbian Medical Association), 2001, *Healthy People 2010: A companion document for LGBT health*, San Francisco, CA: GLMA

GRAI (GLBTI Retirement Association Inc), 2010, *'We don't have any of those people here': Retirement accommodation and aged care issues for non-heterosexual populations*, Perth: GRAI

Green, L and Grant, V, 2008, '"Gagged grief and beleaguered bereavements?" An analysis of multidisciplinary theory and research relating to same sex partnership bereavement', *Sexualities*, 11, 3, 275-300

Harding, R, Epiphaniou, E and Chidgey-Clark, J, 2012, 'Needs, experiences, and preferences of sexual minorities for end-of-life care and palliative care: a systematic review', *Journal of Palliative Medicine*, 15, 5, 602-11

Higgins, A and Glacken, M, 2009, 'Sculpting the distress: easing or exacerbating the grief experience of same-sex couples', *International Journal of Palliative Nursing*, 15, 4, 170-6

Hunt, R and Fish, J, 2008, *Prescription for change: Lesbian and bisexual women's health check*, London: Stonewall

Jones, RL, 2011, Imagining the unimaginable: bisexual roadmaps for ageing, in R Ward, I Rivers and M Sutherland (eds) *Lesbian, gay, bisexual and transgender ageing*, London: Jessica Kingsley Publishers, 21-38

King, M and Nazareth, I, 2006, The health of people classified as lesbian, gay and bisexual attending family practitioners in London: a controlled study, *BMC Public Health*, 6, 127, doi: 10.1186/1471-2458-6-127

King, M, McKeown, E, Warner, J, Ramsay, A, Johnson, K, Cort, C, Wright, L, Blizard, R and Davidson, O, 2003, 'Mental health and quality of life of gay men and lesbians in England and Wales', *British Journal of Psychiatry*, 183, 552-8

Knauer, NJ, 2010, 'Gay and lesbian elders: estate planning and end-of-life decision making', paper presented at a Symposium: Family, Life, and Legacy: Planning for the LGBT Community, Florida Coastal School of Law

Mayer, KH, Bradford, JB, Makadon, HJ, Stall, R, Goldhammer, H and Landers, S, 2008, 'Sexual and gender minority health: what we know and what needs to be done', *American Journal of Public Health*, 98, 6, 989-95

McNeil, J, Bailey, L, Ellis, S, Morton, J and Regan, M, 2012, *Trans Mental Health Survey*, Edinburgh: Scottish Transgender Alliance

Mulé, NJ, Ross, LE, Deeprose, B, Jackson, BE, Daley, A, Travers, A and Moore, D, 2009, 'Promoting LGBT health and wellbeing through inclusive policy development', *International Journal for Equity in Health*, 8, 18, doi: 10.1186/1475-9276-8-18

NCPC (National Council for Palliative Care), 2011, *Open to all? Meeting the needs of lesbian, gay, bisexual and trans people nearing the end of life*, London: NCPC

NEoLCP (National End of Life Care Programme), 2010 *Supporting people to live and die well: A framework for social care at the end of life*, London: NEoLCP

NEoLCP, 2012a, *The route to success in end of life care: Achieving quality for social work*, London: NEoLCP

NEoLCP, 2012b, *The route to success in end of life care: Achieving quality for lesbian, gay, bisexual and transgender people*, London: NEoLCP

Price, E, 2012, 'Gay and lesbian carers: ageing in the shadow of dementia', *Ageing and Society*, 32, 3, 516-32

Röndahl, G, Innala, S and Carlsson, M, 2006, 'Heterosexual assumptions in verbal and non-verbal communication in nursing', *Journal of Advanced Nursing*, 56, 4, 373-81

Rosenfeld, D, Bartlam, B and Smith, R, 2012, 'Out of the closet and into the trenches: gay male baby boomers, aging and HIV/AIDS', *The Gerontologist*, 52, 2, 255-64

Seale, CF, 2004, 'Demographic change and the experience of dying', in D Dickinson, M Johnson and JS Katz (eds) *Death, dying and bereavement*, London: Sage Publications, 35-43

Seymour, J, Almack, K, Bellamy, G, Clarke, A, Crosbie, B, Froggatt, K, Gott, M, Kennedy, S, Sanders, C and Welton, M, 2009, *A peer education programme for end of life care education among older people and their carers: Final report*, Nottingham: University of Nottingham

Social Work Reform Board, 2012, *Professional capabilities framework*, London: Social Work Reform Board

Stall, R, Coates, T and Hoff, C, 1988, 'Behavioral risk reduction for HIV infection among gay and bisexual men: a review of results from the US', *American Psychologist*, 43, 11, 878-85

Stein, G and Almack, K, 2012, 'Care near the end of life: the concerns, needs and experiences of LGBT elders', in R Ward, I Rivers and M Sutherland (eds) *Lesbian, gay, bisexual and transgender ageing: Biographical approaches for inclusive care and support*, London: Jessica Kingsley Publishers, 114-34

Stonewall, 2011, *Lesbian, gay and bisexual people in later life*, London: Stonewall

Whittle, S, Turner, L and Al-Alami, M, 2007, *Engendered penalties: Transgender and transsexual people's experiences of inequality and discrimination*, London: The Equalities Review

Wright, C and Coyle, A, 1996, 'Experiences of AIDS-related bereavement among gay men: implications for care', *Mortality*, 1, 3, 267-82

ELEVEN

LGBT asylum seekers and health inequalities in the UK[1]

Kate Karban and Ala Sirriyeh

VIGNETTE

Jay was born in Nigeria where same-sex behaviour between adults is punishable by up to 14 years' imprisonment. Although she identifies herself as a lesbian, she was pressured into marriage and has one child, now 10 years old, who remains in Nigeria and who she has not seen for seven years. Jay rarely goes out as she is frightened of meeting people from the Nigerian community, fearing harassment or violence if they find out about her sexuality. She has attempted to self-harm on several occasions and is receiving anti-depressant medication from her general practitioner (GP) although she has not disclosed that she is gay.

Introduction

The experiences of lesbian, gay, bisexual and trans (LGBT) asylum seekers have attracted little attention in social work literature in the United Kingdom (UK), reflecting the somewhat marginal status of both asylum seeking and LGBT issues in mainstream practice and literature. However, growing interest in human rights and social work (Cemlyn, 2008; Ife, 2012) has drawn attention to the need for social work to address human rights and social justice issues for LGBT people nationally and internationally.

Globally there are unequal protections for LGBT people in United Nations (UN) member states, despite the UN *Resolution on Human Rights, Sexual Orientation and Gender Identity* (UN Human Rights Council, 2011). The death penalty is in force in six UN member states and same-sex relationships are criminalised in approximately 76 countries (ILGA, 2013). Even with legal protection, homophobia and transphobia are experienced in many countries (Bach, 2013). The case for international human rights for LGBT people has been stressed by the UN Human Rights Office (2012) in the report *Born free and equal*, setting out the core legal obligations to:

- prevent torture and inhuman treatments;
- repeal laws criminalising homosexuality;
- prohibit discrimination based on sexual orientation and gender identity;
- safeguard freedom of expression and association.

It is the lack of these human rights protections for LGBT people in many countries that leads them to the decision to flee persecution and seek safety in another country.

This chapter explores the experiences of LGBT asylum seekers after they have arrived in the UK. Reference will be made to health inequalities and human rights and the significance of these issues for social work practice, relating this back to Jay's story. The chapter draws on literature in this field, while also making reference to the experiences of two lesbian women seeking asylum who participated in an ongoing research study.

The term 'asylum seekers' refers to those who have applied for, but not yet been granted, refugee status according to the criteria embedded within the 1951 Geneva Convention 1951 (Refugee Status) (article 1A(2)). While waiting for the outcome of their asylum application in the UK, people are not permitted to work and rely on weekly cash payments to pay for food and basic necessities (Hynes and Sales, 2010). Concerns regarding the lack of co-ordination and communication in managing asylum applications led to the introduction of the New Asylum Model initially introduced in 2005 and fully implemented in 2007. This was intended to speed up the processing of applications and conclude an increasing proportion of cases within six months, with the introduction of a single case owner who would be responsible for each case (Refugee Council, 2007). However a Refugee Council Report (2010) refers to asylum seekers continuing to experience problems in gaining timely access to legal advice, problems with interpreting services and overall concerns with the implementation of the single case owner system. Additionally there is continuing evidence of increasing delays in initial decisions with a 63% rise in applications waiting for more than six months in 2012 (Home Affairs Committee, 2013).

Background

There is evidence of legislative progress and increasing public acceptance of LGBT people in public life in the UK. A government policy initiative introduced in 2010 made explicit reference to stopping the deportation of asylum seekers who left particular countries because their sexual orientation or gender identification put them at proven risk of imprisonment, torture or execution (HM Government, 2010, p 3). However, many LGBT people continue to experience prejudice and hate crime and fear discrimination at school, work and in health and social care services (Stonewall, 2008, 2013). Together with their experiences in their country of origin this provides the backdrop to the experiences of LGBT people seeking asylum in the UK.

Many LGBT asylum seekers have faced violence and persecution in their country of origin before seeking asylum (Miles, 2010). Bennett's (2013) study of lesbian asylum seekers in the UK found that many had experienced physical and/or sexual violence in their countries of origin and some had been imprisoned. Women spoke of personal struggles in discovering their sexuality within a cultural context where same-sex relationships were not publicly discussed or acknowledged. In attempts to maintain their safety and acceptance, some had married or formed public heterosexual relationships while continuing same-sex relationships in private, leading to considerable personal distress.

Although there are limited data, it is estimated that between 1,200 and 1,800 LGBT asylum seekers come to the UK each year (UKLGIG, 2012, p 10). There is evidence that many face distinct barriers in having their claims for asylum upheld, with higher rates of refusal compared with other groups (UKLGIG, 2010). Gaining entry to the UK and requesting asylum involves an initial screening interview followed by a substantial asylum interview at a later date, when asylum seekers must provide reasons for claiming asylum and evidence for their case. A Supreme Court judgment in 2010, *HJ (Iran) & HT (Cameroon) v Secretary of State for the Home Department*, overturned the practice of refusing permission to stay for LGBT asylum seekers on the basis that they could return to their countries and behave with discretion. This judgment also critiqued a narrow understanding of sexual identity, stating that 'the consequences of sexual identity has wrongly been confined to participation in sexual acts rather than that range of behaviour and activities of life which may be informed or affected by sexual identity' (UKSC, 2010, p 45). Yet those claiming asylum may still have to prove they are genuinely LGBT, often in the face of immigration judges voicing inappropriate and outdated stereotypes of sexuality (ICAR, 2003; Miles, 2010; Bennett, 2013). A ruling from the Court of Justice of the European Union (2013) also stated that asylum can be granted in cases where people are jailed for homosexuality in their own country. However, it is up to each country to determine whether imprisonment is applied in practice when considering any individual claim.

Some women in Bennett's (2013) study struggled with disclosing their sexuality in asylum interviews, having never previously declared this publicly, fearing negative judgements from immigration officers and interpreters. A Stonewall report (Miles, 2010) notes that sexuality is often perceived as a personal and private matter and may be difficult to discuss and disclose in a formal interview. This can be problematic because evidence that is not mentioned in the first substantial asylum interview cannot be added at a later date, unless it is fresh evidence that did not exist at the time of the initial interview (Sirriyeh, 2013a).

Challenges in the processing of asylum applications, discussed earlier, lead to many LGBT asylum applicants failing in their first claim, with accompanying risks of detention and deportation. Detention can also impact on mental and physical health, with LGBT people fearing harassment and abuse from other detainees or disclosure if they are not open about their sexuality (Robjant et al, 2009; MMF, 2012).

In summary, LGBT asylum seekers arriving in the UK may have experienced physical violence and discrimination in their country of origin, culminating in a decision to leave, while others only 'come out', even to themselves, after arriving; still others may continue to conceal their sexuality even after arrival.

In terms of access to services and support within the UK, the Immigration and Asylum Act 1999 removed the previous limited access to welfare benefits and replaced these with the National Asylum Support Service (NASS). The Act introduced a dispersal programme, placing asylum seekers in allocated housing in regions away from London and the South East of England (Hynes and Sales, 2010). Financial support is provided to destitute asylum seekers at a rate of approximately 70% of the benefit entitlement of UK nationals. The National Health Service and Community Care Act 1990 requires that local authorities assess adult asylum seekers who are seen to be in need of social care and there is a duty to provide care established under the National Assistance Act 1948 although the Nationality and Asylum Act 2002 restricts local authorities from providing support to people where asylum has been refused, unless this would constitute a breach of their human rights. In practice, asylum seekers' access to health and social care services varies significantly between areas and separate 'specialist' provision of services may not always be acceptable.

LGBT asylum seekers face particular difficulties in accessing services, support and safe accommodation (Bell and Hanson, 2009; Miles, 2010), with profound effects on their mental and physical wellbeing (Safra Project, 2003; Miles, 2010), compounded by the culture of suspicion that may exist towards all asylum seekers (Fell and Fell, 2013). The use of shared single-sex housing fails to take account of the needs of LGBT people and fails to provide a safe space for lesbians in houses where men are invited in by heterosexual women. Meanwhile, concerns about sexual exploitation and involvement in sex work due to destitution have been raised in a report on LGBT asylum seekers in Scotland (Cowen et al, 2011). This also highlights difficulties in accessing support due to the close links between refugee support organisations and faith-based groups. Attention has also been drawn to difficulties faced by Muslim LGBT asylum-seeking and refugee women in accessing housing, employment, education and mental health services because of their legal status, lack of knowledge about the country, language barriers and limited financial resources (Safra Project, 2003). A report on the Double Jeopardy Project in London (Stuart, 2013) also endorses the need for improving services for LGBT asylum seekers among both refugee and LGBT organisations.

Social work and asylum

Early literature on social work and asylum offered a cautious response to the oppressive and coercive nature of the processes associated with establishing asylum-seeker and refugee status. There was a concern that social workers must avoid collusion with practices that denied human rights (Parker, 2000; Hayes and Humphries, 2004; Humphries, 2004).

A systematic literature review (Newbigging et al, 2010) found few examples of good practice with older asylum seekers and refugees or those with disabilities. There was, however, evidence of complex health needs in refugee and asylum-seeking communities and recognition that women's experiences of rape and sexual violence, pregnancy and childcare responsibilities may be significant. The review called for a person-centred, rights-based and solution-focused approach to the needs of asylum seekers and refugees, including promoting social inclusion and independence within an holistic approach and cross-organisational collaboration. The development of curriculum guidance on migration (Guru, 2013) also reflects the need for greater attention to asylum seekers in social work education.

Fell and Fell (2013) highlight five key aspects of reflective practice as Welcome, Accompaniment, Mediation, Befriending and Advocacy (WAMBA), emphasising that this is neither a linear model nor a method of practice. Their approach also refers to the 'unconditional' nature of hospitality, challenging practice that requires 'interrogation of the foreigner' (Fell and Fell, 2013, p 15; Sirriyeh, 2013b).

The mental health of asylum seekers features strongly in the literature, although there is a risk that over-reliance on a medical model potentially compounds a view of individuals as vulnerable victims, failing to acknowledge strength and resilience (Chantler, 2012; Masocha and Simpson, 2012). Similarly, Tribe (2002, p 244) emphasises that being an asylum seeker is not a defining characteristic and that there is a risk that services may become 'skewed and over-reductionist'. An over-emphasis on pre-migration stress also diverts attention from post-migration stress associated with poor housing, racism, isolation and uncertainty in dealings with the UK Border Agency (UKBA). These concerns have continued despite the abolition of the UKBA in 2013 and its replacement by the UK Visas and Immigration (UKVI) as a Home Office department.

It is noticeable that LGBT asylum seekers are largely invisible within social work literature, with the notable exception of Fish (2012) in a social work text on LGBT people. This provides a valuable review of the legal and policy framework and the challenges facing LGBT asylum seekers.

LGBT asylum seekers

A small-scale unfunded study is being undertaken by the authors in response to the absence of LGBT asylum seekers in social work literature and in collaboration with the Equity Partnership, an LGBT organisation in Bradford, UK.

The study design includes individual interviews and focus groups with 6–12 LGBT asylum seekers and a telephone survey of 12 local agencies. The study is informed by a critical social research perspective and the pursuit of social justice (Mertens and Ginsberg, 2008), seeking to avoid the re-inscription of powerlessness and a 'problem-saturated discourse' (Fell and Fell, 2013, p 5). Instead there is commitment to identify strategies of resilience and survival in the narratives of LGBT asylum seekers. It is intended that this work will form the basis of a good practice guide for local organisations. This study is ongoing (2013–15), with male and female participants over the age of 18 recruited from across Yorkshire.

The discussion that follows explores complex and interlinked issues that emerged from initial interviews conducted with two lesbian women from the study seeking asylum in the UK. The data are presented as four themes of:

- psychological stress;
- a question of safety;
- social isolation;
- resistance and survival.

Psychological stress

Meyer's (2003) conceptual framework recognises how stress, prejudice and discrimination create a hostile environment that impacts on the health and wellbeing of LGBT people. The concept of 'minority stress' is recognised as unique and additional to stresses experienced by the general population. In relation to LGBT asylum seekers, this would identify the minority stress of being LGBT in addition to the stress experienced by all asylum seekers. Additionally, stress is clearly located within the wider environment and is not an intrinsic feature of being LGBT. Aspects of stress also include the objective (distal) experience of prejudice or discrimination as well as the stress processes associated with concealment of identity (proximal). Issues of disclosure and concealment are evident in the following quotes from the two women in this study:

> 'What if the UKBA still gonna turn down my case? If I had to go back home I've already exposed myself, and people back home – they know. It really stress me.... If I have to go back home, that will be the end of me.... So it's a depressing life.' (Participant A)

> 'Because I was [in a] really unusual situation when I came here, so I was so upset, it wasn't normal circumstances. I was hiding, I couldn't tell anyone what was going on. I was in my room and I was looking at the walls. I didn't know how I should go to the doctor, get some help.' (Participant B)

The anxieties expressed here challenge any clear distinction between pre-migration stress, migration stress and post-migration stress (Masocha and Simpson, 2012), demonstrating how these are not discrete but overlapping, interconnecting and multi-layered. Meyer's (2003) concept of 'minority stress' also assists in understanding psychological stress associated with LGBT asylum seekers' experiences of uncertainty, fear of detention, removal and forced return to the country of origin.

A question of safety

Many LGBT asylum seekers have fled to the UK without their sexuality being public knowledge or known by their families. However, use of social media enables continuing communication between communities in the country of origin and the UK. This may include the disclosure of information about LGBT individuals. As participant A stated:

> 'Indeed there's a list in [country] as well where people put in the Facebook ... the names of the people in [country], or the UK, they put their names down so you should know they are lesbians or gay men ... but when their relatives, their family find out they will be in trouble. They are not allowed to be alive.'

Social media and other forms of contact and communication undermine the expectation that arrival in the UK, for LGBT asylum seekers, can be equated with safety, reflecting wider critiques of dichotomies of 'safe' and 'unsafe' locations in the context of asylum seeking (Fiddian-Qasmiyeh, 2006).

Social isolation

Strategies adopted by LGBT asylum seekers to avoid being 'discovered' by others from their country of origin can lead to social isolation. This may include avoiding places where people may know them or their family and, consequently, being unable to build supportive relationships among others from their country of origin. Participant B commented:

> 'My situation here is a bit different here because there is a lot of [country] community ... I need to be really careful, very careful, so this is the first place I just joined. I normally avoid the gay places because if someone noticed me there, what's going to happen? And the other thing, it happened with me ... they just came to know about my orientation. They just told my family, and now I am cut off from my family. It's a really big problem for me.'

This extract also highlights the potential double jeopardy that, in addition to restricted contact with people from their country of origin, there is also a fear of being seen to be involved publicly with LGBT organisations. Additionally, there may be challenges in finding information or accessing LGBT-friendly support. This calls for LGBT organisations to develop appropriate asylum-seeker-friendly events as well as greater awareness of the needs of LGBT people among organisations supporting asylum seekers (Cowen et al, 2011; Stuart, 2013). The combination of social isolation, the stress and uncertainty of asylum status and previous experiences of harassment and persecution, can have damaging effects on health and wellbeing.

Resistance and survival

Despite the difficulties expressed by Participants A and B, they also were able to share stories of resistance and survival. Participant A referred to her experiences of living in one UK city as being in a 'cage', but hoped eventually she would be free. The future was seen as a 'paradise' where she would be able to be herself, seek work and live as she wanted to: "I don't want to be somewhere where people don't want me to be. A good quality of life for myself, without fear, without someone going to tell me about this or that ... free from something which I was afraid for, for the rest of my life." Participant A also referred to her decision to live openly as a lesbian: "I've decided to just maybe talk about me. I know they talk a lot about me, okay I just block my ears and move on." This was after the UKBA told her that if she was to live in hiding, she might as well go back and hide in her country of origin. Participant B referred to the need to assess the environment and people before being open. Her advice to others in her situation would be to be cautious about disclosing that they were LGBT.

There was a shared acknowledgement of the benefits of having a good circle of friends. Participant B said: "The main problem was my emotional health, and for your emotional health, your friends are really very important." She stated that joining an LGBT organisation was important as part of her increasing confidence: "I just started, to understand society, the UK society, I just make myself realise, one will harm you if you say anything if you are gay or anything, so now I'm very very confident, now I go to the gatherings, like, here, I just joined the centre."

These views offer an important counterpoint to a discourse of vulnerability and the tendency to see LGBT asylum seekers pathologised as 'victims' of oppression and discrimination, as noted in the literature on asylum seekers (Chantler, 2012; Masocha and Simpson, 2012; Fell and Fell, 2013), as well as reflecting a critical social research perspective.

Human rights and health inequalities

The two women in this study were positive about access to good-quality healthcare, compared with what they might have received in their country of origin. Educational opportunities were valued and there was a sense of security obtained from the UK protective legislation for LGBT people.

However, notwithstanding basic access to healthcare and other services, a social work perspective on human rights points to the importance of being safe and protected from harm, being treated fairly and with dignity, having autonomy and taking an active role in local communities and wider society (Fish, 2012). Furthermore, the Yogyakarta Principles (International Service for Human Rights, 2007) – concerning the application of universal human rights on the basis of sexual orientation and gender identity – locate sexual orientation and gender identity as essential aspects of self-determination, dignity and freedom.

These issues can also be viewed within an 'upstream–downstream' model of health inequalities (Cameron et al, 2003), where attention is drawn to 'the causes of the causes' of ill-health (Marmot, 2005, p 1102), including the general socioeconomic, cultural and environmental conditions of people's lives. Krieger (1999, p 331) points to the differential impact of health caused by the 'daily wear-and-tear of everyday discrimination', including that based on racial/ethnic difference and anti-gay/lesbian discrimination, leading to exposure to physical, chemical, biological and psychosocial insults, which are literally 'embodied'. For example, social trauma such as anticipation and experience of discrimination may provoke fear and anger, triggering physiological changes in the body impacting on both physical and mental wellbeing. For LGBT asylum seekers, the double stress of being an asylum seeker and being LGBT as well as oppression in terms of gender, ethnicity and immigration status, may also contribute to economic and social disadvantage and limit access to healthcare.

These perspectives can provide a framework for challenging LGBT human rights abuses worldwide as well as supporting changes in the way that LGBT asylum seekers are treated in the UK. In particular, health and social care service providers and community organisations need to ensure that staff are adequately trained to respect diversity and address the ways in which prejudice and discrimination may impact on the health and wellbeing of LGBT asylum seekers and their access to support.

What does this mean for practice?

Returning to the vignette at the beginning of this chapter, from a human rights perspective Jay does not feel safe, despite the protection afforded by national legislation and her status as a member of a protected group as a result of her sexual orientation. Her experiences with the UKBA continue to undermine her dignity and she is uncertain about how to access support or engage in community networks. She lacks the basic conditions, economically, socially and emotionally, that underpin health, including a sustainable and health-promoting environment.

Involvement with social work might take place in a range of contexts, including statutory and non-statutory services, family support, mental health or adult social care. Initial contact could build on the basic principles of hospitality-based practice (Fell and Fell, 2013), developing these to be sensitive to the experiences of LGBT asylum seekers, including a welcoming and accepting approach grounded in collaboration and recognition that being an LGBT asylum seeker is not *the* defining characteristic of an individual's life (Tribe, 2002). For Jay this could mean allowing her time to tell her own personal narrative, acknowledging strengths and resilience as well as challenges.

A holistic approach to Jay's life would include recognising her past experiences and the impact of these on her mental health and general wellbeing. Where appropriate, and with Jay's consent, referral and/or access to specialist mental health or trauma services may help. Jay may also choose to have some support in talking more openly with her GP about her mental health. It is also important to acknowledge that Jay has a child and may wish to explore strategies for contact that do not jeopardise her or her child's safety.

Access to LGBT-friendly advocacy may be necessary for legal expertise to support Jay's asylum claim, ensuring that this is addressed without unnecessary intrusion into her private life and relationships and pressure to 'prove' her sexuality. Importantly, the work will also recognise the need to combat Jay's social isolation. This could include putting her in touch with trusted organisations and services where she can meet other LGBT asylum seekers and begin to build new friendships. As her basic needs for support are met and Jay's situation becomes less precarious, she may also choose to disclose other concerns, including hate crime, recognising that LGBT asylum seekers may not wish to draw attention to themselves.

Effective social work practice with LGBT asylum seekers requires building up knowledge and contacts with local organisations in both statutory and non-statutory sectors, and in the longer term developing sustainable and trusting relationships to support partnership working. Developing human rights-based practice may also entail challenging restrictive immigration legislation and systems and their accompanying ethos.

Conclusion

This chapter has drawn attention to how an awareness of health inequalities can assist in understanding and responding to LGBT people seeking asylum, with reference to the concept of 'minority stress' (Meyer, 2003) and both the psychological and social stressors that may be encountered. Dichotomies of being 'safe' and 'unsafe', 'pre' and 'post' migration have been questioned and the portrayal of LGBT asylum seekers as victims has been challenged. These issues are seen as reinforcing the need for social work practice to be grounded in social justice and located within an emancipatory human rights perspective.

What we know about this already
- LGBT asylum seekers are frequently fleeing from persecution and oppression in their countries of origin.
- LGBT asylum seekers may face particular difficulties in seeking asylum on the grounds of their sexuality.
- LGBT asylum seekers will also experience the challenges faced by all asylum seekers.

What this chapter adds
- It emphasises the need to consider the needs of LGBT asylum seekers while they await the outcome of their application for asylum.
- It highlights LGBT asylum seekers' experiences of fear, loneliness and isolation and locates these experiences within a framework of human rights and health inequalities.
- It recognises the strength and resilience of many LGBT asylum seekers in telling their stories of survival.

How this is relevant for social work and LGBT health inequalities
- There is a need to recognise particular issues affecting LGBT asylum seekers and the importance of social contacts and networks and for sensitivity in assessment and the provision of support.
- There is a need to develop knowledge of local LGBT services and carry out partnership work with social work, health and social care services and other statutory and non-statutory agencies.
- There is value in a perspective grounded in human rights and an understanding of the social determinants of health in working to recognise strengths and resilience.

Note
[1] We would like to thank the Equity Partnership for their support in this work: www.equitypartnership.org.uk

References

Bach, J, 2013, 'Sexual orientation and gender identity and the protection of forced migrants', *Forced Migration Review*, www.fmreview.org/sogi/bach

Bell, M and Hanson, C, 2009, *Over not out: The housing and homelessness issues specific to lesbian, gay, bisexual and transgender asylum seekers*, www.metropolitan.org.uk/images/Over-Not-Out.pdf

Bennett, C, 2013, 'Claiming asylum on the basis of your sexuality: the views of lesbians in the UK', *Women's Asylum News*, 115

Cameron, M, Edman, T, Greatley, A and Morris, D, 2003, *Community renewal and mental health*, London: The King's Fund

Cemlyn, S, 2008, 'Human rights practice: possibilities and pitfalls for developing emancipatory social work', *Ethics and Social Welfare*, 2, 3, 222-42

Chantler, K, 2012, 'Gender, asylum seekers and mental distress: challenges for mental health social work', *British Journal of Social Work*, 42, 2, 318-34

Court of Justice of the European Union, 2013, *Press release no 145/13*, Luxembourg, 7 November, http://europa.eu/rapid/press-release_CJE-13-145_en.htm

Cowen, T, Stella, F, Magahy, K, Strauss, K and Morton, J, 2011, *Sanctuary, safety and solidarity: Lesbian, gay, bisexual, transgender asylum seekers and refugees in Scotland*, Glasgow: Equality Network, BEMIS and GRAMNet, www.gla.ac.uk/media/media_195792_en.pdf

Fell, B and Fell, P, 2013, 'Welfare across borders: a social work process with adult asylum seekers', *British Journal of Social Work*, advance access, doi: 10.1093/bjsw/bct003

Fiddian-Qasmiyeh, E, 2006, 'Relocating: the asylum experience in Cairo', *Interventions: International Journal of Postcolonial Studies*, 8, 2, 295-318

Fish, J, 2012, *Social work and lesbian, gay, bisexual and trans people: Making a difference*, Bristol: Policy Press

Guru, S, 2013, *Curriculum guide: Migration and refugees*, London: The College of Social Work, www.tcsw.org.uk/uploadedFiles/TheCollege/Media_centre/CG_Migrationrefugees.pdf

Hayes, D and Humphries, B, 2004, *Social work, immigration and asylum: Debates, dilemmas and ethical issues for social work and social care practice*, London: Jessica Kingsley Publishers

HM Government, 2010, *Working for lesbian, gay, bisexual and transgender equality*, London: Government Equalities Office, https://www.gov.uk/government/uploads/system/uploads/attachment_data/file/85483/lgbt-work-plan.pdf

Home Affairs Committee, 2013, *Report on asylum*, /www.publications.parliament.uk/pa/cm201314/cmselect/cmhaff/71/7104.htm

Humphries, B, 2004, 'An unacceptable role for social work: implementing immigration policy', *British Journal of Social Work*, 34, 1, 93-107

Hynes, P and Sales, R, 2010, 'New communities: asylum-seekers and dispersal', in A Bloch and J Solomos (eds) *Race and ethnicity in the 21st century*, Basingstoke: Palgrave Macmillan, 39-61

ICAR (Information Centre about Asylum and Refugees), 2003, *Lesbian, gay, bisexual and transgender (LGBT), refugees and asylum seekers*, London: ICAR

Ife, J, 2012, *Human rights and social work towards rights-based practice* (3rd edn), Cambridge: Cambridge University Press

ILGA (International Lesbian Gay Bisexual Trans and Intersex Association), 2013, *State sponsored homophobia* (8th edn), ILGA, http://old.ilga.org/Statehomophobia/ILGA_State_Sponsored_Homophobia_2013.pdf

International Service for Human Rights, 2007, *Yogyakarta Principles on the application of international human rights law in relation to sexual orientation and gender identity*, www.yogyakartaprinciples.org/principles_en.htm

Krieger, N, 1999, Embodying inequality: a review of concepts, measures, and methods for studying health consequences of discrimination, *International Journal of Health Services*, 29, 2, 295-352

Marmot, M, 2005, 'Social determinants of health inequalities', *The Lancet*, 365, 1099-104

Masocha, S and Simpson, M, 2012, 'Developing mental health social work for asylum seekers: a proposed model for practice', *Journal of Social Work*, 12, 4, 421-43

Mertens, DM and Ginsberg, PE, 2008, 'Deep in ethical waters: transformative perspectives for qualitative social work research', *Qualitative Social Work*, 7, 4, 484-503

Meyer, IH, 2003, 'Prejudice, social stress, and mental health in lesbian, gay, and bisexual populations: conceptual issues and research evidence', *Psychological Bulletin*, 129, 5, 674-97

Miles, N, 2010, *Going back: Lesbian and gay people and the asylum system*, London: Stonewall

MMF (Metropolitan Migration Foundation), 2012, *Over Not Out Refreshed: Refreshed 2012*, London: MMF, www.metropolitan.org.uk/images/Metropolitan-MF-LGBT-Over-Not-Out2012-final1.pdf

Newbigging, K, Thomas, N, Couple, J, Habte-Mariam, Z, Ahmed, N, Shah, A and Hicks, J, 2010, *Good practice in social care with refugees and asylum seekers*, London: Social Care Institute for Excellence

Parker, J, 2000, 'Social work with refugees and asylum seekers: a rationale for developing practice', *Social Work in Action*, 12, 3, 61-76

Refugee Council, 2007, *The new asylum model*, policy briefing, London: Refugee Council

Robjant, K, Hassan, H and Katona, C, 2009, 'Mental health implications of detaining asylum seekers: systematic review', *British Journal of Psychiatry*, 194, 306-12

Refugee Council, 2010, *Refugee Council client experiences in the asylum process*, research report, London: Refugee Council

Safra Project, 2003, *Identifying the difficulties experienced by Muslim lesbian, bisexual and transgender women in accessing social and legal services*, London: Safra Project, www.safraproject.org/Reports/Safra_Project-Initial_findings-2002.pdf

Sirriyeh, A, 2013a, *Inhabiting borders, routes home: Youth, gender, asylum*, Farnham: Ashgate

Sirriyeh, A, 2013b, 'Hosting strangers: hospitality and family practices in fostering unaccompanied refugee young people', *Child and Family Social Work*, 18, 1, 5-14

Stonewall, 2008, *Homophobic hate crime: The Gay British Crime Survey*, London: Stonewall, www.stonewall.org.uk/

Stonewall, 2013, *Gay in Britain: Lesbian, gay and bisexual people's expectations of discrimination*, London: Stonewall, https://www.stonewall.org.uk/

Stuart, A, 2013, *A final report on the Trust for London funded Double Jeopardy Project*, London: MBARC

Tribe, R, 2002, 'Mental health of refugees and asylum seekers', *Advances in Psychiatric Treatment*, 8, 240-8

UKLGIG (United Kingdom Lesbian and Gay Immigration Group), 2010, *Failing the grade: Home Office initial decisions on lesbian and gay claims for asylum*, London: UKLGOG_

UKLGIG, 2012, *Annual report*, London: UKLGIG

UKSC, 2010, *HJ (Iran) and HT (Cameroon) v Secretary of State for the Home Department*, UKSC 31

UN (United Nations) Human Rights Council, 2011, *Resolution on Human Rights, Sexual Orientation and Gender Identity, Resolution 17/19*, New York, NY: UN

UN (United Nations) Human Rights Office, 2012, *Born free and equal: Sexual orientation and gender identity in international human rights law*, New York, NY: UN, www.ohchr.org/Documents/Publications/BornFreeAndEqualLowRes.pdf

PART THREE

Social work education and research

Pedagogy for unpacking heterosexist and cisgender bias in social work education in the United States

Susan Saltzburg

Introduction

Reflecting the profession's values to promote social justice, policies and standards on health established by United States (US) national (NASW, 2005) and international (Bywaters and Napier, 2009) social work associations serve as maps for leading the profession's mission across the globe. Explicit commitments recognise that health is fundamental to human rights and that social work training plays a key role in educating students about the need to mitigate the impact of social and health inequalities among the marginalised communities they serve. Social work has an 'obligation to challenge social conditions that contribute to social exclusion, stigmatisation or subjugation, and to work towards an inclusive society' (IFSW, section 4.2 (5)). Notions of what is meant by an inclusive society include recognising diversity across individual characteristics, traditions and identities based on race, ethnicity, sexual orientation, gender identity, religion, ability and so on (Van Soest, 2003). While social work educators are charged with instilling these values in students, embracing these ideals may create unique challenges for students socialised to view lesbian, gay, bisexual and trans (LGBT) lives through the lens of heteronormative morality versus 'cultural diversity' (Van Den Bergh and Crisp, 2004).

Many social work students still harbour lingering vestiges of prejudice, with and without their conscious knowledge (Raiz and Saltzburg, 2008). As internalised beliefs derived from dominant heterosexist/cisgender discourses carry over into direct practice (Schope and Eliason, 2000), LGBT clients are at risk of having their lives evaluated and prescribed by using heterosexual and cisgender norms. Such lack of understanding creates barriers to culturally responsive and effective services. Social work education plays a critical role in dispelling inequalities in healthcare for LGBT people by preparing students for ethical and culturally affirmative practice.

Helping students to gain needed cultural-diversity competences (CSWE, 2008) for LGBT practice calls for cultivating a cognisant departure from assumptions instilled by heterosexist/cisgender socialisation. There have been a number of teaching strategies for practice courses suggested in the social work literature for decreasing heterosexist/cisgender bias (for example, LGBT guest speakers: Black et al, 1999; the 'infusion method': Basset and Day, 2003); however, efficacy of outcomes has been inconsistent. Teaching self-reflection as a means for instilling values is well established in social work pedagogy (for example Healy, 2000). However, given the religious–moral issues for some students related to same-sex attraction and behaviours and non-conforming gender expression, these topics may be experienced as too highly sensitive and provocative for transparent self-reflection. Herein lies a set of pedagogical challenges; distinct from other cultural groups, practice with LGBT people is impacted by the socially constructed, moral order of traditional religious culture.

Moving social work students forward in 'unpacking' heterosexist/ cisgender assumptions calls for creative teaching methods. This chapter describes one educator's approach to positioning students in a reflexive stance to explore and examine biases that may stand in the way of becoming LGBT-affirmative practitioners. While developed for teaching an LGBT-focused practice course, the pedagogy could be readily integrated into other courses.

Pedagogy for self-reflective learning

Forging pathways to transformative learning experiences requires a benevolent environment and meaningful tools to bring the person-of-the-student into the folds of learning in genuine, reflexive and transparent ways (Shor, 1992). Drawing from tenets of critical pedagogy (CP) and narrative therapy and community practice (NTCP), the author proposes innovative pedagogy using critical self-reflection in the context of dialogue for repositioning students in LGBT culturally affirmative locations for practice. The discussion that follows describes the theory and application of the proposed pedagogy, highlighting:

- mutual learning environments;
- dialogue as transformative space;
- the narrative and Foucaultian theory undergirding NTCP;

- the practices of 'deconstruction inquiry', 'discursive repositioning' and 'definitional ceremony' as tools for engaging students in reflexive work.

Interspersed are brief pedagogic reflections by the author, highlighting observations that evolved through several iterations of using this approach.

Mutual learning environments

Using the democratising principles of CP (Shor, 1992) and NTCP (White and Epston, 1990) establishes a 'mutual learning' environment through collaboration. Teaching becomes transformed into a collective and dynamic process between instructor, student and peers. Viewing students as the experts on how learning becomes meaningful for them (much like how NTCP considers clients to be the experts on their own lives), the teaching experience becomes shared in ways that empower students to help shape the trajectory and constitutive elements of instruction (Shor, 1992).

> Students would arrive to class spinning with new ideas, lingering assumptions, strong or unexpected reactions, and questions triggered by readings; they were looking for expanded dialogue tied to these responses. Achieving this often meant that students' voices locked into meaningful dialogue, guided classroom focus in unforeseen directions, necessitating shifting gears to meet learning needs. (Saltzburg, reflective notes, 2013)

In NTCP we refer to this as 'abiding with' clients in conversation (White, 2007), rather than legislating what conversations should be based on our perceived expertise. Using the NTCP lens in similar ways, we strive as instructors to abide with students where they find themselves positioned in critical learning spaces, remaining attentive to the discourses lending their weight in creating this space. Given the subject matter and unfamiliarity that many students have with LGBT lives, *abiding with* them as they discover or grapple with new ways of thinking about sexual attraction and behaviours, romantic relationships and gender expression/identity will serve as a pedagogic scaffold in supporting students' growth.

As LGBT topics may challenge assumptions or touch on students' own experiences of sexuality and gender, there can be initial uneasiness and reluctance to respond authentically to readings and discussion. Recognising the importance of lowering students' guard, it is vital to forge a sense of connection among class members and instructor of ethnic, sexual and gender diversity. The collaborative learning environment, respect for everyone's starting point and exercises conducive for sparking spontaneous dialogue contribute to engaging students in critical reflection.

Dialogue as transformative space

In CP, teaching and learning are conceptualised as co-occurring through the organising structure of 'dialogue' (Shor, 1992).

> Early on, as I reflected on instances of too much silence and too little substance in students' participation, I recognized the need to expand and structure pathways for meaningful open dialogue. By incorporating more of this into the class, the back and forth exchange drew students down different pathways than what was happening in the isolation of their own univocal space. (Saltzburg, reflective notes, 2013)

The crux of the pedagogic process in this model lies in creating dialogue through shifting formats and interpersonal configurations, using self-reflexive and reflective writing and verbal discussion for the basis of dialogical exchange. Staying open to the spontaneous emergence of conversations further reinforces the generative process. Lectures transcend to dynamic, poly-vocal conversations, forging new directions and unplanned pathways of inquiry and exploration.

Dialogues as posited in CP (Shor, 1992) and 'conversations' in NTCP (White, 2007) become the mechanism for transformative change by prompting shifts in 'situational' understanding and meaning. In the author's course, content for the dialogic work rested on locating students in the narratives of LGBT lives; this emic experience was captured through immersion in readings, films and videos presenting personal and historical testimonies (for example, *Last Call at Maud's*, Kiss, 1993; *American experience: Stonewall uprising*, DiGiacomo, 2011). Positioning students in such a way provided opportunities for them to 'hold up' internalised messages about being LGBT to the life-accounts they became intimately a part of. Dialogues that transpired in class discussions, peer dyads and reflexive assignments for students (with instructor and peers engaging in exchange of reflective comments), and between student and (the reading of) texts or (viewing of) films, created the critical learning space.

Theoretical lens of narrative therapy and community practice

Steeped in the theoretical perspectives of social constructionism and post-structuralism, NTCP establishes groundbreaking pathways to effect change. Particularly relevant are the epistemological assumptions that these theories lend to the vision of practice, positing reality as subjective and fluid in nature, socially constructed through language and maintained through social discourse (Freedman and Combs, 1996). In keeping with these perspectival views, the interpretive turn of language is perceived as creating multiple and shifting perspectives of meaning-making (Strong and Pare, 1995). This has important implications in viewing conversations (and student–instructor conversational configurations) as the loci for change.

Treatises of Foucault

Influenced by Foucault, NTCP is attentive to the processes by which 'practices of power' (White, 1993, p 50) become unknowingly internalised by people in their everyday lives. These 'techniques of social control' (White, 1993, p 50) that wield their influence as binding truths, permeate at collective and individual levels, recruiting people into certain ways of evaluating and judging themselves and others (Saltzburg, 2008). The workings of power and its by-product of privilege, influence societal institutions and professional knowledges as well as individual lives; so that, privileged statuses such as white privilege, male privilege, heterosexual privilege, cisgender privilege and so on become enacted at all levels of our day-to-day existence. Social discourses permeate our thinking by way of such privilege, creating a sense of 'absoluteness' by virtue of their seeming omnipotence. Often we do not recognise or challenge such influences because of their canonic familiarity (White and Epston, 1990). Assuming the NTCP stance instils a mindfulness of how social discourses position each of us in the narratives we tell about ourselves and others (the practice of 'discourse repositioning' is explicated in the next section). NTCP practitioners are always examining the influences of power and privilege on the lives of the people they work with and joining with them in conversation to discover and reinforce resistance and resilience in the face of these constraints (White and Epston, 1990). In this way, the spirit of social justice activism characterising NTCP closely matches the ideals of social work. NTCP integrates the philosophical treatises of Foucault with the *re-authoring* metaphor to create transformative experiences for people and communities (White and Epston, 1990).

The re-authoring metaphor

Shedding modernist, structural thinking, the change-effecting practices of NTCP are built on the premises of the generative capacity of conversations in re-authoring narratives that shape identity and outlook for individuals and communities (White and Epston, 1990). It is within these understandings that NTCP ideas seemed particularly relevant for engaging students in re-authoring assumptions by developing increased self-awareness of internalised messages that may shape biases towards LGBT people.

> Early on, I speculated over the sense of distance I was experiencing in students' work. There was a lack of depth and critical complexity, conveying the absence of praxis in self-reflection. Students were reading about the effects of heterosexism and cisgender expectations on well-being, yet there seemed a gap in capturing what this meant to them. I felt the absence of 'situated vulnerability' in our work together, and looked for pedagogic ways to structure this learning. (Saltzburg, reflective notes, 2013)

Given the sensitivity in talking about LGBT issues for some students, designing meaningful ways to get students to share 'inner talk' associated with LGBT topics required consideration as to 'process'.

> Through the silence or thin responses in class discussion and assignments, students reflected fears of appearing uninformed, genuine struggles to reconcile conflicting values, and concerns of offending others (especially LGBT instructor and peers). Worry of how transparency might be judged weighed heavily on students' minds. Vulnerabilities existed for LGBT students as well as heterosexual and gender-conforming peers, as everyone, including instructor, stood at the margins of others' sub-categories of sexual and gender diversity. (Saltzburg, reflective notes, 2013)

Breaking down barriers to self-reflection and opening space for grappling with heterosexist/cisgender norms required awareness of students' sense of vulnerability. Three of the NTCP practices of NTCP described below seemed particularly relevant in engaging students in the self-awareness work needed for 'unpacking' heterosexist/cisgender assumptions.

Praxis and practices of NTCP

Consistent with NTCP, the author strived to create an 'experience-near' learning process with students. In NTCP terminology, 'experience-near' depictions suggest thick descriptions from those located in the eye of the experience. This helps practitioners (or in our case, students) to step inside the circle of first-hand knowing of their clients (White, 2003). As previously mentioned, this 'insider' experience was captured for students by their immersion in the LGBT personal and historical testimonies of readings and films, and created the context for critical and reflexive thinking.

In NTCP, we start out establishing moments of 'lived experience' that contradict the 'problem stories' (or presumed 'truths') that are interfering with clients' or communities' lives (White and Epston, 1990). Relative to student learning, the concept of 'problem story' may be thought of as the heterosexist/cisgender assumptions standing in the way of students' capacity to approach LGBT lives without biases. The unique practices of NTCP rely on the composition of critical questions across various categories of inquiry to move people (students) forward in re-authoring narratives (or internalised discourses, such as heterosexism) that better fit with how they prefer to be known and to live their lives, as people (and as social workers) (White, 1993). To support students in re-authoring through engaging in critical self-reflection, the following practices proved extremely useful for transformative change:

- making meaning in discursive positioning;
- deconstruction inquiry;
- a re-authoring through 'definitional ceremony'.

Meaning-making in discourse positioning

The significance of the concept 'discourse' and its role in creating positions that people stand in in their beliefs and assumptions (Davies and Harre, 1990) is fundamental to the workings of NTCP, and relevant in shaping students' competences for practice with LGBT populations. Constituting a set of socially constructed assumptions, discourse represents the values, beliefs and ideologies of particular groups of people and the ways they live out their lives (Sinclair and Monk, 2005). The language and assumptions of specific discourses establish set ways to think about phenomena of the lived experience and the bodies of knowledge that purport to explain them. Through a Foucaultian lens, dominant discourses are those whose authority are legitimised through positions of power and propagated through privilege, convincing their audiences of the absoluteness of their assertions (White and Epston, 1990).

Of particular relevance for drawing students into self-awareness exercises, discourse positioning is an iterative, reflexive praxis using critical questions to unravel insightfulness about the discourses influencing people's assumptions. Positing that discourse persuasion occurs within the conversational dynamics of people and their 'languaged' realities, NTCP views the possibilities for discourse repositioning to take place through the reconstitutive properties of new and shifting conversations (Winslade, 2005). This can only transpire when there is awareness of contradictions to these seemingly immutable truths (such as internalised heterosexist/cisgender arguments). Hence, the critical pedagogic thrust is aimed at helping students to locate themselves within the social discourses that are directing their assumptions and attitudes.

Instructors and class peers serve as anchors in helping students to examine their discursive positioning, using dialogical means. These dialogical responses take shape through in-class conversations or written comments provided for reflective writings (and then students' responses to the comments). Locating discursive positioning rests on the understanding that people establish a position in relation to certain meanings in social discourse with others; such positioning reflects a set of beliefs or assumptions without one necessarily recognising their origin or by-products (Winslade, 2005). Employing techniques of deconstruction (a method of inquiry) provides the vehicle for discourse positioning analysis (Sinclair and Monk, 2005), and ties into self-reflective work. Deconstruction questioning will be expounded on in the next subsection.

Deconstruction inquiry

> I recognized early on that asking traditional questions to spark self-reflection was not helping students get at internalized discourses shaping assumptions. Instead, students were either missing or avoiding relevant issues.

There was 'thinness' to the self-reflections and critical discussions, particularly in how they linked assumptions with thoughts and feelings that were emerging as they interfaced with the stories of LGBT lives. (Saltzburg, reflective notes, 2013)

Helping students to detect discourse positioning employs practices of 'deconstruction inquiry'. The concept of 'deconstruction' is used in this sense to signify the dismantling of culturally embedded, essentialist assumptions internalised as immutable truths (White, 1993; Saltzburg, 2008). Derived from the post-structuralist theory of Derrida (1981) and translated to NTCP, this process of disassembling texts or discourses in order to expose 'to-be-discovered' meanings, raises awareness of what lies outside the words of privileged conversations (White, 1993).

Premises for how this metaphoric practice congruently fits with the theoretical designs of NTCP rest within the idea of 'scrutinising' mindsets about ways of being that have been afforded privilege (White, 1993). For purposes of teaching practice with LGBT populations, we are talking about 'gender' ways of being, 'sexual' ways of being, 'in relationships' ways of being. These scrutinising exercises create opportunities for students to figuratively take apart knowledges and understandings that have come to constitute fixed ways of knowing life (for instance heterosexist), in order to open space for the mining of new perspectives (White, 1993). The NTCP concept of 're-authoring' (stepping into preferred narratives) becomes first realised within the context of 'deconstruction conversations'. Such conversations exist as a co-determinate set of processes in which discourses suggesting constraining knowledges get taken apart and within the context of disassembling, other storylines and meaning-making emerge.

The ideas of repositioning and re-authoring seem highly relevant for creating transformative learning experiences for students who come into social work bogged down by dominant politics of sexuality and gender, preventing other ways of being from being accorded equal value. In recognising that the meanings attached to heterosexist/cisgender discourse signify much more than sexual behaviours or gender roles, we are looking for students to understand how sexual and gender minority identities represent a nuanced complexity of 'whole lives' and 'lived experiences', intersecting with other ways of knowing self. Raising this kind of awareness (through group conversation and interactive written reflections) necessitates both an analytical lens and a critical process. Herein lies the invaluable contributions of deconstruction listening and questioning, providing the scaffold to support students in exploring unfamiliar territory (White, 2003).

Deconstruction listening involves the two-fold process of attentive listening for the discourses undergirding current assumptions, and 'double-listening' (White, 2003), or listening for other possible understandings. The latter detects openings through which we can begin asking questions that will get at critical thinking about current assumptions. For the work with our students, such questions might be:

- where existing ideas might have come from;
- what they represent;
- how they found their way into the student's life;
- how it is they became relevant or useful;
- how they were able to recruit the student into evaluating others' worth;
- how they fit into the student's identity as a social worker;
- how the student might strip these essentialising ideas of their status of absoluteness (adapted from White, 1993).

Crafted in creative ways, these questions are asked in a manner that positions the discursive influences external to students' sense of personhood; this concept of metaphoric 'externalising' is central to NTCP and the way in which effecting change is understood (White, 1993). As questions are posed, the critical thinking involved in shaping responses begins the process of destabilising the strength of standing discourses. Taking the NTCP perspective, instructors are posing questions that allow room for students to subvert familiar storylines that underlie assumptions. In time, other students in the class are brought into this role as well. Instructors model this process by raising their own assumptions and bringing students into the dialogue with their questions.

In cultivating cultural-diversity awareness, we engage in deconstruction questions that will connect heterosexist/cisgender bias to the psychological distress and resilience of the LGBT people who students come to know in their immersion readings and films (and who they will meet in practice). Herein lie the 'listening for' emergent narratives of other ways of understanding and knowing. In a series of autobiographical essays assigned for reading (for example Jensen, 1999), lesbian women talked about grappling with coming out, hiding significant relationships for fear of repercussions and discovering the unique dynamics in forming intimate relationships with other women. Students' responses to these readings reflected internalised assumptions regarding normative sexual identity and intimate relationship functionality and health. Deconstruction questions to get at these biases (adapted from White, 1993) might include those posed below pertaining to the vignette of Kit – a woman struggling with publically 'coming out' after leaving a 20-year marriage to be with a woman she is just getting to know. Questions such as these challenge heterosexist assumptions that situate sexuality as static, discount same-sex ways of 'being in relationship', and overlook the weight of internalised homophobia:

- How does coming to know Kit fit with these assumptions?
- After having stepped into Kit's life, what new conclusions might you have reached about her as a person and perhaps others who are lesbian and struggling with internalised homophobia?
- Whose ideas are coming forth when describing lesbian relationships as being 'fused' or 'enmeshed'?
- Where do these ideas come from?
- Based on whose definition of relationship health or closeness?
- How might these conclusions enter how you work with lesbian couples?

Using NTCP practices, we are striving to tie psychological and sociological effects of social prejudice on the lives of LGBT people with students' up-close and personal knowing of LGBT life narratives (through readings and films) and students' prevailing internalised assumptions. For instance, if we are talking about non-monogamous relationships of gay men, how can we deconstruct the judgement attached to this discussion, and begin to refocus on the idea that perhaps healthy and caring relationships can show up in many different ways. Or, how might we come to understand the trajectory of a woman who at mid-life discovers her lesbian identity without judging or pathologising decisions that she then makes in order to claim this identity. It is within the cultivation of these questions and students' responses that fixed assumptions dissolve and new narratives take shape, creating pathways for students' understanding and support of LGBT clients.

As instructors, our role in the processes of deconstruction listening and questioning establishes a co-authoring relationship in uncovering the budding narratives and new conclusions that emerge. We do this work in the context of reflexive/reflective assignments, posing questions for students to consider and respond to through written dialogue (both on paper and in online written exchange) and in the classroom (through large group, small group and dyadic dialogue). As instructors, we are looking to join our students in co-constructing new storylines steeped in the intentions of LGBT culturally competent, affirmative practice.

A re-authoring through definitional ceremony

Drawing from the anthropologic practices of Myerhoff (1982), NTCP borrowed the metaphoric process of 'definitional ceremony' for creating 'outsider witnesses' to re-authoring and change (White, 2007). It is the intentional staging of having others stand-in-witness of personal testimonies and narratives as people step into new ways of knowing and preferred storylines of identity. Preferred stances become constituted through these 'events of acknowledgement' as speaker and observer(s) join in reflective dialogue (White, 2007). The process for definitional ceremony as adapted to NTCP (White, 2007) unfolds as a round of 'tellings':

- tellings (by the person at the centre of the definitional ceremony, in other words, the person who is telling the narrative – about their lives, assumptions, understandings) as witnesses listen;
- retellings (by witnesses, reflecting on noticed developments in the teller's narrative) as the teller listens;
- 'retellings of retellings' (by the original teller), incorporating the ideas of others into their own discourse.

The process creates a generative conversation. Particularly important is the set of structured questions that NTCP asks witnesses to guide reflective thinking in their retelling of what they heard. These questions focus on bringing out and amplifying new developments in the storyline, and purport to link the tellings of one person to the lives of others (witnesses) around shared themes, values and commitments (White, 1993). It is within the communion of these tellings and retellings that new storylines are defined and internalised. This is especially relevant for social work students in recognising the limitations of heterosexist/cisgender assumptions and creating LGBT-affirmative communities of practice.

As the author applies definitional ceremony to repositioning students from their heterosexist/cisgender discourses, these witnessing practices are conceptualised transpiring in two ways. The first involves the students' themselves, bearing witness to the 'tellings' of the LGBT people they come to know in the readings and films. Using the lens of definitional ceremony, students reflect on these LGBT tellings (taking the position of the audience providing reflective retellings) through writing assignments, dyadic and group conversations, and class discussion. Bearing witness, so to speak, of personal hardship and resilience from this more personal position aids students in viewing LGBT people's lives from a different vantage point; such positioning provides new knowledges about the local context of LGBT lives. The 'retelling of students' retellings' would then entail a reflective assignment about what students might imagine the people in the readings and films would say in response to students' thoughts about their lives.

The second way in which witnessing would occur involves the tellings, retellings and 'retellings of retellings' that emerge dynamically between students, instructor and classmates. As students take risks with their questions, expressing confusion or tentative understanding, they would be invited to reflect about these questions/thoughts - taking the position of the person doing the 'telling'. Instructor and class-peers then serve as the audience, listening to the tellings and then engaging in their 'retellings' of these accounts through several means:

- the instructor's reflective comments on students' papers, opening space for dialogue;
- the instructor's in-class comments anonymously addressing thoughts raised in students' papers, eliciting peer-discussion;
- small group dialogue in response to one another's conversations.

Finally, in terms of translating these practices to the classroom, the 'retelling of retellings' may be viewed as the shifts, growth and expansion of discourses that come out of these generative conversations, facilitating students' re-authoring of heterosexist/cisgender discourses.

CASE VIGNETTE

> Judy (51) and Barbara (50) have been in an undisclosed, one-year relationship. While Judy has been out for many years, Barbara was in a twenty-year marriage with three adolescent children when they met. Doubt and guilt flood Barbara's conscience as family and friends reel at her disclosure with accusations of abandoning her husband and children when she leaves the family home.... Despite the rejection and guilt, Barbara cannot deny the sense of finally feeling 'whole'. (*Transitions: Discovering my lesbian soul*, Laherty, 1998)

As students reflected on the storyline, many reacted similarly to Barbara's family. Using the structured mode of inquiry involved in bringing forth 'outsider witness' retellings' (White, 2007) (students witnessing Barbara and Judy's story), the instructor/peers might ask questions such as:

- What words were you drawn to as you heard Barbara and Judy talk in their relationship narrative?
- How do the ways that they move through life together make sense to you?
- What images come forward for you when they talk about how their identities are honoured through their relationship?
- How does this strike a chord with you?
- How does this knowledge tie in with what you look for or experience in your own significant relationships?
- How do these ways inspire you?
- Is this a new development in how you thought about yourself in relationships?
- How have you been moved by being witness to this telling?
- How might having witnessed the conversation make a difference in your own life?

As responses to these questions unfold, stirrings of new narratives begin to take root, tying new conclusions about LGBT lives back to the assumptions of the teller (the person of the student). Hearing the retellings through the lens of the structured questions is critical to shifting students' narratives. Witnesses act as a 'reflecting team', contributing to the construction of discourse repositioning (White, 2007).

Conclusion

Helping social work students to grapple with internalised heterosexist/ cisgender assumptions is essential in preparing social workers to address inequalities in healthcare. Forging pedagogical pathways to engage students in critical self-reflection is important in helping them to recognise the role of privilege in social disparities. Critical reflection provides the means for students to identify their internalised assumptions and the discursive positioning that underlies 'taken-for-granted' beliefs. Such learning exercises aid students in challenging these assumptions. Thoughtful selection of reading and video materials is essential for creating an immersion experience that reflects the diversity of LGBT lives, particularly those who are most marginalised within our communities. The integrative use of CP, NTCP and Foucault's theory as a conceptually cohesive means for structuring learning has shown promising results and positive student feedback.

What we know about this already
- LGBT clients are at higher risk for disparate services because of heterosexist/ cisgender bias.
- Many students are unaware of how their heterosexist/cisgender assumptions carry over into practice.
- Achieving LGBT cultural competence includes addressing heterosexist/ cisgender bias.

What this chapter adds
- It illustrates innovative pedagogy for teaching LGBT cultural-diversity competence.
- It describes the use of NTCP practices as tools for engaging students in self-awareness of heterosexist/cisgender bias.
- It contributes to social work education literature for preparing students for LGBT practice.

How this is relevant for social work and LGBT health inequalities
- It underscores the values of the social work profession.
- It contributes an innovative pedagogic approach to social work education literature.
- It recognises the critical role that social work education plays in breaking down barriers to students' overcoming heterosexist/cisgender bias.

References

Bassett, J and Day, K, 2003, 'A test of the infusion method: emphatic inclusion of material on gay men in a core course', *Journal of Teaching in Social Work*, 23, 3/4, 29–41

Black, B, Oles, T, Cramer, E and Bennett, CK, 1999, 'Attitudes and behaviors of social work students toward lesbian and gay male clients: can panel presentations make a difference?', *Journal of Gay and Lesbian Social Services*, 9, 47–68

Bywaters, P and Napier, L, 2009, 'Revising international social work's policy statement on health', *International Social Work*, 52, 4, 447-57

CSWE (Council on Social Work Education), 2008, *Educational policy and accreditation standards*, Alexandria, VA: CSWE

Davies, B and Harre, R, 1990, 'Positioning: the discursive production of selves', *Journal for the Theory of Social Behavior*, 20, 1, 43-63

DiGiacomo, DG (producer), 2011, *American experience: Stonewall uprising*, Boston, MA: Public Broadcasting Service

Freedman, J and Combs, G, 1996, *Narrative therapy*, New York, NY: Norton

Healy, K, 2000, *Social work practices: Perspectives on change*, London: Sage Publications

IFSW (International Federation of Social Workers), 2012, Statement of ethical principles, http://ifsw.org/policies/statement-of-ethical-principles/

Jensen, K, 1999, *Lesbian epiphanies: Women coming out in later life*, New York, NY: Harrington Park Press

Kiss, K (producer), 1993, *Last call at Maud's*, Charlottesville, VA: Water Bearer Films

Laherty, C (producer), 1998, *Transitions: Discovering my lesbian soul*, private distribution

Myerhoff, B, 1982, 'Life history among the elderly: performance, visibility and remembering', in J Ruby (ed) *A crack in the mirror*, Philadelphia, PA: University of Pennsylvania

NASW (National Association of Social Workers), 2005, *Standards for social work practice in health care settings*, Washington, DC: NASW

Raiz, L and Saltzburg, S, 2007, 'Tolerance, but with conditions.... Developing awareness of subtleties of heterosexism and homophobia among undergraduate, heterosexual social work majors', *Journal of Baccalaureate Social Work*, 12, 2, 53-69

Saltzburg, S, 2008, 'Mentoring beyond homophobia', *Journal of Baccalaureate Social Work*, 13, 2, 35-53

Schope, R and Eliason, M, 2000, 'Thinking versus acting: assessing the relationship between heterosexual attitudes and behaviors toward homosexuals', *Journal of Gay and Lesbian Social Services*, 11, 4, 69-92

Shor, I, 1992, *Empowering education: Critical teaching for social change*, Chicago, IL: University of Chicago

Sinclair, SL and Monk, G, 2005, 'Discursive empathy: a new foundation for therapeutic practice', *British Journal of Guidance and Counselling*, 33, 3, 333-49

Strong, T and Pare, D, 1995, 'Striving for perspicuity: talking our way forward', in T, Strong and D, Pare (eds) *Furthuring talk*, New York, NY: Kluwer Academic/Plenum, 1-14

Van Den Bergh, N and Crisp, C, 2004, 'Defining culturally competent practice with sexual minorities: implications for social work education and practice', *Journal of Social Work Education*, 40, 2, 221-38

Van Soest, D, 2003, 'Advancing social and economic justice', in D Lum (ed) *Culturally competent practice*, Belmont, CA: Brooks Cole, 345-76

White, M, 1993, 'Deconstruction and therapy', in S, Gilligan and R, Price (eds) *Therapeutic conversations*, New York: Norton, 22-61

White, M, 2003, 'Narrative practice and community assignments', *International Journal of Narrative Therapy and Community Work*, 2, 17-36

White, M, 2007, *Definitional ceremony: Maps of narrative practice*, New York, NY: Norton, 165-218

White, M and Epston, D, 1990, *Narrative means to therapeutic ends*, New York, NY: Norton

Winslade, J, 2005, 'Utilising discursive positioning in counselling', *British Journal of Guidance and Counselling*, 33, 3, 351-64

Maximising research outcomes for trans children and their families in Canada: using social action and other participatory methods of inquiry

Annie Pullen Sansfaçon and Kimberley Ens Manning

Introduction

'To me it's really that, it's that the person who has a gender creative child or trans child or fluid or whatnot, is not going to be shoved or pushed by the medical community or the school community or social services and get their kid taken away. Like that was my biggest fear at that point when I started out, was that my kid was going to be taken away.' (Akiko Asano, President of Gender Creative Kids Canada, 8 May 2013)

Akiko Asano is a single parent of two children, the youngest of whom, Mat, who was born a biological boy, identifies as trans. Now aged 15, Mat was just two when she began to show a strong preference for wearing dresses and playing with dolls, and began to live as a girl full time at the age of four. Although many in Akiko's community were supportive of her parenting, not all were, and when Mat was about six, Akiko was briefly investigated by social services. The complaint? That Akiko was trying to change her child's 'sexual orientation'. Although the case was quickly dismissed, many other North American families have not been so lucky. Indeed, although there is still limited evidence, some children have been forcibly removed from the care of parents who allow their children to live in accordance with their felt sense of gender (see Manning et al, forthcoming, for a discussion of child apprehension prompted by a child's gender non-conformity).

A growing body of scholarship suggests that childhood gender non-conformity is a natural part of human diversity. Indeed, research suggests that between 2.3% and 8.3% of children (Moller et al, 2009, pp 118-19) engage in varying degrees of cross-gender dress and behaviour, and of those, a small number will end up following through with gender change interventions later on in their lives (Meyer, 2012). The problem is, Western society continues to be structured on the basis of a gender binary in which a child's failure to conform to their assigned birth sex, has often resulted in the pathologisation of parent and child (Langer and Martin, 2004). The fact that another member of Akiko's community viewed her parenting as 'harmful' and thus requiring state intervention, suggests the degree to which gross misunderstandings about gender identity continue to prevail.

In Canada, two broad directions for intervention are currently available: reparative treatments and trans-affirmative interventions. Reparative treatments include those promoted by Kenneth Zucker, a psychologist at the Centre for Addiction and Mental Health Gender Identity Clinic in Toronto, who has undertaken therapy with some 500 children over the last 25 years, in order to make them conform with their anatomical sex (Zucker and Bradley, 1995; Zucker, 2008). However, Zucker's work in Canada has been considered controversial for a number of years. Indeed, the form of reparative therapy he and his colleagues employ has been criticised for being homophobic, transphobic and misogynistic (Isay, 1997; Feder, 1999; Bryant, 2008; Wallace and Russell, 2013; Tosh, 2014). Furthermore, the social work profession is now beginning to recognise the long-term damage produced through forcing children to live in accordance with what psychologist Ehrensaft (2011, 2012) calls a 'false gender self'. Thus, new practices, such as trans-affirmative interventions, that is, interventions that support the child to live according to their true gender self, are being encouraged. This specific orientation is increasingly present in the social work literature (see, for example, Morrow, 2004; Mallon and DeCrescenzo, 2006; Mallon, 2009).

That said, social work should have an extra duty, over and beyond the provision of trans-affirmative interventions. Professionals should also work toward the emancipation, the liberation and the empowerment of people (IFSW, 2013). Guidelines for practice should therefore not only avoid reproducing the violence to which so many parents and children are already subject, but also provide these families with new tools for self-empowerment and advocacy.

In this chapter we explore how social work research and practice can be used as an important means of offsetting the health inequalities faced by so many gender non-conforming children and their families. Based on our experience of organising a participatory action research project, we illustrate how the development of knowledge can also be used as a means to challenge the very structures that give rise to gender-based and other intersecting oppressions in childhood. Specifically, we argue that the social work values and principles (IFSW, 2013) must be the driver of social work research and practice. To this end we chose to employ a participatory action research methodology because it is consistent with the profession's principles and offer practical tools to articulate values and realise anti-oppressive and empowering goals.

The first section of the chapter describes legal and medical obstacles to accessing care currently faced by gender non-conforming young people and their families in Canada. Next, we explore some of the ethical principles that guided our research and the methodology that underpinned the project. Third, and paying particular attention to dimensions of health and inequalities, we explore some of the components of the research and describe some of the effects it had, in terms of development of services for young people, their families and the broader community. The chapter concludes with a proposal of guidelines for research with trans young people, in Canada and beyond.

Gender-creative children, trans youth and their families: experiences of health inequalities

At present, two major factors promote and maintain health inequalities among gender non-conforming children and young people in Canada: insufficient political and legal protections, and inconsistent healthcare delivery and access. At the political level in Canada, there has been almost no discussion focused on the real need to protect gender non-conforming children and young people. Indeed, despite two recent attempts to pass legislation (Bill 279 – an Act to amend the Canadian Human Rights Act and the Criminal Code (gender identity)), which would provide recognition and protection of transgender people, children have only entered the discussion as possible 'victims' of the proposed Bill In a twisted vision of childhood vulnerability, the Campaign Life Coalition (2010) has argued that providing legal protection for gender identity will jeopardise the safety of young girls by subjecting them to leering paedophiles dressed up as women. In fact, however, it is gender non-conforming and trans young people who face the threat of violence in school bathrooms (Public Health Agency of Canada, 2010).

A lack of legal protections, we argue, increases the level of vulnerability of young people with regard to discrimination and oppression. A mounting body of research has shown that trans individuals are subject to high levels of discrimination and violence and face grave difficulties gaining access to employment, housing and basic services (Lombardi et al, 2001; Bauer et al, 2009; Grant et al, 2011; Pyne, 2011). Moreover, and with the exceptions of Ontario, British Columbia and Alberta, it is impossible to change one's sex designation on official documents without undergoing surgery and/or hormone therapy. As a result, some children and young people are subject to misunderstandings and even abuse. One young British Columbian trans girl considers the interrogation she encounters every time she travels to the United States to see her grandmother as a form of 'border bullying'. Indeed, border officials question why she has an 'm' designation on her passport when she presents as a girl (Smart, 2013).

In Canada, insufficient legal protections are compounded by the uneven provision of care across the country. Few options exist to support the needs of young people residing outside of major urban centres. Indeed, only Montreal, Toronto, Vancouver and Winnipeg offer any kind of comprehensive support for pre-pubescent and pubescent trans and gender-independent children. Families who live in rural areas and who are also already subject to intersecting oppressions, such as some First Nations peoples, are far less likely to receive the services they require. Moreover, given that Canadian young people are required to be at least 14 years of age to access care without parental consent, and given that not all parents are as supportive as Akiko, many children and young people are unable to access the limited resources that are available. Indeed, 50% of parents confuse gender non-conformity and homosexuality as the same phenomenon (Wells et al, 2012). Many children do not get access to care, therefore, because their primary caregivers do not understand what is happening or are too frightened to seek help.

Not all **gender-creative** young people desire a medical transition: indeed, some grow into adolescence asserting a gender queer identity, a development that many providers have difficulty understanding. Among parents who have attempted to find affirming services for their children, for example, some have complained about their lack of accessibility because they were developed according to a binary model that is geared towards 'male or female', with little understanding of gender fluidity in children and young people. They also noted that most paediatricians they encountered were not very attuned to the realities of gender creativity in children (Pullen Sansfaçon, 2012). In cases where access to some form of physical transition is desired, trans people need a diagnosis of gender dysphoria. While gender dysphoria is an improvement on gender identity disorder (the classifications of diagnoses as published previously in the *Diagnostic statistical manual: DSM 4-TR*), the diagnosis is not without its issues. The very need for a 'diagnosis' leads to the unnecessary medicalisation of identity, which may lead to perverse effects on those who seek to access services by increasing levels of stigmatisation (Vooris, 2013).

This is not to say that medicine and psychiatry have no place in the lives of gender-creative children. In some cases, it is necessary to access medical or psychiatric help. A recent research report on parents shows that affirmative medical interventions are needed in some cases because 'they bring their children's bodies and selves into greater alignment' (Pullen Sansfaçon, 2012, p 38). This underlines a paradox: in order to receive care and receive appropriate health and social services in the current context, gender non-conforming children must be given a medical label. Yet, this very medical label can also contribute to the stigmatisation, oppression and discrimination of gender non-conforming children and young people, and to a sense that there is something wrong with their very identity.

Similar to many other groups experiencing oppression and discrimination, gender-creative children and trans young people have poorer health outcomes than cisgender youth (Fish, 2007). Indeed, gender non-conforming children who are pressured to conform to their assigned sex at birth are more 'prone to anxiety, sadness, social withdrawal, self deprecation, and other signs of internalized distress' (Carver et al, cited in Pyne, 2014, p 4) as well as self-harm, including suicide (Spack et al, 2012). Recent research suggests that young people's mental health outcomes are worse in families where they are not supported. Trans young people who are not supported by their families are significantly more likely to have poor mental health outcomes, to self-harm, to experience depression and anxiety and to be at risk of suicide than those who experience parental support (Travers et al, 2012).

Researching the social worlds of gender-creative children: participatory and emancipatory led approaches to inquiry

Social work is a discipline that is underpinned and recognised by a specific set of values and principles that should drive practice. Indeed, social work is a profession that highlights respect for the equality, worth and dignity of all people and in which human rights and social justice are central to the justification for social work action (IFSW, 2013). These values and principles should not only be fundamental to social work practice, however, but also be integrated in social work research (Butler, 2002; Shannon, 2013). As Finn (1994, p 25, cited in Shannon, 2013, p 103) argues: 'Social work must develop change-oriented, value-based models of knowledge development that address people, power, and praxis.' Accordingly, social work research has a responsibility to move away from research ethics frameworks that are passive (avoid harm, obtain informed consent and so on) to a more active form, that is to say, a framework that is empowering and enables participants to find a means to tackle the issues they may face.

The starting point of the research project on which this chapter is based was to begin to analyse the social, educational and activist worlds of gender non-conforming children in Canada. Specifically, the project aimed to gain a better understanding of various actors' experience as well as the context in which gender-creative children grow in Canada, and ultimately, to develop new research questions regarding the rights, needs and wellbeing of children, young people and their families. In line with our underlying research principles, we wanted to shift the focus away from the child as patient, to one in which children and young people and their families have a greater voice in the policy-making process that is currently failing to protect their 'difference' (Scott-Dixon, 2006, p 15).

Given our collective background as feminist, queer studies, ethics and anti-oppression scholars, and given that two members of the research team belong to families with gender-creative children, we were keenly attuned to the complex intersectionality of power operating in families, society and politics. Our decision to draw on participatory action research methodology was informed precisely by the desire to understand the linkages between what happens in the personal lives of people and in Parliament, for example, and what meanings children, their parents and their advocates make of them, as well as to effect change. Our decision to draw from this methodology was also underpinned by a concern about embedding social work values in research and practice to offset inequalities experienced by this group, and thus contribute to challenging the very structures that give rise to the oppression faced by so many of these children and their families. Participatory action research methodologies are recognised as helpful for effecting change while simultaneously embedding social work values in research (Shannon, 2013). As discussed above, there is a lack of knowledge and as a consequence, resources to support young people are scarce. Guidelines for practice are also rare. Developing knowledge, without reproducing structures of power and oppression and the violence to which young people, their families and, sometimes, their allies are already subject, is essential.

More specifically, self-directed groupwork (Fleming and Ward, 2004) was applied as a method of data collection to the project. Self-directed groupwork applied to research allows for data collection while addressing problems, taking action for change and empowering specific groups of participants, in this case, parents, professionals and other allies working with 'trans children'. Self-directed groupwork applied to research involves a research process aimed not only at discovering, interpreting and revising human knowledge on different aspects of the world (Pullen Sansfaçon et al, 2014a), but also addressing a problem and taking action for change. In self-directed groupwork, stakeholders are viewed as 'knowers' (Fleming and Ward, 2004), which we felt was compatible with our underlying research principles.

The project was organised into several strands:

- an action research project with families of gender-creative children;
- two pieces of qualitative research: one with educators and other professionals working with gender-creative children, and one with parent activists;
- the organisation of a national conference to establish a platform for national networking;
- producing and sharing knowledge among stakeholders through publications and the development of a website.

The following section focuses specifically on research components that we feel have most fully integrated the principles and values of social work, and the process of Social Action Research (SAR). To do so, the research strand is briefly described before there is a focus on the outcomes, in terms of both knowledge and social change.

Researching the family and the social environment in which gender-creative children grow

In order to gain an understanding of the experiences of gender-creative children as well as the context in which they grow, we developed a self-directed group (Mullender and Ward, 1991) that met over a period of 14 weeks. Self-directed groupwork is an approach for working with people who experience oppression, aimed at the development of empowerment. In the context of this research, self-directed groupwork was used as our tool for data collection. Indeed, after securing ethics clearance and circulating invitations to participate among key organisations in Montreal, we began the research-intervention group. The research group met for a period of 14 weeks, exploring the key questions pertaining to the approach. The data were gathered through open notes taken by the research assistants, on flip charts, and on paper that was left on the table for participants to check at the end of each session (see Pullen Sansfaçon et al, 2014a for further detail on the methodology). Throughout the process of self-directed groupwork, parents and caregivers were invited to share their experiences as well as to define strategies to tackle barriers and thus effect change at the personal, cultural and policy levels. The experience discussed during the 14 sessions-long group meeting constituted the data that were then analysed and collated into a research report. Akiko Asano, one of the participants in the self-directed groupwork, also collaborated in presenting some of the findings at the TransHealth conference in Philadelphia in spring 2013.

While the research component ended in October 2012, the group has formalised and continues to work together. Indeed, in the months following the completion of the research, the host organisation (Famijeunes, Montreal) and the parents' group facilitated a new partnership, and the parents were allowed to continue meeting at Famijeunes over and beyond the formal ending of the research. At the time of writing this chapter, the group continues to meet on a monthly basis. At the same time, the parents' association, which has now formally registered with the Québec government (Gender Creative Kids/Enfants transgenres Canada), also offers a new support group for gender-creative children and their siblings, under the age of 14, with the help of Famijeunes staff and allied from the broader community. Before the launch of this new children's group, no such service was provided in the area for children and young people. Finally, the parents' group has created a Facebook page, organised two petitions in support of changes in federal legislation (see context above – Canadian Charter of Rights and Freedoms) and sent personalised letters to senators urging the passing of the gender identity Bill.

At the time of writing this chapter, the parent-led organisation had also been invited to join Comité Trans, made up of half a dozen organisations that work to improve the lives of trans individuals in Québec. As a result, they participated in reviewing a formal document that was presented at the National Assembly to modify the Civil Code so that it will become easier for trans individuals to change their names and sex marker on official identification papers without having to undergo surgery or any other form of medical treatment. Gender

Creative Kids/*Enfants transgenres Canada* has also actively participated in transpride events and other LGBT community days. Finally, the group has also begun to develop a short training (with the support of the researchers) to provide to schools that have gender-creative children as their pupils. The course was delivered successfully for the first time in spring 2013 in the region of Montreal. Providing support to parents at meetings and other informal gatherings continues to be central to this work as well.

A National Workshop on Gender Creative Kids *and* Gendercreativekids.ca

As noted at the beginning of the chapter, the project was designed in such a way as to facilitate new research and social change beyond our own particular research projects. To this end, we sought to build a national network of stakeholders who would continue, beyond the research project, to develop further knowledge and services for gender-creative children and their parents. With the support of a Social Sciences and Humanities Research Grant, we were able to undertake two additional initiatives: (a) the organisation of the first National Workshop on Gender Creative Kids and (b) the design and launch of a new national website: Gendercreativekids.ca. In October 2012, over 70 scholars, parents, clinicians, activists, artists and educators gathered in Montreal for two and a half days of presentations, discussions and debates. The event was free of charge, and many participants were able to have their travel expenses covered. As such, the workshop provided a voice for a broad range of stakeholders concerned with the wellbeing of young people and their families. The concluding session of the workshop also included a facilitated activity of SAR that produced a broad orientation for future research with and for gender-creative children in Canada (see Pullen Sansfaçon et al, 2014b).

In keeping with participatory action research principles, Gendercreativekids.ca, launched in September 2013, enables service providers across the country to upload information about their services so that young people, parents and other involved adults can access informed care quickly and easily. As part of a broader effort to increase the visibility of gender-creative young people in Canada, the website also houses a wide array of resources, research, information and means of community building. Again, the website development was inspired by social action and social work principles and values in so far that a democratic process was central to its construction and its organisation: members of the public, for example, are able to upload relevant resources to the website on an ongoing basis. Furthermore, maintenance and translation of the website into French is coordinated by the Gender Creative Kids group members. Finally, a 'locating function' allows families to find one another in their own communities – a tool we hope will enable otherwise isolated families to connect with one another.

Conclusion

Parents such as Akiko should not have to fear social workers. Indeed, just the opposite: social workers should be working as allies of parents and children struggling to realise change in their home communities. As increasing numbers of children and young people begin to socially transition, social workers will also be increasingly called on to support and educate parents, medical providers and educators, not to mention to children and young people themselves. By speaking up and serving as advocates for children and young people, and by carrying out SAR in areas of their own domains, social workers can play a powerful role in reducing the serious social and health inequalities faced by gender-creative young people today.

Participatory action research holds promise for social work scholars seeking to both learn about and transform the social conditions of gender non-conforming children and their families. In a recently published piece, Singh et al (2013) have developed a useful checklist for participatory action research with trans communities. We recommend that social work scholars consult this checklist while attending to the following broad guidelines:

- embed social work values in the research process;
- incorporate families as co-researchers who contribute to all steps of the research design, implementation and dissemination;
- endeavour to create tangible outcomes through which both knowledge and social change are immediately affected.

In sum, we believe that social workers are in a unique position to foster inclusive and affirmative communities for gender-creative children and their families. Indeed, standing on the interstices of family, school, community and social service institutions, social work practitioners can play a key role in promoting social and health equalities in the lives of gender-creative children. We hope that social workers will soon begin to play a leading role in transforming our communities into safe and affirmative sites of belonging, and thus enabling children such as Mat to more easily thrive as they mature into adulthood.

What we know about this already
- As a consequence of serious social discrimination, gender non-conforming children and young people are at risk of anxiety, depression, self-harm and suicide.
- However, many of these risks are reduced through positive social support – especially parental acceptance.

What this chapter adds
- Social action research can be a powerful model for tackling social discrimination and creating new understanding about the lives of gender non-conforming children and young people.

How this is relevant for social work and LGBT health inequalities
- As the most vulnerable population to suicide (within and beyond the LGBT community), the challenges faced by gender non-conforming young people require urgent attention by social work professionals.
- Through their strategic location in many institutions (including schools, hospitals, community clinics and the courts), social workers have the potential to play a powerful role in creating the affirming environments necessary so that all children and young people can thrive.

References

Campaign Life Coalition, 2010, 'Campaign Life Coalition is Concerned that the "Bathroom Bill" C-389 Could Pass in Parliament', *Canada News Wire*, 16 November, www.campaignlifecoalition.com/index.php?p=Press+Room&id=44, last accessed 19 November 2013

Bauer, GR, Hammond, R, Travers, R, Kaay, M, Hohenadel, KM, Boyce, M, 2009, '"I don't think this is theoretical; this is our lives": how erasure impacts health care for transgender people', *Journal of Assoc Nurses AIDS Care*, 20, 5, 348-61

Bryant, K, 2008, 'In defense of gay children? "Progay" homophobia and the production of homonormativity', *Sexualities*, 11, 4, 455-75

Butler, I, 2002, 'A Code of Ethics for Social Work and Social Care Research', *British Journal of Social Work*, 32, 2, 239-48

Ehrensaft, D, 2011, *Gender Born, Gender Made: Raising Healthy Gender-Nonconforming Children*, New York, NY: The Experiment

Ehrensaft, D, 2012, 'From gender identity disorder to gender identity creativity: true gender self child therapy', *Journal of Homosexuality*, 59, 337-56

Feder, EK, 1999, 'Regulating sexuality: gender identity disorder, children's rights, and the state', in U Narayan and JJ Bartowiak (eds) *Having and raising children: Unconventional families, hard choices, and the social good*, University Park, PA: The Pennsylvania State University Press, 163-76

Fish, J, 2007, *Reducing health inequalities for lesbian, gay, bisexual and trans people: Briefing papers for health and social care staff*, London: Department of Health

Fleming, J, and Ward, D, 2004, 'Methodology and practical applications of the social action research model', in F. Maggs-Report (ed) *New qualitative methodologies in health and social care: Putting ideas into practice*, London: Routledge, 162-78

Grant, JM, Mottet, LA, Tanis, J, Harrison, T, Herman, JL, and Keisling, M, 2011, *Injustice at every turn: A report of the National Transgender Discrimination Survey*, Washington, DC: National Center for Transgender Equality and the National Gay and Lesbian Task Force

IFSW – International Federation of Social Workers, 2013, *Global definition of social work*, http://ifsw.org/get-involved/global-definition-of-social-work/, last accessed 23 September 2013

Isay, RA, 1997, 'Remove gender identity disorder from DSM', *Psychiatric News*, 32, 9, 13

Langer, S, and Martin, J, 2004, 'How dresses can make you mentally ill: Examining gender identity disorder in children', *Child and Adolescent Social Work Journal*, 23,5/6, 533-55

Lombardi, E, Wilchins, RA, Priesing, D, and Malouf, D, 2001, 'Gender violence: transgender experiences with violence and discrimination', *Journal of Homosexuality*, 42, 1, 89-101

Mallon GP, (ed), 2009, *Social work practice with transgender and gender variant youth* , London: Routledge, 104-14

Mallon, GP, and DeCrescenzo, T, 2006, 'Transgender children and youth: a child welfare practice perspective', *Child Welfare*, 85, 2, 215-41

Manning, K, Pullen Sansfaçon, A and Meyer, EJ, 2014, 'Introduction', in EJ Meyer and A Pullen Sansfaçon(eds), *Supporting transgender and gender creative youth: Schools, families, and communities in action*, California: Peter Lang, 1-12

Meyer, WJ, 2012, 'Gender identity disorder: an emerging problem for pediatricians', *Pediatrics*, 129, 3, 571-73

Moller, B, Schreier, H, Li, A and Romer, G, 2009, 'Gender identity disorder in children and adolescent', *Current Problems in Pediatric and Adolescent Health Care*, 39, 117-43

Morrow, DF, 2004, 'Social work practice with gay, lesbian, bisexual and transgender adolescents', *Families in Society*, 85, 91-9

Mullender, A, and Ward, D, 1991, *Self-directed groupwork: Users take action for empowerment*, London: Within and Birch

Public Health Agency of Canada, 2010, *Questions and answers: Gender identity in schools*, Ottawa: The Minister of Health

Pullen-Sansfaçon, A, 2012, *Princess Boys, Trans Girls, Queer Youth: Social Action Research Project: Parenting a "gender creative" child in today's society*, Research report, University of Montreal, Canada

Pullen-Sansfaçon, A, Ward, D, Robichaud, MJ, Dumais-Michaud, A and Clegg, A, 2014a, 'Working with parents of gender-variant children: using social action as an emancipatory research framework', *Journal of Professive Human Services, Journal of Progressive Human Services*, 25, 3, 214-29, doi: 10.1080/10428232.2014.939938

Pullen Sansfaçon, A, Manning, K, Meyer, EJ and Robichaud, MJ (2014b) 'Conclusion: looking back, looking forward', in E Meyer, and A Pullen Sansfaçon (eds) *Supporting gender creative and transgender youths : Family, schools and community in action*, Peter Lang Press : California

Pyne, J, 2011, 'Unsuitable bodies: Trans people and cisnormativity in shelter services', *Canadian Social Work Review*, 28, 1, 129-37

Pyne, J (2014) 'Gender independent kids: A paradigm shift in approaches to gender non-conforming children', *Canadian Journal of Human Sexuality*, 23, 1, 1–8; doi:10.3138/cjhs.23.1.CO1

Scott-Dixon, S (ed), 2006, *Trans/forming feminisms: Trans-feminist voices speak out*, Toronto: Sumach Press

Shannon, P, 2013, 'Value-base social work research: Strategies for connecting research to the mission of social work', *Critical Social Work*, 14, 1, www1.uwindsor.ca/criticalsocialwork/valuebasedSWresearch

Singh, AA, Richmond K, and Burnes, TR 2013, 'Feminist participatory action research with transgender communities: fostering the practice of ethical and empowering research design', *International Journal of Transgenderism*, 14, 93-104

Smart, A, 2013, '10-year-old transgender girl wages battle against border "bullying"', *Times Colonist*, September 15

Spack, N, Edwards-Leeper, L, Feldman, H, Leibowitz,S, Mandel, F, Diamond, D and Vance, S, 2012, 'Children and adolescents with gender identity disorder referred to a pediatric medical center', *Pediatrics*, 129, 3, 418-25

Tosh, G, (2014) 'Working together for an inclusive and gender creative future: a critical lens on "gender dysphoria"', in E Meyer and A Pullen Sansfaçon (eds), Supporting transgender and gender creative youth: schools, families, and communities in action', Peter Lang: California, 41-53

Travers R, Bauer G, Pyne J, Bradley K, 2012, for the Trans PULSE Project; L Gale, M Papadimitriou, *Impacts of Strong Parental Support for Trans Youth: A Report Prepared for Children's Aid Society of Toronto and Delisle Youth Services,* 2 October

Vooris, JA, 2013, 'Trapped in the wrong body and life uncharted: anticipation and identity within narratives of parenting transgender/gender non-conforming children', in FJ Green and M Friedman (eds), *Chasing rainbows: Exploring gender fluid parenting practices,* Bradford, ON: Demeter Press

Wallace, R and Russell, H, 2013, 'Attachment and shame in gender-nonconforming children and their families: toward a theoretical framework for evaluating clinical interventions', *International Journal of Transgenderism,* 14, 3, 113-26

Wells, K, Roberts, G, and Allan, C, 2012, *Supporting transgender and transsexual students in K-12 schools: A guide for educators,* Ottawa: ON: Canadian Teachers' Federation

Zucker, KJ, 2008, 'Children with gender identity disorder: Is there a best practice?' *Neuropsychiatrie de l'enfance et de l'adolescence,* 56, 358-64

Zucker, KJ and Bradley, SJ, 1995, *Gender identity disorder and psychosexual problems in children and adolescents,* New York, NY: Guilford Press

Mental health inequalities among LGBT older people in the United States: curricula developments

Valerie Lester Leyva

Introduction

Large-scale studies and national population-based surveys have been used to explore the interactions between sexual orientation, gender identity and mental health outcomes in the United States (US), Canada, and other English-speaking countries. These studies illuminate the ways in which lesbian, gay, bisexual and trans (LGBT) adults experience inequalities in mental health outcomes when compared with their heterosexual peers. For example, lesbians and bisexual women are at greater lifetime risk for substance abuse and dependence than heterosexual men and women (King et al, 2008). Gay men experience higher rates of mood and anxiety disorders than their heterosexual male peers or lesbians (Bostwick et al, 2010). Bisexual women are more likely to report poorer outcomes related to mood, anxiety, and suicide than their heterosexual, lesbian or gay counterparts (Steele et al, 2009). Trans individuals cite discrimination, negative body image and the complexity of intimate partner relationships as significant factors affecting mental health (Bockting et al, 2006).

One additional factor not included in these studies is the effects of ageing on mental health outcomes within the LGBT population. While Fredriksen-Goldsen and Muraco (2010) specify the need to focus on the additional factors of age, cohort affect, culture and individual life experiences when studying any aspect of the LGBT population, few studies have utilised these when exploring mental health inequalities among LGBT adults. This chapter describes how incorporating these factors will illuminate ways in which LGBT mental health inequalities may shift over the lifecourse and offers suggestions for developing best practices.

Sexual orientation, gender identity and mental health outcomes

Despite enjoying access to similar economic resources than their heterosexual counterparts, LGBT adults living in the US experience significant inequalities in mental health outcomes when compared with their heterosexual peers. Numerous studies explore the rates of depression, anxiety, suicidality, substance abuse and self-harm in the LGBT population (Cochrane and Mays, 2006; Herek and Garnets, 2007; Institutes of Medicine, 2011). In a meta-analysis of lesbian, gay and bisexual (LGB) mental health studies published worldwide, King et al (2008) compared these rates to existing data on non–LGB populations. They determined that the risk for depression and anxiety were 1.5 times more likely in LGB individuals, that lesbians and bisexual women experienced a higher risk of substance dependence and the lifetime prevalence of suicide rates was substantially higher in gay and bisexual men. Studies of mental health and trans adults are few. However, existing studies suggest that the prevalence of adverse mental health outcomes is higher for trans adults than in the LGB population (Institutes of Medicine, 2011). For example, one study of 571 trans women in New York City reported a lifetime prevalence of depression at 52.4%, and a lifetime prevalence of suicidal ideation, planning and attempts at 53.5% (Nuttbrock et al, 2010). A review of the extant studies of trans mental health cites the rate of suicidal ideation as ranging from 38% to 65% (US Department of Health and Human Services, 2012). While actual rates of suicide completion within the LGBT population are historically difficult to obtain, recent governmental efforts in the United Kingdom (UK) encourage coroners to monitor the gender identity and sexual orientation of deceased persons so that suicidality and other health trends may be explored (DH, 2013).

It is clear from these studies that LGBT adults experience mental health inequalities when compared with their non–LGBT peers, but few studies hypothesise the reasons behind these differences. The effects of discrimination and stigma over the lifecourse are a significant factor leading to depression and anxiety, including the classification of 'homosexuality' as a mental illness, are well documented (Spence et al, 2011). These are in addition to the deleterious effects of internalised homophobia and its effect on overall health and wellness (Newcomb and Mustanski, 2010). It is important to note that while accessing health and mental healthcare in the US has been problematic for significant portions of the general population (57.4 million individuals in the US were without health insurance in the first three months of 2013), this statistic is amplified for LGBT adults, who have been barred from spousal healthcare benefits due to the lack of legal recognition for same-sex marriages (Cohen and Martinez, 2013).

The social benefits of marriage or legal domestic partnership may also play a role in mental health outcomes for LGBT adults. It is well established that marriage has a positive impact on mental health outcomes (King and Bartlett, 2006). It is associated with increased coping skills (Kessler and Essex, 1982), decreased depression (Simon, 2002) and generally good mental health (Liu et al, 2010). Recent studies confirm that these outcomes are replicated in legally recognised same-sex relationships (Gorman et al, 2013). Despite the 2013 changes to the Defence of Marriage Act, laws in 25 US states specifically deny legal recognition of same-sex couples (Millstone, 2013). The denial of access to the legal, social and protective mental health benefits of marriage continues to affect the lives of LGBT adults in the US.

The combined effects of lifelong discrimination, past victimisation in the name of 'curing' homosexuality, inadequate services and exclusion from the benefits of marriage have created an environment in which LGBT adults experience inequalities in mental health outcomes, particularly with regard to depression, substance misuse, coping skills and suicidal thoughts. These factors demonstrate the need for a dual approach. Development of service delivery systems and evidence-based practice models cognisant of the particular needs of LGBT individuals will likely improve mental health outcomes for this population (National Resource Center, 2013; Gendron et al, 2013; Leyva et al, 2014). However, a response focusing on the eradication of systematic exclusion experienced by this population is another valid pathway to achieving these outcomes. With their focus on individual and societal challenges to health and wellbeing, social workers are well placed to respond to this complex set of factors at play in the lives of LGBT adults.

Social determinants of health and social exclusion

While discrimination, stigma and legal barriers appear to negatively influence mental health outcomes for LGBT adults in the US, consideration of other theories may identify additional pervasive patterns. The World Health Organization (WHO) has adopted the social determinants of health (SDoH) as a framework for addressing inequalities in physical and mental healthcare. These are defined by the WHO (2013) as 'the conditions in which people are born, grow, live, work and age'. A burgeoning body of research identifies the SDoH as the primary set of factors underlying physical and mental health inequalities (Marmot, 2005). Social exclusion, one feature of the SDoH, describes a complex process of marginalisation affecting those who do not possess economic or social status, such as people living in poverty, those whose age results in isolation or individuals who identify as ethnically different from the majority of residents in a given community (WHO, 2008). This marginalisation results in exclusion from cultural, civic, social and physical assets that might improve one's lifecourse or mental health status. Social exclusion and marginalisation have also been hypothesised as a significant factor in the adverse health outcomes of LGBT populations (Fish, 2010).

When considering mental health outcomes for LGBT adults, social exclusion based on age provides a useful framework for conceptualising how the SDoH influence the inequalities experienced by this population. Fredriksen-Goldsen and Muraco (2010) examined this phenomenon in their review of ageing and sexual orientation literature published between 1984 and 2008 in the US. They considered age, cohort affect, culture and individual life experiences in their construction of multiple lifecourse trajectories of LGB adults. Their focus on dividing the LGB adult population into age-related cohorts leads to consideration of multiple factors related to mental health outcomes. Primary among these is the interaction between age, sexual orientation, gender identity and the socio–historical contexts related to each resulting cohort of LGBT adults. To illustrate, they cite Parks' 1999 study that divided LGB adults into cohorts roughly corresponding to three eras of the LGB experience in the US:

- the era of LGB invisibility and intolerance (those who are aged 60 and older);
- LGB liberation (those aged 45 to 60 years old);
- LGB rights (those aged 30 to 45 years old).

The lived experience of someone who came of age during a time of extreme homophobia versus the experience of one who came of age during the era of same-sex marriage will differ in relationship to attitudes regarding mental healthcare (see Chapter Fifteen, this volume, for further discussion). LGB adults in the oldest cohort experienced the pathologising of LGB status, victimisation at the hands of those trying to 'cure' their homosexuality, substantial discrimination and harassment and violence in employment, housing and the delivery of healthcare services. This negatively impacts the likelihood that those in the older cohort will seek mental health services (Butler and Hope,

1999), while those in the youngest cohort may view access to mental healthcare as a right.

Fredriksen-Goldsen and Muraco (2010, p 400) call for additional research exploring the lived experience of LGB adults in more detail, acknowledging that 'a single, uniform life course for gay men and lesbians does not exist'. They specifically recommend further delineating the older two cohorts into subgroups based on age. This will direct further investigation into the interaction between age and other factors related to the social exclusion of LGBT older adults, particularly in relation to mental health outcomes. One result will be an improvement in evidence-based best practices for this population. A parallel initiative should be infusion of these best practices into social work curricula.

Best practices for LGBT older adults and mental healthcare

Recognising that LGBT adults do not constitute a monolithic bloc and have diverse experiences of mental health services calls for the development of practice behaviours that will meet these individualised needs. Acknowledging the differences in age and cohort will enable service providers to deliver mental healthcare in ways that are sensitive to the needs of LGBT adults, especially those who have experienced discrimination or victimisation from past mental health service providers.

Several organisations in the US have developed training curricula to improve the knowledge, skills and attitudes of those providing services to LGBT older adults. The most visible of these is the National Resource Centre on LGBT Aging (NRC). The NRC (2013) has developed a training curriculum that has been adopted for use by multiple service agencies across the US. Other organisations have replicated or independently developed similar programmes (US Department of Health and Human Services, 2001; Pearson, 2003; Brotman et al, 2007; Greytak and Kosciw, 2010; Landers et al, 2010; Knochel et al, 2012). Most have arrived at the following themes for inclusion in training programmes for those serving LGBT older adults:

- creating safe and inclusive service environments;
- developing knowledge of the inequalities experienced by LGBT older adults;
- exploring and overcoming one's biases about this population;
- creating tools for improving service delivery.

While most of these training seminars were developed for a broad range of service providers (doctors, nurses, medical aides and others) these best practices are also suitable for inclusion in social work curricula.

Many of these suggested best practices require small changes, although knowing where to start can be challenging. An excellent tool for exploring suggested changes is the SAGE (2012) publication *Inclusive services for LGBT older adults: A practical guide to creating welcoming agencies.* It provides practical guidance for beginning the process of making service environments sensitive to the needs of LGBT older adults. Another invaluable publication listing internet-based resources is the *Top health issues for LGBT populations information and resource kit* (US Department of Health and Human Services, 2012). Reviewing one's social work curriculum for these practice resources is another useful avenue for ensuring their inclusion.

A more challenging aspect of initiating these changes is the social environment that contributed to the development of mental health inequalities for LGBT older adults. Service providers will need to assess their service organisation to effectively target areas in which changes are attainable. For many, this will mean taking a visible leadership role to advocate for a historically marginalised population. In the US this should be feasible under the rubric of overall best practices in mental healthcare. However, social exclusion has heretofore been a nearly eradicable element of the lived experience of LGBT older adults in the US. While social acceptance has shifted considerably over the lifecourse of this population, it will take determined persistence to sustain these changes in many practice settings.

Additional research is needed to assess how these best practices may influence mental health inequalities with LGBT older adults. Many of these recommendations have already been initiated in consideration of other marginalised populations (based on ethnicity, economic status and other factors). Nursing has taken the lead in developing and measuring these best practices and offers sophisticated models for implementation. For example, Kahan (2012) offers an ethical approach to nursing best practices that incorporates many of the suggestions listed previously. Chin et al (2010) review the outcomes from a Robert Wood Johnson Foundation initiative to identify promising practices to reduce health inequalities among marginalised populations. These similar approaches offer a roadmap for developing and assessing best practices for working with LGBT older adults.

Mental health inequalities develop over many years and will take significant efforts and time to diminish. Called for now are studies of the long-term effects of competent service environments on mental health inequalities across multiple domains of the LGBT lived experience. Determining which factors have a successful impact on reducing inequalities will enhance the training curricula of mental health service providers, including social work.

LGBT diversity training in the social work curriculum: the mandate for inclusion

Given the human rights and social justice focus of social workers across the globe, social work is an ideal discipline for developing curricula regarding LGBT older adults. Numerous accrediting bodies guide these approaches. Central among these is the International Association of Schools of Social Work (IASSW). The IASSW is a confederation of schools of social work and holds United Nations consultative status regarding human rights issues. It subscribes to international human rights declarations, and articulates common ethical guidelines in its *Ethics in social work, statement of principles* (IASSW, 2004). Principle 4.2 calls on social workers to 'challenge negative discrimination on the basis of characteristics such as ... sexual orientation' (IASSW, 2004, p 2). This sets the stage for global adoption of social work curricula that challenge the inequalities and social exclusion experienced by LGBT individuals. A review of the accreditation standards in various English-speaking countries follows a similar pattern. While accrediting organisations for social work curricula in the US, UK, Canada and Australia address inclusion of LGBT specific curricula with varying degrees of specificity, none is as clear as the mandate in the IASSW *Statement of principles* to challenge negative discrimination.

The Council on Social Work Education (2008) developed the *Educational policy and accreditation standards*, regulating content in social work degree programmes in the US. Standard 2.1.4 requires social workers to 'understand how diversity characterises and shapes the human experience and is critical to the formation of identity' (2008, p 4). It further indicates that 'dimensions of diversity are understood as the intersectionality of multiple factors including ... gender identity and expression ... [and] sexual orientation' (p 5). The explicit inclusion of gender identity and sexual orientation is a step forward for raising the visibility of this population. However, understanding that gender identity and sexual orientation are dimensions of diversity in itself falls short of the IASSW mandate to challenge negative discrimination.

In the UK, the Health and Care Professions Council's (2008) *Standards of conduct, performance and ethics* articulate the expectations of social workers' professional practices. Duty #1 states that one's attitudes about sexuality (among many other factors) should not 'affect the way you deal with them [service users] or the professional advice you give' (2008, p 8). The vague reference to *sexuality*, however, can be misunderstood to include heterosexual sexuality. The *Standards of conduct, performance and ethics* also fail to include the IASSW mandate.

The Canadian Association for Social Work Education (CASWE) accredits social work education programmes in Canada. Principle #9 of its *Standards for accreditation* (CASWE, 2012, p 4) specifically states that diversity includes gender and sexual identities. Its Core Learning Objective for Students #1.1 further states that 'students acquire ability for self-reflection as it relates to engaging in professional practice through a comprehensive understanding and consciousness of the complex nature of their own social locations and identities' (2012, p 9). Additionally, Core Learning Objective #4.2 states that 'social work students have knowledge of how discrimination, oppression, poverty, exclusion, exploitation, and marginalisation have a negative impact on particular individuals and groups and strive to end these and other forms of social injustice' (2012, p 10). By specifically identifying gender and sexual identities, asking students to develop reflection skills to address their internal biases, increasing knowledge of the effects of social exclusion, and '*striving to end ... social injustice*', the CASWE comes closest to meeting the mandate of the IASSW.

The Australian Association of Social Work's (2008) *Education and accreditation standards* delineate expectations regarding professional practice with marginalised populations. It contains an entire section on cross-cultural curriculum content. This section lays out learning tasks related to universal human rights, the complexities of diverse identities and experiences, and the differential positions of power across different cultural groups. However, it too fails to specifically identify sexual orientation and gender identity or mandate their inclusion in social work curricula.

Inclusion of LGBT issues in the social work curriculum

While the accreditation standards in these English-speaking countries affirm ethical practices in general, few do so specifically with LGBT individuals. Given this environment, it is not surprising that few studies review the implementation of appropriate best practices with LGBT populations. Those that do, indicate that there are significant challenges regarding faculty attitudes and knowledge. Fredricksen–Goldsen et al (2011) surveyed a random sample of US and English–

speaking Canadian social work faculty ($n = 327$) regarding support for use of LGBT content in social work courses. Similar to findings for social work education in Italy delineated in Chapter Three, they found that, while supportive of LGBT content in general, many social work faculty believed that content on all aspects of the experiences of LGBT oppression was not an essential aspect of their curriculum. For example, approximately 38% ($n = 67$) of the US and 28% ($n = 43$) of the Canadian faculty reported that inclusion of content about transphobia is 'less than important' (p 25). Additionally, 29% ($n = 51$) of the US and 24% ($n = 37$) of the Canadian faculty did not know if their degree programmes possessed gender identity-related teaching resources. One additional study notes the lack of cultural competency training regarding LGBT individuals available to social work students in the US (Logie et al, 2007).

These studies point to significant gaps in implementation of social work education regarding best practices in serving LGBT older adults. If social work education is to have an impact on mental health inequalities for this population, it will need to employ strategies to raise faculty awareness of LGBT social exclusion and historical discrimination, particularly for trans individuals. Although several training modules on best practices for social work services with LGBT individuals do exist (Hunter, 2005; Morrow and Messinger, 2006; Mallon, 2008; Cosis-Brown and Cocker, 2011), Logie et al (2007) and Fredricksen-Goldsen et al (2011) demonstrate the limited faculty knowledge on the inclusion of these materials in social work curricula.

Clearly, additional efforts are needed to develop increased awareness and adoption of specific curricula regarding LGBT adults, as is further research to measure their effectiveness in social work education. Most importantly, however, a call for leadership is needed among social work faculty. Recognition that the LGBT population experiences significant inequalities and marginalisation is not uniform across any country or region, despite the many studies that attest to this reality. It is incumbent upon social work faculty to raise their peers' awareness of this fact, insist on implementation of the IASSW mandate to challenge negative discrimination, and develop and include curricula to help social workers achieve the goal of social justice for this population.

Conclusion

Mental health inequalities among LGBT older adults are a complex and multifaceted phenomenon. Educating social workers to be competent mental health providers for this population is one pathway to reversing this historical trend. Uncovering and dismantling discriminatory attitudes and practices, however, is no easy task. While most accrediting bodies for social work education in English-speaking countries affirms this (albeit weakly) as central to ethical practice, operationalising it presents significant challenges to social work faculty. A growing body of scholarship exists regarding best practices for providing services to this population. However, it is not adequately included in social work curricula, with some social work faculty not viewing it as an important element of social work education. Developing faculty leadership to advocate for these actions is a crucial next step in building a workforce of informed and inclusive social work service providers.

What we know about this already
- Many LGBT older people experience inequalities in mental health outcomes.
- Some LGBT older people have experienced victimisation and mistreatment in the name of 'curing' homosexuality.
- LGBT older people have diverse experiences of and attitudes towards mental health services.

What this chapter adds
- It considers various age-related cohorts of LGBT older people and their differential mental health experiences and needs.
- It offers guidelines for best practices for creating safe, inclusive and informed service environments.
- It describes the challenges in developing and implementing social work curricula regarding LGBT oppression, and alternatively, best practices for service delivery.

How this is relevant for social work and LGBT health inequalities
- Organisations accrediting social work education programmes require inclusion of the differential effects of age, gender identity and sexual orientation on the human experience.
- Developing competence in serving all individuals regardless of age, gender and sexual orientation is an ethical requirement of all social workers.
- Social workers are included in the professions offering mental health services and have the opportunity to provide leadership in reducing mental health inequalities.

References

Australian Association of Social Workers, 2008, *Australian Social Work Education and Accreditation Standards*, www.aasw.asn.au/document/item/100

Bockting, W, Knudsen, G and Goldberg, J, 2006, *Counselling and mental health care of transgender adults and loved ones*, www.vch.ca/transhealth

Bostwick, W, Boyd, C, Hughes, T and McCabe, S, 2010, 'Dimensions of sexual orientation and the prevalence of mood and anxiety disorders in the United States', *American Journal of Public Health*, 100, 3, 468-75

Brotman, S, Ryan, B, Collins, S, Chamberland, L, Cormier, R, Julien, D, Meyer, E, Peterkin, A, Richard, B, 2007, 'Coming out to care: Caregivers of gay and lesbian seniors in Canada', *The Gerontologist*, 47, 4, 490-503

Butler, SS and Hope, B, 1999, 'Health and well-being for late middle-aged and old lesbians in a rural area', *Journal of Gay and Lesbian Social Services*, 9, 4, 27-46

CASWE (Canadian Association for Social Work Education) (2012) *Standards for Accreditation*, www.caswe-acfts.ca/vm/newvisual/attachments/866/Media/CASWEStandardsAccreditation2012.pdf

Chin, N, Chiplin, A, Dayton, K, and Rowen, M, 2010, 'Asserting choice: Health care, housing, and property-planning for lesbian, gay, bisexual, and transgender older adults', *Clearinghouse Review: Journal of Poverty Law and Policy*, 43, 11-12, 552-33

Cochrane, SD and Mays, VM, 2006, 'Estimating prevalence of mental and substance-using disorders among lesbians and gay men from existing national health data', in *Sexual orientation and mental health*, AM Omoto and HS Kurtzman (eds), Washington, DC: American Psychological Association, 143-65

Cohen, R and Martinez, M, 2013, 'Health insurance coverage: early release of estimates from the National Health Interview Survey, January–March 2013', Centers for Disease Control, www.cdc.gov/nchs/data/nhis/earlyrelease/insur201309.pdf

Cosis-Brown, H and Cocker, C, 2011, *Social work with lesbians and gay men*, London: Sage

Council on Social Work Education, 2008, *Educational Policy and accreditation standards*, www.cswe.org/File.aspx?id=41861

Department of Health, 2013, 'The LGBT public health outcomes framework companion document', www.lgf.org.uk/policy-research/the-lgbt-public-health-outcomes-framework-companion-document/

Fish, J, 2010, 'Conceptualising social exclusion and lesbian, gay, bisexual, and transgender people: The implications for promoting equity in nursing policy and practice', *Journal of Research in Nursing*, 15, 4, 303-12

Fredriksen-Goldsen, K and Muraco, A, 2010, 'Aging and sexual orientation: A 25-year review of the literature', *Research on Aging*, 32, 3, 372-413

Fredriksen-Goldsen, K, Woodford, M, Luke, K and Gutierrez, L, 2011, 'Support of sexual orientation and gender identity content in social work education: Results from national surveys of US and anglophone Canadian faculty', *Journal of Social Work Education*, 47, 1, 19-35

Gendron, T, Maddux, S, Krinsky, L, White, J, Lockeman, K, Metcalfe, Y and Aggarwal, S, 2013, 'Cultural competence training for health care professional working with LGBT older adults', *Educational Gerontology*, 39, 6, 454-63

Gorman, B, Denney, J and Barrera, C, 2013, 'Families, resources, and adult health: Where do sexual minorities fit?', *Journal of Health and Social Behavior*, 54, 1, 46-63

Greytak, E and Kosciw, J, 2010, 'Year One evaluation of the New York City Department of Education "Respect for All" training program', www.glsen.org/research

Health and Care Professions Council, 2008, *Standards of Conduct, Performance and Ethics*, www.hpc-uk.org/assets/documents/10003B6EStandardsofconduct,performanceandethics.pdf

Herek, GM and Garnets, LD, 2007, 'Sexual orientation and mental health', *Annual Review of Clinical Psychology*, 3, April, 353-75

Hunter, S, 2005, *Midlife and older LGBT adults: Knowledge and affirmative practice for the social services*, New York, NY: Routledge

Institutes of Medicine, 2011, *The health of lesbian, gay, bisexual, and transgender people: Building a foundation for better understanding*, www.iom.edu/Reports/2011/The-Health-of-Lesbian-Gay-Bisexual-and-Transgender-People.aspx

IASSW (International Association of Schools of Social Work), 2004, *Ethics in Social Work, Statement of Principles*, www.iassw-aiets.org/ethics-in-social-work-statement-of-principles

Kahan, B, 2012, 'Using a comprehensive best practices approach to strengthen ethical health-related practice', *Health Promotion Practice*, 13, 4, 431-37

Kessler, R and Essex, M, 1982, 'Marital status and depression: the importance of coping resources', *Social Forces*, 61, 2, 484-507

King, M and Bartlett, A, 2006, 'What same sex civil partnerships may mean for health', *Journal of Epidemiology and Community Health*, 60, 3, 188-91

King, M, Semlyen, J, Tai, SS, Killaspy, H, Osborn, D, Popelyuk, D and Nazareth, I, 2008, 'A systematic review of mental disorder, suicide, and deliberate self harm in lesbian, gay and bisexual people', *BMC Psychiatry*, 8, 1, 70

Knochel, K, Croghan, C, Moone, R, and Quam, J, 2012, 'Training, geography, and provision of aging services to lesbian, gay, bisexual, and transgender older adults', *Journal of Gerontological Social Work*, 55, 5, 426-43

Landers, S, Mimiaga, M and Krinsky, L, 2010, 'The Open Door project task force: A qualitative study on LGBT aging', *Journal of Gay and Lesbian Social Services*, 22, 3, 316-36

Leyva, VL, Breshears, E and Ringstad, R (2014) 'Assessing the efficacy of LGBT cultural competency training for aging services providers in California's Central Valley', *Journal of Gerontological Social Work*, 57, 1-2, 335-48

Liu, H, Elliott, S and Umberson, D, 2010, 'Marriage in young adulthood', in JE Grant and MN Potenza (eds) *Young adult mental health*, New York, NY: Oxford University Press, 169–80

Logie, C, Bridge, T and Bridge, P, 2007, 'Evaluating the phobias, attitudes, and cultural competence of master of social work students toward the LGBT populations', *Journal of Homosexuality*, 53, 4, 201-21

Mallon, G, 2008, *Social work practice with lesbian, gay, bisexual, and transgender people*, New York, NY: Routledge

Marmot, M, 2005, 'Social determinants of health inequalities', *The Lancet*, 365, 9464, 1099-104

Millstone, K, 2013, *Where gay marriage stands in all 50 states*, http://news.msn.com/us/where-gay-marriage-stands-in-all-50-states

Morrow, D and Messinger, L, 2006, *Sexual orientation and gender expression in social work practice: Working with gay, lesbian, bisexual, and transgender people*, New York, NY: Columbia University Press.

National Resource Center, 2013, *About our training curricula*, www. lgbtagingcenter.org/about/training.cfm

Newcomb, M and Mustanski, B, 2010, 'Internalized homophobia and internalizing mental health problems: A meta-analytic review', *Clinical Psychology Review*, 30, 8, 1019-29

Nuttbrock, L, Hwahng, S, Bockting, W, Rosenblum, A, Mason, M, Macri, M, Becker, J, 2010, 'Psychiatric impact of gender-related abuse across the life course of male-to-female transgender persons', *Journal of Sex Research*, 47, 1, 12–23

Parks, CA, 1999, 'Lesbian identity development: An examination of differences across generations', *American Journal of Orthopsychiatry*, 69, 3, 347-61

Pearson, Q, 2003, 'Breaking the silence in the counselor education classroom: A training seminar on counseling sexual minority clients', *Journal of Counseling and Development*, 81, summer, 292-300

SAGE, 2012, *Inclusive services for LGBT older adults: A practical guide to creating welcoming agencies*, www.sageusa.org/resources/publications. cfm?ID=107

Simon, R, 2002, 'Revisiting the relationships among gender, marital status, and mental health', *American Journal of Sociology*, 107, 1065–98

Spence, N, Adkins, D and Dupre, M, 2011, 'Racial differences in depression trajectories among older women: Socioeconomic, family, and health influences', *Journal of Health and Social Behavior*, 54, 444-59

Steele, LS, Ross, LE, Dobinson, C, Veldhuizen, S and Tinmouth, J, M, 2009, 'Women's sexual orientation and health: Results from a Canadian population-based survey', *Women and Health*, 49, 5, 353-67

US Department of Health and Human Services, Substance Abuse and Mental Health Services Administration, 2001, *A provider's introduction to substance abuse treatment for lesbian, gay, bisexual, and transgender individuals*, http://store.samhsa.gov/product/A-Provider-s-Introduction-to-Substance-Abuse-Treatment-for-Lesbian-Gay-Bisexual-and-Transgender-Individuals/SMA12-4104

US Department of Health and Human Services, Substance Abuse and Mental Health Services Administration, 2012, *Top health issues for LGBT populations information and resource kit,* http://store.samhsa. gov/shin/content//SMA12-4684/SMA12-4684.pdf

WHO (World Health Organization), 2008, *Understanding and tackling social exclusion,* www.who.int/social_determinants/knowledge_ networks/final_reports/sekn_final%20report_042008.pdf

WHO, 2013, *Social determinants of health,* www.who.int/social_determinants/sdh_definition/en/index.html

Strategies for maximising participation from LGB people in internet surveying in the United States

Andy Dunlap

Introduction

Just as social work practice is infused with empowering and collaborative ways of helping, social workers who conduct research can find ways to partner with those who are participating in their research and create projects that enrich the communities that they study. In order to better understand the experiences of lesbian, gay or bisexual (LGB) people within the healthcare and social services systems, and to fully explore health inequalities related to sexual orientation, social work researchers must overcome important difficulties inherent in trying to query these populations.

One widely used strategy for reaching these populations is non-probability internet surveying. In general, internet-based surveying has been noted for its ability to increase participation because of its ease of access, relative privacy and convenience for the participant (Dillman et al, 2009). Additionally, some researchers (Harris Interactive, 2010; Lever et al, 2008) have suggested that LGB populations are more likely to be active users of the internet than other populations. This argument focuses on the likelihood that LGB people may be more likely to seek personal information in the seeming privacy of their home than their heterosexual peers.

In 2011, I completed my doctoral degree with the successful defence of my dissertation: 'Changes in the coming-out process over time' (Dunlap, 2011). For this study, I defined *coming out* as the process that same-sex attracted people go through in order to develop a healthy sense of sexual orientation identity. Because same-sex attracted people often live in communities that are not fully validating of this aspect of identity, this process often involves understanding an important difference, incorporating that difference and often finding ways to detoxify this stigmatised difference (Cohler and Galatzer-Levy, 1996). Consistent with earlier researchers (for example Drasin et al, 2008), I also identified five age cohorts based on cultural events within the United States (US) that had influenced the degree of social stigma attached to same-sex attraction (see Figure 15.1).

Figure 15.1: Historical frame of reference for cohort distribution

Cohort distribution (*n* = 1,131)

	Years born	Current ages	Historical frame of reference	Female	Male
Cohort A	Before 1951	60 +	Pre-Stonewall generation	47	80
Cohort B	1951–62	59 to 49	Stonewall generation	113	124
Cohort C	1963–69	48 to 42	AIDS crisis generation	68	51
Cohort D	1970–88	41 to 23	Post AIDS crisis and millennial generation	282	151
Cohort E	After 1988	18*-22	Youngest cohort	140	75
Total				650	481

* Respondents under the age of 18 were screened out.

I used an internet survey hosted on Surveymonkey.com. I chose a mixed-method study and collected demographic data, self-labels for sexual orientation, information about family support, narratives of coming out and data related to the ages that individuals experienced important milestones in the coming-out process (for example, How old were you when you first realised you had a same-sex attraction? How old were you when you first told someone inside your family about your same-sex attraction?). I also invited participants to complete the Lesbian, Gay and Bisexual Identity Scale (LGBIS) (Mohr and Fassinger, 2000). This scale is designed to evaluate various outcomes of the coming-out process (for example, internalised homo/bi negativity, difficult process, etc). My goal was to elicit multiple data points that would help to answer three interrelated research questions:

- What is the coming-out experience of today's same-sex attracted young people?
- What are the personal theories about coming out that LGB people have about themselves?

- Have the ages changed at which important milestones in the coming-out process are reached?

The survey was designed to be completed in 30 to 45 minutes.

Conceptual and definitional issues

One challenge in researching the experiences of LGB people is deciding who is to be queried. Researchers have approached this question in several ways. Some researchers rely on behaviours as a way to establish who LGB people are (see, for example, Kinsey et al, 1948). Other researchers ask LGB people to self-select themselves for inclusion or exclusion from the study (for example, Shelton and Delgado-Romero, 2011). By asking LGB-targeted questions to a broad population, this strategy has the advantage of allowing LGB people to respond without being singled out for attention. Each of these strategies has advantages and disadvantages, and researchers should decide how to frame their sample based on fit with the research question and available resources.

In my study, I wanted to understand what my participants' experience of coming out was from their point of view. Because of this, I targeted for inclusion in the study anyone who identified as a member of the LGB community. Adult participants who did not identify as exclusively heterosexual or straight were invited to screen themselves in to the survey. Thus, my study relied on a very broad and inclusive definition of same-sex attracted minorities.

Tailored design method with LGB people

One generic concern in crafting successful survey instruments is in finding ways to hook potential participants into the process. How can the researcher maximise the likelihood that participants will complete the instrument? This problem is magnified when attempting to survey members of the LGB community. People who have been historically oppressed may be careful about sharing information with researchers. The LGB community is not one, but many communities made of up of diverse groups. LGB people may be sensitive to the fact that the experiences of white men have too often been targeted without much consideration of the diversity within the communities and reluctance to participate. Similarly, LGB people have often been the subject of studies that have objectified and pathologised their experiences.

Dillman et al (2009) describe a tailored design method in creating survey instruments. They recommend careful word choice to invite the person considering participating in the research into a collaborative role with the researcher. Word choice leads participants to recognise that they are experts on the information that they are providing, thus encouraging them to feel greater motivation to complete the survey. This approach is consistent with strengths–based research commitments (Sallebey, 2008) as well as post–modern ways of helping that privilege the voice of the person seeking assistance rather than the voice of the expert (see, for instance, White and Epston, 1990). Drewery et al (2000) have described *position calls*, which invite the subject of the inquiry into a more active stance than traditional methods of helping or research.

In my study, after inquiring about what label (if any) the participant used for their sexual orientation, I then asked what the impact, positive and negative, of their sexual orientation had been in their life. This kind of question immediately invites the participant to enter a space that has multiple possibilities and asks them to account for their individual experience.

While tailoring survey instruments, researchers are wise to carefully consider the motivations for participation of members of the LGB community and to pitch their request for participation accordingly. Many LGB people are motivated by the simple desire to give back to the community. For those LGB people who have made a life despite little family or social support, the idea of helping to make someone else's life a little easier may be appealing. Because of the great diversity within the LGB community, many people are interested in sharing their experiences as a way to strengthen the community. For instance, many older LGB people are motivated to share their experiences with younger generations: the notion of the 'love that dare not speak its name' (Douglas, 1894) has meant that many members of sexual and gender minority groups have been unseen and unheard for many years. Members of LGB communities are often very ready to participate in research because there is power in having one's voice heard.

The benefit of such a carefully worded survey and plea is not merely that the researcher is likely to obtain richer data, but the researcher is likely to obtain more participation. LGB communities hold a wealth of understanding and experience that has historically run ahead of commonly held and historically valid 'facts'. Gay and lesbian people knew that they were not sick long before homosexuality was declassified as an illness. Simply put, when treated as experts of their own experiences, members of LGB communities are often interested in contributing to research. Careful use of language in the service of framing the study, crafting the survey and executing the plea is crucial in this endeavour.

The plea for participation in my study in the first stage of recruitment included several carefully selected features, all designed to position participants as experts (see Figure 15.2).

Figure 15.2: Initial survey plea

Coming Out Survey

Anonymous!   Make your voice count!
Help others!

My name is Andy Dunlap. I'm a gay man and a PhD student at Smith College School for Social Work researching changes in the coming out process. As a human rights activist and an assistant professor of social work, I think it's crucial to tap in to the wisdom of the lgbtq community in order understand our issues, struggles and strengths.

If you identify as a same-sex attracted individual (lesbian, gay, bisexual, homosexual, queer, etc.) and are 18 years of age or older, please share your experience of coming out by taking this anonymous survey. This is truly a unique opportunity to have your story count and to be able to share your experiences in an anonymous way.

This study, An Investigation into Changes in the Coming Out Process Over Time, explores how today's experiences of coming out are different than they used to be and how they are different or the same by gender.

Your participation in this study will help other LGB folks who may struggle with the coming out process. The results of this study will contribute to a growing body of research that will help to design support targeted to different age groups of same-sex attracted people.

To take the survey, follow this link online: [link no longer active]

And don't forget to pass it on to your friends, family and colleagues who might want to help too!

Thank you for your participation

Andy
[Contact information and full credentials provided here]

Within six months, roughly 600 people responded to the survey. This provided the opportunity to evaluate the developing dataset for under-represented groups and then to target more individual pleas towards likely participants.

Sampling frame

One of the difficulties in surveying LGB populations is establishing a sampling frame from which to draw. The sampling frame describes the characteristics of the individuals from which the researcher's sample will be drawn, and like other aspects of research design is a question that should be addressed early in the project. Similar to other choices in research design (for example, what measure to use; quantitative versus qualitative; etc) the sampling frame should be calibrated to the research question. This is often an evident process, but when conducting research about LGB people the researcher would do well to avoid infusing their research with a heterosexist and/or gender bias that prevents them from carefully targeting their research population. Historically, research into same-sex attraction has tended to sample white, middle-class, non-disabled men living in urban environments. In short, viewing the LGB community as having little within-group differences is one way that researcher might stereotype these experiences. An important question to determine when establishing a useful sampling frame is simply what part of the known LGB communities does one want to query?

Establishing a useful sampling frame is greatly complicated by the simple question of how many LGB people there are. Foundational research on LGB people has estimated that roughly 10% of the population expresses some degree of same-sex attraction (Kinsey et al, 1948). A more recent study (Gates and Newport, 2012) has suggested that 3.4% of the US population identifies as LGB. Clearly this problem is compounded by differences in defining what is meant by sexual orientation and gender identity. Given the lack of demographic statistics describing the size and nature of LGB populations, it is not possible to reliably determine what percentage of any given part of the LGB community any piece of research has captured.

One way that researchers can attempt to obtain a comprehensive view of the LGB experience is to cultivate a sample that reflects the general population of the society in which the community is embedded. Race/ethnicity, socioeconomic status, gender, age and religious backgrounds should all be considered and evaluated, ideally as the sample is coming together. In this fashion, researchers may hope to capture as diverse a sample as is possible in order to address their research questions.

Since I was interested in understanding the experience of establishing a positive identity in the face of social stigma (that is, the internal coming-out process), I wanted to target people who self-identified with a label that designated them as other than heterosexual (for example, gay, lesbian, queer) and therefore targeted my sample to reflect the diversity within North American society writ large. Further, I was very interested in comparing the experiences of different age cohorts and knew that I would need diverse subsamples in each of the age categories that I settled on. I also wanted to evaluate the experiences of men and women within these age cohorts, and so further divided my subsamples into those two categories.

Challenges of international sampling

Difficulties establishing a sampling frame are only compounded when researchers begin to examine international experiences of LGB people. The expression of sexual orientation, like many aspects of identity, is mediated by culture. Individuals from different cultural backgrounds with similar experiences may view their sexual identities quite differently. Assaying international LGB communities can be a complex task. Despite this complexity, it has been argued that the internet may create previously unknown potential for a global bi-cultural experience (Arnett, 2002). Local cultures may now exist side by side with a global culture that may allow researchers to find common cultural ground between themselves and their subjects.

Language also plays an important role in cross-cultural/international sampling. Researchers must recognise that the language(s) of a survey will limit participation. Restricting the language of the survey may be a way to usefully narrow the sampling frame. Conversely, if you want to survey a society in which multiple languages are utilised, your survey should be available in multiple languages.

Beyond culture and language, legal and safety issues for participants may be of concern as well. In many nations same-sex attraction is criminalised (Office of the United Nations High Commissioner, 2012) and subjects may be putting themselves at risk simply by participating in research. Beyond the usual procedures for assuring privacy of data, it is incumbent upon the researcher to understand the potential risks of participating and to make them transparent to the participants. This includes, but is not limited to, encouraging participants who may be concerned about privacy to erase cookies and to clear their internet cache. Additionally, a researcher may be able to strip data of identifying information, including ISP identification numbers, but little can be done to ensure privacy of data that may be monitored as it is uploaded. In countries where homosexuality is criminalised, this may be an important concern.

Finally, another important limit to encouraging participation in internet surveying for any population is the goodness of fit with this method of data gathering. Some individuals may simply be reluctant to share personal information online. The perceived privacy that may encourage some participants will be a barrier to others. Alternative data gathering strategies should be developed for cultural groups that find internet surveying to be a barrier. Further, people who do not have access to a computer or internet will be ruled out of the study by default and are another important group to consider.

Encouraging participation from diverse quarters

Despite these barriers, researchers have several strategies at their disposal for maximising participation. Many studies have funding, which makes it possible to target online communities by purchasing advertisement space on web pages. Some researchers may have the support of the government behind them, perhaps increasing their legitimacy.

Researchers who are members of LGB communities have a careful decision to make about *outing* themselves or not. Sharing with participants that the researcher is a member of an LGB community can increase confidence in the hope that the research is legitimate and will not be used against the community. Some researchers who are more philosophically committed to the importance of the role of the researcher as neutral expert may find this suggestion problematic. These researchers may be concerned that sharing this information may bias the results. I would suggest that a carefully crafted survey can avoid bias by the rigour of its questions. Regardless, the outing of the researcher should be viewed as one option among many for increasing participation by LGB people.

While the one-way filter of the internet may provide a sense of discretion for the individual user, it has become clear that internet privacy is a relative term (see, for instance, American Civil Liberties Union, 2013). Regardless of the reality of internet privacy, the perception of privacy may increase the likeliness of internet use for people experiencing a degree of social stigma. In all stages of research with these populations, careful consideration of issues around privacy must be addressed. I would argue that a thorough and straightforward summary of how privacy is addressed in the survey can also increase participation by increasing confidence in the researcher. The vital need for maintaining participants' privacy should not be underestimated and it should be communicated clearly and openly to potential participants.

One final strategy for maximising participation of LGB populations is communicating with community leaders. In many cases it can be easier to convince an individual of the value of your research than to attempt to convince a group of people. When community leaders see the value of the research, you may then rely on their influence within the community to increase participation. It has been my experience that many leaders will actively participate in the distribution of survey materials and in a manner that efficiently targets their group better than the researcher could hope to. Community leaders should be carefully selected to maximise diversity within the sample and to target parts of the LGB community that are slow to respond to research.

In my study, the second round of recruitment was targeted to community leaders at 115 LGB community centres (both online and brick and mortar). This list was generated by investigating LGB community news sources and community web pages. Additionally, community centres that served groups that were under-represented in the sample were also selected for the second round of solicitation. The second plea was very similar to the first in tone and language. As a way to share information about the study, I developed a web page that included a running total of the number of participants by age category and gender. My hope was that by providing this information, it would encourage potential participants in hard-to-reach groups to complete the survey and to pass it on. When technical glitches necessitated that I resend mass emails to clarify what the problems were, I endeavoured to do this with as much grace as possible. In the end, I think the way that I handled these problems helped to instil more confidence in the participants. It also served to emphasise the pleas presence in their inboxes! In the end about 21% of all participants identified as non-White/European descent. Once the goal of 100 respondents (approximately 50 men and 50 women) in each of the target age cohorts was achieved, the survey was closed and the dataset ($n = 1,131$) was complete.

Ethical review boards

The final issue for consideration in maximising participation has to do with navigating potentially heteronormative Human Subject Review Boards (HSRBs). The important purpose of the HSRB process is to ensure the protection of human subjects who are participants in research. In the US, these bodies act as safeguards against abuses by researchers towards research participants who are designated 'vulnerable'. Vulnerable, in this case, indicates that they are not able to make free decisions about consent or may be unduly vulnerable to coercion. Children, prisoners, pregnant women, and people with impairment in their cognitive processes are examples of vulnerable populations. Additionally, the US Department of Health and Human Services (1993) charges that researchers minimise the risk to all participants and mediate risk where they can. The government guidelines go a step further to recommend heightened scrutiny for questions related to 'sexual practices, substance abuse, or illegal behavior' (1993) because these questions might cause the subject undue distress or otherwise put the subject at risk for public exposure.

Unfortunately, this important guideline may be interpreted by some HSRBs through a heteronormative lens. Do questions related to sexual identity (and not about sexual practices) cause undue distress to LGB people and merit extra scrutiny from review boards? Who decides what is an upsetting question and what standards do they apply? Is the question *'At what age did you first have a crush on a member of the opposite sex?'* more upsetting if it asked about a *crush on a member of the same sex*? If so, to whom? Extra scrutiny in the service of protecting research participants is an important aim, and one that should not unreasonably inhibit research about these vulnerable populations. Researchers querying LGB populations should be aware of the guidelines and laws that are designed to minimise risk to participants and be prepared to advocate for their projects if heteronormative standards are being applied. Researchers should be proactive with institutional review boards and provide accurate information about how sexual and gender minorities are viewed in their local regulations. Researchers might also find themselves in the position of needing to advocate for themselves (and by extension the people they are researching) and challenge heteronormative practices that might inhibit the development of research into the experiences of LGB people.

Because of my multiple affiliations at the time, my study went through three HSRBs with very different results. The first was a perfunctory expedited review. The questions in my survey were not viewed as troubling to participants and LGB adults were not viewed as a vulnerable population. The second was an expedited review with specific feedback on tightening the language of the survey and with a specific note that LGB people were not considered vulnerable populations. The final review was not expedited and involved some confusion on the question of whether or not LGB people were considered vulnerable populations. Consultation with the regulators at the national level cleared up this question, and resulted in the recommendation that I modify the survey to include online support resources for participants who might be troubled by questions about their sexual orientation. These supports included general resources such as the International Lesbian, Gay, Bisexual, Trans, and Intersex Association (www.ilga.org) and suicide intervention resources such as The Trevor Project (www.thetrevorproject.org). This extra scrutiny was troublesome at the time, but in the end, netted a stronger survey.

Limitations of the study

As with all research, my study was not perfect and had several limitations. One difficulty I encountered was balancing the desire to create a survey that was inclusive of all members of the LGB community while maintaining a focus on the coming-out experience. As the data were collected, I realised that the coming-out experience of trans respondents seemed more complex than my research design was able to evaluate. This seemed consistent with research on the experiences of trans people (see, for instance, Lev, 2004). Rather than dilute the input of the 59 trans-identified participants in the larger dataset, and in consultation with other researchers, their data were set aside for later analysis and subsequent publication.

With hindsight, another limitation to the study was neglecting to offer the survey in any language other than English. I was also not prepared for the survey to reach participants outside of the US. I was surprised when international responses began to come in ($n = 53$) and chagrined when I realised that the racial and/ethnic categories were very North America-centric. These respondents were included in the analysis.

A final limitation of my study was related to its greatest strength: the tailored design method. For some members of the LGB community the collaborative tone, the tailored design, of the plea and survey were offputting. I received feedback that the project did not inspire enough confidence in me as a researcher to garner participation. Gender and age cohort also became important cultural variables in the rate at which the survey was completed. While I did have adequate participation from each cohort to conduct analysis, the response rates were uneven (see Figure 15.2). In particular, women over the age of 60 seemed much less willing to complete the survey. Feedback that I received from members of this cohort seemed to indicate that participating in male-led research in an online format was a barrier for some of these members. Further, several social work researchers from this cohort noted that for this cultural group, a history of actively working against patriarchy for many years, might foster less confidence in an unknown male researcher.

Conclusion

One of the reasons for differences in healthcare outcomes between LGB people and heterosexuals is the often hidden and isolating nature of homophobia. Social inclusion is an important part of health. Also, when people are able to be open and clear about their experiences and needs, the possibility for competent healthcare is increased. In order to understand the nature of health inequalities for partially hidden populations such as LGB people, researchers must continue to develop strategies for eliciting participation from these sometimes hidden groups. This chapter argues for a thoughtful and strategic use of language in order to encourage participation. The use of collaborative research techniques can be an effective tool for increasing participation. Also, collaborating with community leaders can be an effective way to extend the call for participation to larger and more diverse groups. My study taught me that there is an enormous amount of good will towards researchers who seem competent, friendly and reasonable.

After a project is completed, researchers are also encouraged to complete the loop by sharing information with participants. In my case, this meant answering their questions about the study, interpreting findings alongside participants, and disseminating the findings along the same channels of communication that I distributed my pleas.

The project was very successful in several ways. A large number of people participated in the research ($n = 1,131$). The five open-ended questions embedded in the survey netted a large qualitative sample ($n = 870$). The study was successful as an example of my academic work and was the capstone of my degree. Further, the study received recognition for excellence in doctoral research by being awarded the Smith College Roger Miller Dissertation Grant for 2011. The final, and most meaningful, measure of success of my project was the feedback that I received from community leaders, other researchers and participants about the supportive and thought-provoking nature of the survey.

What we know about this already

• LGB people are a difficult population to research. Internet surveys are one way to sample these populations.

What this chapter adds
- It provides guidance about conducting internet research with LGB people. A tailored design method, which encourages participatory research, can enhance recruitment efforts with LGB populations.

How this is relevant for social work and LGBT health inequalities
- In order to understand the causes of health inequalities between LGB people and heterosexuals, we must be able to produce research that effectively samples this population.

References

American Civil Liberties Union, 2013, *Internet privacy*, www.aclu.org/technology-and-liberty/internet-privacy on 6/14/13

Arnett, JJ, 2002, 'The psychology of globalization', *American Psychologist*, 57, 10, 774-83

Cohler, BJ and Galatzer-Levy, R, 1996, 'Self psychology and homosexuality; Sexual orientation and maintenance of personal integrity', in RP Cabaj and TS Stein (eds), *Textbook of homosexuality and mental health*, Washington, DC: American Psychiatric Association, 207-23

Dillman, D, Smyth, J and Christian, LM, 2009, *Internet, mail and mixed-mode surveys: The tailored design method*, Hoboken, NJ: John Wiley and Sons

Douglas, Lord Alfred, 1894, *Two loves*, www.poets.org/viewmedia.php/prmMID/19366

Drasin, H, Beals, KP, Elliott, MN, Lever, J, Klein, DJ and Schuster, MA, 2008, 'Age cohort differences in the developmental milestones of gay men', *Journal of Homosexuality*, 54, 4, 381-99

Drewery, W, Winslade, J and Monk, G, 2000, 'Resisting the dominating story: Toward a deeper understanding of narrative therapy', in W Drewery, J Winslade and G Monk (eds), *Constructions of disorder: Meaning-making frameworks for psychotherapy*, Washington, DC: American Psychological Association

Dunlap, A, 2011, *Changes in the coming out process over time*, unpublished doctoral dissertation, Northampton, MA: Smith College School of Social Work

Elford, J, McKeown, E, Doemer, R, Nelson, S, Low, N and Anderson, J, 2010, 'Sexual health of ethnic minority MSM in Britain (MESH project): Design and methods', *BMC Public Health*, 10, 419

Gates, GJ and Newport, F, 2012, *Special report: 3.4% of US adults identify as LGBT*, www.gallup.com/poll/158066/special-report-adults-identiry-lgbt.aspx on 6/14/13

Harris Interactive, 2010, 'Gay and lesbian adults are more likely and more frequent blog readers', www.prnewswire.com/news-releases/gay-and-lesbian-adults-are-more-likely-and-more-frequent-blog-readers-98317299.html

Kinsey, AC, Pomeroy, WB and Martin, CE, 1948, *Sexual behavior in the human male*, Philadelphia, PA: W.B. Saunders

Lev, AI, 2004, *Transgender emergence: Therapeutic guidelines for working with gender-variant people and their families*, Binghamton, NY: Hawthorn Press

Lever, J, Grov, C, Royce, T and Gillespie, BJ, 2008, 'Searching for love in all the "write" places: Exploring internet personals use by sexual orientation, gender, and age', *International Journal of Sexual Health*, 20, 4, 233-46

Mohr, JJ and Fassinger, RE, 2000, 'Measuring dimensions of lesbian and gay male experience', *Measurement and Evaluation in Counseling and Development*, 33, 2, 66-90

Office of the United Nations High Commissioner for Human Rights, 2012, *Born free and equal: Sexual orientation and gender identity in international human rights law*, UN publication number HR/PUB/12/06, New York, NY: United Nations

Russell, ST and Joyner, K, 2001, 'Adolescent sexual orientation and suicide risk: Evidence from a national study', *American Journal of Public Health*, 91, 8, 1276-281

Shelton, K and Delgado-Romero, E, 2011, 'Sexual orientation microaggressions: The experience of lesbian, gay, bisexual, and queer clients in psychotherapy', *Journal of Counseling Psychology*, 58, 2, 210–21, doi: 10.1037/a0022251

United States Department of Health and Human Services, 1993, *Office of Human Research Protections: Institution Review Guidebook*, www.hhs.gov/ohrp/archive/irb/irb_guidebook.htm on 6/14/13

White, M and Epston, D, 1990, *Narrative means to therapeutic ends*, Adelaide, South Australia: Dulwich Centre

SIXTEEN

Gay and bisexual men raped by men: an invisible group in social work in Sweden

Hans Knutagård

Introduction: the phenomenon of male rape

Gay and bisexual men who have been raped by men are an invisible group in social work worldwide. Abdullah-Khan (2008, p 3) claims that through a 'combination of cultural, social, legal, and psychological issues, male rape remains one of the most unaddressed issues in our society'. The untreated experience of rape renders men silent and prevents them from their rightful access to health and social services, social inclusion and justice. For many men, it triggers a destructive trajectory, especially in the area of sexual behaviour. This chapter explores the phenomenon of male rape and considers the implications for sensitive interventions with this group of survivors in social work practice. The chapter argues that violence and lack of choice in sex or sexual relationships should be recognised as a health inequality. There is supporting evidence for this view. The World Health Organization acknowledges that:

> Sexual health requires a positive and respectful approach to sexuality and sexual relationships, as well as the possibility of having pleasurable and safe sexual experiences, free of coercion, discrimination and violence. For sexual health to be attained and maintained, the sexual rights of all persons must be respected, protected and fulfilled. (WHO, 2006, p 5)

Internationally, there is a growing number of English language research studies about men who are raped by men. Pioneering works include *Men behind bars: Sexual exploitation in prison* (Wooden and Parker, 1982). International research ranges from rape in the criminal justice system (Lehrer, 2001; Gear, 2007), in wartime (Stener Carlson, 1997;

DelZotto and Jones, 2002), among male college students (Scarce, 1997), sexual abuse and rape in various religious denominations (for example, John Jay Report, 2004) and sexual abuse and rape of gay men (Robertson, 2006). Few studies about this phenomenon were published in Sweden until 2013, with Knutagård (2009) being the first paper published in Swedish. What characterises all these studies is that:

- the abuse takes place in more or less closed groups, where men should expect to be protected;
- it is framed as a kind of a ritual, like a rite of passage;
- it involves the lack of access to health and social services for men, a health inequality.

Knowing about the circumstances and events surrounding male rape helps us to comprehend men's experiences.

In my 30-year career as a professional social worker I have met men (straight, gay and bisexual) who have been raped by men. This study focuses on gay and bisexual men. These men have also appeared, but only in the margins, in other studies that I have conducted in recent years about sexuality in social work. For instance, I have studied gay victims of hate crimes (Knutagård, 2003), honour-related violence against young people because of their sexual orientation (Knutagård and Nidsjö, 2004) and men who sell sex to other men via the internet (Eriksson and Knutagård, 2005). The different studies, as well as the various individual life histories, are linked to each other in numerous ways. I then decided to focus on this vulnerable group in a separate study (Knutagård, 2009), which serves as the basis for this chapter. This study involved 18 qualitative semi-structured interviews with victims of non-consensual sex (I contacted 28 men, but 10 of them decided not to proceed with an interview after an initial conversation). The oldest was 70 years and the youngest 20. In addition, I conducted written interviews with another five men and the data are also reported here, bringing the total sample to 23 men. But let us first look at what rape means.

Introducing the concept of 'rape'

Male rape challenges common understandings of rape. Until 1984 in Sweden, rape was considered to be the forcible carnal knowledge of a woman by a man. A man could therefore not be raped. This is still the case, for example, in the State of Israel. In current Swedish law, it is possible to rape a man. Rape is regulated by the Penal Code, Chapter 6, which provides that a person shall be sentenced for rape 'who by violence or threat which involves, or appears to the threatened person to involve an imminent danger, forces another person to have sexual intercourse or to engage in a comparable sexual act' (Swedish Statute Book, 2013, p 365). England and Wales use the concept of 'rape' and include male victims within the purview of the Sexual Offences Act 2003. While the Canadian Criminal Code does not use the term 'rape', the law uses the concept of 'sexual assault' to include a variety of acts, from unwanted sexual touching to forced penetration. By contrast, the United States (US) has no national rape or sexual assault law, as these crimes are defined at the state level. The new anti-gay laws of 2013 in Russia, make it nearly impossible for citizens to report male rape.

In Sweden, there are currently discussions of how to define rape as 'without that person's consent' and of what constitutes penetration (for example, does it include a male perpetrator performing oral sex on a male victim). The absence of a universal agreement on these and other terms renders the use of the term 'rape' as problematic, nationally and internationally. This is particularly the case when same-sex male rape is being discussed. Feminist researcher, Liz Kelly (1988), has been influential in empowering women to name their own experiences and in framing broad questions about sexual violence. In a similar vein, I pose the question, 'have you been a victim of non-consensual sex or sexual violence?' and thus take the participant's meanings of rape as the starting point of my research. In the study I found that rape is embedded in Western society's social construction in three areas: masculinities, sexualities and homosexuality, which I will explain below.

Masculinities

I have found Collins' (2005) concept of 'interaction ritual chains' helpful in acquiring an understanding of the phenomenon of male rape. Using a theoretical approach, he describes a process whereby a person develops culturally, as well as sexually, first on a social level and then on an individual level. I argue that the person experiences the event as a link in a ritual chain, with the raped man becoming a product of previous interactions of masculinities.

During the interviews, each of the respondents was unable to find words for the experiences they had gone through, as Hampus' story reveals: Hampus (a pseudonym), one of the respondents, told me about something that happened to him when he was 15 years old and living in a small town in Sweden. He had been bullied as a young boy because he was overweight. He lost weight by playing soccer, and became like all his classmates, except that he was sexually attracted to other boys. When his classmates in high school each described how they lost their virginity and how fabulous this experience was, Hampus felt an increasing urge to have his first experience of sexual intercourse. Due to the stigma of being a young gay man in a small town, he could not share his feelings for boys with his friends, nor seek a boyfriend among them. He felt trapped. Instead he started to use different gay communities on the internet for dating, and soon he found a man who claimed to be about his age. They chatted for a couple of months before they decided to meet in a grove near Hampus' home.

Once there, Hampus discovered that the man was 20 years older than he had claimed to be, but Hampus was determined to "lose his virginity", as he said in the interview. The men took off their clothes and they fondled and kissed. Suddenly the man changed his behaviour and threw Hampus to the ground and started to penetrate him harshly, while shouting humiliations in his ear. "It was very painful," Hampus said, and he cut off his emotions as he had trained himself to do all the years when he had been bullied. Hampus was ambivalent about his feelings after the incident, as it should have been, but was not, the fabulous experience of sexual intercourse his friends had talked about. He described, to me, that he went home, had no appetite, could not sleep and felt depressed. The next day his sister telephoned him. Hampus, who had a close friendship with her, told her that he had had his first sexual experience. "You don't sound happy about that," she said. Hampus told her what had happened and she said tearfully: "but you've been raped".

Since the concept 'men who have been raped by men' is not included in mainstream discourse in Sweden, the phenomenon does not exist in world of the men in the study. Social constructions of masculinities posit that men can penetrate but not be penetrated, and consequently, cannot be raped. The language at their disposal did not help them to describe, or to come to terms with, their experiences: 'What is not named is invisible and, in a social sense, non–existent' (Kelly, 1988, p 114). The men in the study, as Hampus, were unable to protect themselves or seek help, as they could not explain what had happened and found themselves in a vulnerable position. Some will argue that Hampus had not been raped as he wanted to have sex. No stranger attacked him or threatened to kill him. However, the 'date rape' that Hampus experienced is actually the most common form of rape (Scarce, 1997).

A common reaction expressed on the topic of male rape is why the victim did not fight back, as 'violence is often the most evident marker of manhood' (Kimmel, 2005, p 278). Instead, the men I interviewed experienced what Rentoul and Appleboom (1997, p 270) have described as 'frozen helplessness and submission'. Gabriel said in the interview:

> 'I was very aware. When I lay there, it's like I'm asleep or dead. Inside, a process is going on. It feels like there's just a big room from your toes up to your head and where it bounces off things. It's not like there are any bones, guts or such things. Then there are just feelings, thoughts, emotions, things like that just flying around everywhere in the body. Then you have your eyes. I closed my eyes, but it feels like they were seeing anyway. I wanted to tear him to pieces. Be angry, and react by hitting him in the face, whatever, but I didn't. Actually, *I couldn't.*'

Gabriel described the feeling of being both totally powerless and dominated and also being unable to communicate. This experience challenged the men's idea about their own masculinity.

Let me interpose an interesting perspective that Collins (2008, p 83) adds by introducing the notion of 'forward panic'. The concept derives from the panic that makes soldiers run away during war, but also makes them run forward towards the enemy. The soldiers go into an emotional tunnel of violent attack, which occurs in an atmosphere of superiority. As a result of the perpetrator's sudden attack, known as an asymmetric synchronisation, the victim is paralysed, as Gabriel's story shows. Collins uses an historical example to illustrate the concept. At the Battle of the Granicus in 334 BC, the Macedonians trapped the Persians' mercenary infantry. The latter were 'rooted to the spot by the unexpected catastrophe rather than from being out-manoeuvred' and this 'is a phenomenon reported time and again from battlefields: the rabbit-like paralysis of soldiers in the face of a predator's unanticipated onslaught. They were soon surrounded and hacked down on the spot' (Collins, 2008, p 103). This passivity, by the men in the study, contradicts the core of their masculinities, since this puts the men in what might be described as an effeminate position.

Applying the same concept to male rape, the perpetrator's dominance ruptures the victim's manhood. Research shows that 'male rape is used by the perpetrator to enhance his own masculinity, which is done by exerting power and control over another man' (Abdullah-Khan, 2008, p 221). This is a social interaction with a dominant and a subordinate: the relationship is composed of two elements, as 'it occurs through emotional processes that pump some individuals up while depressing others' (Collins, 2005, p xiii). Because hegemonic masculinity has been associated with power and dominance, when a man is unable to defend himself or is overpowered, his self-concept as a man is questioned and he may believe that he is less of a man and therefore effeminate. Such beliefs may lead a man to question his sexuality or sexual orientation.

Gender and power are therefore important elements in the social construction of masculinities, a dynamic process that is constantly shifting and in motion. I found that paramount to understanding male rape are the ways these perceptions of masculinities are developed and how men perceive themselves. These perceptions include male invulnerability, male superiority, male violent and aggressive behaviour and homophobia. Consequently, 'the construction of masculinity is central to understanding male rape because the problem of rape is a problem of masculinity' (Abdullah-Khan, 2008, p 71). In these cases, 'the gendering of men only exists in the intersections with other social divisions and social differences' (Connell et al, 2005, p 3), like age, class, ethnicity, sexuality and ability.

Research shows that dominant masculinity sees homosexuality as a threat and as a double defining action, the homophobic performance of men 'consolidates the heterosexual masculinity of Self and the homosexual femininity of Other' (Kehily and Nayak, 1997, p 82). Therefore we have to understand that 'homophobia is a foundational factor in the formation of masculine identities' (Mac an Ghaill and Haywood, 2012a, p 76). Gay survivors I interviewed experience the antithesis of masculinities, since 'if men are expected to be masculine and thereby powerful, dominant, and in control, they cannot be discursively produced as victims (Sundaram et al, 2004, p 66).

Sexuality

The concept 'sexuality' is a complex notion, often understood as the experience of our body, desires and pleasures, as well as our sexual identity. It is closely intertwined with sex and gender. Most of us have an image of how to engage in sexual behaviour by proceeding step by step, like a ritual guided by scripts, to hugging, kissing, caressing and so on. Sexual scripts (Gagnon and Simon, 2005) can be described as internalised social conventions that make us think and act in a certain way when it comes to sexual practice. They consist of intrapsychic, interpersonal and cultural scripts that intertwine like a cord of three strands.

Most of the men in the study believed they knew about sexual activity through previous conventional sexual scripts. Instead, they now faced an unexpected break in that script. Isaac, aged 70, described his experience as a 24-year-old man for the first time in a large European city:

> 'I was really romantic and stupid, naive and innocent, when I was younger. I saw a guy on a street who made contact with me. I jumped on the bandwagon. I thought it was all about love. We had a beer and then we went up to my little room at the hotel and undressed. He raped me straight away. It really hurt. I was totally shocked that he could do so. I had no thoughts that it could happen. What I experienced then was the degradation and humiliation inherent in his lack of respect for me when I said, "NO". This experience hurts. This is not fun. This is not what I want. This is being subjected to violence. It is not love. I believe that sex and love between two people means hugging and kissing and caressing and having sex. Rape is just the opposite. In addition to this, you lower the guard, and open to the other, in all ways, physically as well as mentally. So the other bastard used this to injure me, to get something I didn't want to give him.' (Isaac)

Isaac's response is typical: his expectation of love was violated. There was no clue about what was going to happen. The break of sexual scripts is so powerful and seemed to hit the respondents at their core of identity, in their trust towards other people. Daniel stated: "I don't trust anyone. I didn't trust my family and so I left them long ago. I don't trust my boyfriend." Their life trajectories became self-destructive. In addition, their perception of time and place was affected. They experienced blackouts, difficulties in relating to people, the need to be in control, a sense of detachment from people and emotional and physical withdrawal.

It becomes particularly shameful to ejaculate during rape. Adam said:

> 'I've always felt tremendous guilt just because he made me come. If you have sex with someone, then a part of it is that the person probably gets satisfaction. We know that those who get satisfied provide some kind of confirmation. If you do so in such a situation, it becomes cruel. It's not what you want. It felt like a pain, because he made me come. I felt

like it shouldn't be that way. Afterwards, I learned that it's actually just a chemical reaction, that whether you're tied or nailed, you can probably get an erection. So that does not imply that you feel something for the other person. It's just a physical response, not an emotional response. That's how you have to think. That's how I have to think. I can't think of any other way.' (Adam)

Adam had to remind himself a few times that it was just a physical response. Because male ejaculation is linked to sexual gratification, he felt that his desires and emotions were involved in the rape. Rentoul and Appleboom (1997, p 270) state: 'research demonstrates that getting the victim to ejaculate is a major strategy, which symbolises the extent of the offender's sexual control over the victim'. Rape, as we know, is not about sex: it is about power. Sam put it this way: "For some reason he thought I was excited that he hit me, he hit even more and even harder and even started to bite me while he ripped and tore my clothes." The same feeling was experienced by Neo who got raped in a same-sex relationship over five years, but felt he "had to take it in order to be loved". The violence victims experience is later turned inward.

Homosexuality

One consequence of the rape for men in the study was that their sexual orientation became a source of stigma, discrimination, taboo and shame. Rubin (2007/1984) claims that there is a sex hierarchy, where homosexuals are in the outer part of the circle with 'damned sexuality', like the respondents, instead of being in the inner part with 'blessed sexuality', where heterosexuals are located. Connected to 'damned sexuality' is the use of rape myths, where the men in the study described a stigmatising 'myth' that if a man gets raped it is because he likes it, which makes him a de facto homosexual. Although the perpetrator's sexual identity may be questioned, because he retains the power and dominance, his identity is not threatened to the same degree. However, research from the US and England shows that, on the contrary, most perpetrators are heterosexuals and that the survivors are fragile heterosexuals or homosexuals (Mezey and King, 2004).

In the interviews, the gay and bisexual men felt society's condemnation and stigmatisation of homosexuality and some of them did not want to 'come out of the closet'. For example, Eddie, after having been raped, was so afraid of being discovered as a homosexual that he married, had children, separated and started to live more and more isolated for 30 years until I interviewed him. "I did not talk to anybody about it. None of my friends knew anything about it. As a matter of fact, my whole life was changed that moment." Eddie mentioned the stigmatisation of homosexuals in society as a reason why he could not say he was raped, because in doing so he would have also come out as gay to his parents.

> 'I didn't dare say anything then either. Thirty years ago, it was a shame. Because I know, mom has a cousin who was [gay], and there was never anyone who talked about him and no one hung out with him or anything. It's the reason why I don't want to talk about me being gay. Because I knew that I would be excluded. Then, my whole family would exclude me and my siblings and all. Because I knew what they thought about it.' (Eddie)

The respondents reported feeling intense guilt about being a gay or bisexual man. One man who contacted me over the internet wrote:

> Tom wrote: I was raped by a guy on my thirteenth birthday

> *Hans wrote: Is this something you are able to talk about? Have you reported and searched for help?*

> Tom wrote: No way, didn't dare to report to the Police because then my dad would know that I am gay, so I kept quiet about it.

This young boy felt more fear of his father finding out he is gay, then the knowledge of the rape itself. Time and again the fear of someone else knowing one is a homosexual was revealed in the interviews. Because of this, the respondents could not process their experiences of rape by seeking professional help. The social oppression that the men were embedded in made them therefore invisible in the public sphere.

Still invisible and without words

To conclude, the shame of rape due to the stigma of homosexuality drove some of the respondents to practise unsafe sex, to cut themselves and to develop eating disorders. Many of these symptoms could be related to post-traumatic stress disorder, but are not disclosed since the trauma of rape is never mentioned (Ruchkin et al, 1998). In addition, the internalised shame prevents the men from talking about the rape, reporting it or to seeking help and support. There seems to be a reciprocal connection between society's lack of words and the respondents' vulnerability. Only two of the 23 respondents had reported the rape incident to the police. Five of the men sought and received help after a number of failed attempts along the way. The other 18 had never sought help.

The impact on men's lives of not seeking help is exemplified by Timmy's experience. He is 27 years old, was raped, sold sex to other men, served time in a juvenile detention centre, was the target of hate crimes due to his being gay and is now HIV-positive. During the interview, he stated that the worst aspect for him was the untreated anxiety from being raped. He struggled with the shame of it and all the questions. What did I do? Am I worth anything? Am I so sexually violated that there is no reason to live? By addressing the trauma of male rape, the social worker is then able to provide support for other social and health problems.

What can we do as social workers? We have to start making male rape visible and put it on the national and international agenda. This will facilitate a discourse for men and enable them to articulate their experiences. We also have to provide a good health service, social inclusion and social justice for male survivors. Doing so, requires us to challenge the stigmatisation and discrimination that are associated with male rape and homosexuality. For example, Mac an Ghaill and Haywood (2012b, p 581) argue that a shift to a 'broader cultural perception of homosexuality is leading to a recalibration of masculinities that is based upon inclusivity'. Therefore we have to develop non-oppressive social work practices that are inclusive of LGBT people. In order to accomplish this, many social workers need training in developing *attitudes* (for example, reflecting on one's own sexual orientation), greater *knowledge* in relation to LGBT people and enhanced *skills*, such as in creating an LGBT-friendly environment (Fish, 2012). In the longer term, we must take part in the work of reconstructing masculinities.

In Sweden, the national resource for men who have been raped by men is located at the National Centre for Knowledge on Men's Violence against Women, Uppsala University. This institution highlights the contradictions and barriers faced in Sweden in recognising men as victims. There are, as yet, no non-governmental organisations targeting this group of men, as there are in England or the US, and local social work and health services have not developed any relevant resources. Men, especially gay and bisexual men, who are raped by men are indeed an invisible group in Sweden and, unfortunately, in many other countries as well.

What we know about this already
- Gay and bisexual men raped by men are an invisible group.
- They rarely seek or receive help, and this is still an unaddressed issue in social work.

What this chapter adds
- Social work and health practices with this group of survivors could use the concepts of 'interaction ritual chains' and 'sexual scripts' in order to address issues relating to masculinities, sexuality and homosexuality.

How this is relevant for social work and LGBT health inequalities
- Due to stigmatisation and discrimination, LGBT people need non-oppressive social work practices that provide support and help.

References

Abdullah-Khan, N, 2008, *Male rape: The emergence of a social and legal issue*, Hampshire and New York: Palgrave Macmillan

Connell, RW, Hearn, J and Kimmel, MS, 2005, Introduction, in MS Kimmel, J Hearn and RW Connell (eds), *Handbook of studies on men and masculinities*, Thousand Oaks, CA: Sage Publications.

Collins, R, 2005, *Interaction Ritual Chains*, Princeton, NJ: Princeton University Press

Collins, R, 2008, *Violence: A micro-sociological theory*, Princeton, NJ: Princeton University Press

DelZotto, A and Jones, A, 2002, *Male-on-male sexual violence in wartime: Human rights' last taboo?*, Paper presented to the Annual Convention of the International Studies Association (ISA), New Orleans, LA, 23–27 March

Eriksson, N and Knutagård, H, 2005, *Sixmenselling.se/x. – pleasure becomes functional*, (in Swedish) Malmö: RFSL Rådgivningen Skåne.

Fish, J, 2012, *Social work and lesbian, gay, bisexual and trans people: Making a difference*, Bristol: Policy Press

Gagnon, JH and Simon, W, 2005, *Sexual conduct: The social sources of human sexuality*, New Brunswick and London: Aldine Transaction

Gear, S, 2007, 'Behind the bars of masculinity: male rape and homophobia in and about South African men's prisons', *Sexualities*, 10, 2, 209-27

John Jay Report, 2004, *The nature and scope of sexual abuse of minors by catholic priest and deacons in United States 1950-2002*, The John Jay College of Criminal Justice, The City University of New York, Washington DC: United States Conference of Catholic Bishops

Kehily, MJ and Nayak, A, 1997, 'Lads and laughter: Humour and production of heterosexual hierarchies', *Gender and Education*, 9, 69-87

Kelly, L, 1988, 'How women define their experiences of violence', in K Yllö and M Bograd (eds) *Feminist perspectives on wife abuse*, Newbury Park, CA: Sage Publications

Kimmel, MS, 2005, 'Masculinity as homophobia: Fear, shame, and silence in the construction of gender identity', in SM Whithead and FJ Barrett, *The masculinities reader*, Cambridge: Polity Press

Knutagård, H, 2003, *"... It was just a fagot". Towards a strategy to prevent and counteract hostile gay violence*, (in Swedish) Rapportserie 2003:1. Malmö: RFSL Rådgivningen Skåne

Knutagård, H and Nidsjö, E, 2004, *Honour-related violence against young people because of their sexual orientation*, (in Swedish) Skåne i utveckling 2004:24. Malmö: Länsstyrelsen i Skåne län

Knutagård, H, 2009, *"But you have been raped" – about the lack of words for men who have been raped*, Lund: Lund University

Lehrer, E, 2001, 'Hell behind bars', *National Review*, February 5

Mac an Ghaill, M and Haywood, C, 2012a, 'The queer in masculinity: schooling, boys, and identity formation', in JC Landreau and N Rodriguez (eds), *Queer masculinities: A critical reader in education*, New York, NY: NYU Press

Mac an Ghaill, M and Haywood, C, 2012b, 'What next for masculinity? Reflexive directions for theory and research on masculinity and education', *Gender and Education*, 24, 6, 577-92

Mezey, GC and King, MB, 2004, *Male victims of sexual assault* (2nd ed), Oxford: Oxford University Press

Rentoul, L and Appleboom, N, 1997, 'Understanding the psychological impact of rape and serious sexual assault of men: a literature review', *Journal of Psychiatric and Mental Health Nursing*, 4, 267-74

Robertson, S, 2006, 'Boys, of course, cannot be raped: age, homosexuality and the redefinition of sexual violence in New York City, 1880–1955', *Gender & History*, 18, 2, 357-79

Rubin, GS, 2007/1984, 'Thinking sex: notes for a radical politics of sexuality', in R Parker and P Aggleton, *Culture, society and sexuality. A reader*, London and New York: Routledge

Ruchkin, VV, Eisemann, M and Hägglöf, B, 1998, J'uvenile male rape victims: is the level of post-traumatic stress related to personality and parenting?', *Child Abuse & Neglect*, 22, 9, 889-99

Scarce, M, 1997, 'Same-sex rape of male college students', *Journal of American College Health*, Section: Clinical & Program Notes

Stener Carlson, E, 1997, 'Sexual assault on men in war', *Lancet*, January 11, Section: Health and Human Rights

Sundaram, V, Helweg-Larsen, K, Laursen, B and Bjerregaard, P, 2004, 'Physical violence, self rated health, and morbidity: is gender significant for victimisation?', *Journal of Epidemiology and Community Health*, 58, 65-70

Swedish Statute Book 2013: 365 Amendments to the Criminal Code, Stockholm: Department of Justice

Wooden, WS and Parker, J, 1982, *Men behind bars: Sexual exploitation in prison*, New York, NY: Da Capo Press

WHO (World Health Organization), 2006, *Defining sexual health*, Report of a technical consultation on sexual health, 28–31 January 2002, Geneva

Queering social work methods in health disparities and health promotion in the United States

Tyler M. Argüello

Introduction

Identity-based interventions continue to dominate social work's involvement with queer (male) publics. Ironically, queer publics are not readily contained in many dominant categories available to health research and clinical practice, as these publics are indefinite networks of variously identified and behaving men. Within a critical frame, queer publics – or 'counterpublics' – are not static; instead they are produced discursively. Counterpublics exist always in relation to dominant culture, and are evidenced through mediated communication. Accordingly, the objects of communication, rather than its privileged subjects, deserve increased attention in health promotion and -disparities research. This requires a transdisciplinary approach, one that can account for communicative practices while simultaneously making them accountable to the ideological work that they do in lived- and shared experiences. To that end, presented herein is a methodology animated by commitments to social justice and critical theory, and architected through two interrelated critical communication methodologies: critical discourse analysis and social semiotics. This transdisciplinary approach apprehends how micro processes normalise and produce meanings for macro social processes. One case study is provided as an example of this methodology deployed in the field of HIV prevention.

Theoretical framework for LGBT health and social care

Just as the transmission of HIV involves varying amounts of human agency, so do the processes of developing knowledge and distributing information about the pandemic from 'us professionals' to 'those people out there' in the social world. Health communication is predicated on production and promotion; the production relates to the *how*, the processes of making discourse, and the *promotion* is the *what*, or the discourse itself. In other words, the production and promotion of health (from incipient ideas through the evaluation of goods and services) involve authority, discriminating choices, access and, especially in the case of HIV/AIDS, outcomes related to the quality and sustainability of life proper. Simply, health promotion and production involve power – and, more critically, *biopower* or technologies through the human body – and have influence over ways of thinking, self-identification and ways of behaving in social and sexual contexts (Foucault, 1978, 1985, 1986).

Gay men and men who have sex with men (MSM) continue to evince disproportionate rates of HIV infection across the world, and, therefore, receive targeted attention by health authorities. Ironically, such *publics* are not readily contained in many prevailing dominant categories available to health research, which rely heavily on identitarian-based, behaviourally entrenched, and essentialising notions of sex/uality, gender and health status: gay/straight, male/female, top/bottom, HIV-negative/-positive. In fact, there exists no easily identifiable demo- or psycho-graphic that cements securely our knowledge of one's sex/uality and gender and, in turn, eschews doubt in regards to risk.

Alternatively, *queer publics – or counterpublics –* can be better understood as discursive, that is, produced in discourse (Warner, 2002). Within a critical frame, queer publics are indefinite networks of strangers connected through and evidenced by mediated communication, such as words, icons, aesthetics, webpages and the built environment. For example, via smartphone applications for social/sexual networking, queer men simultaneously construct real-world connections *as well as* a network of fellow 'queer' men. And, this ideological and material communication is mediated by the app itself, utilising the multiple components of (mediated) communication and technology. As such, it is the representation, dissemination and repetition of knowledge and information about sex/uality and gender through mediated communication that provides the channels and opportunities with which individuals and communities self-/identify and (sexually) network. This is also always under constraint, as queer publics continuously sit in opposition to the oppressive disciplining of mainstream public spheres. In order to know what or who is 'queer', therefore, requires increased attention to the *objects* of media, rather than predominantly the subjects; the former of which is the stuff that constructs communication, the latter of which are the self-proclaimed or imposed social locations within a given culture that people perform.

Research problem

HIV has become a singularly powerful mediated object that articulates queer; and queer has become an integral part of the matrix of institutional and linguistic discourses wherever 'HIV' is. Thus, queer and HIV discursively as well as materially continually re-infect each other at each keystroke, utterance, representation and deployment of material resources by everyday people and privileged healthcare professionals. The social implications and consequent behaviours of this synergising relationship are minimally understood.

Simultaneously, the globalising world has become increasingly *technologised* and *semioticised*, that is, infused with, constituted by and reliant on multi-media and their varied content, networks, formats and discourses (Appadurai, 1996; Fairclough, 1999; Kress and van Leeuwen, 2006). *What* and *how* we communicate is of utmost importance in public and private lives. Mass and interpersonal communication involve multiple material resources, which develop and sustain connections and multiplicities of relationships within/-out social networks. Examples of these material resources include visual symbols, written and spoken language, sounds, way-finding signs, photographs and advertisements.

In critical language and visual studies terms, these material resources can be understood as *semiotic resources*. In fact, semiotic resources are central to the functioning of our post-Fordist society (opposed to our mass production labour society of previous generations), where signs/symbols, information itself, their packaging and their management are of great import in sustaining modern life and new capitalism (Fairclough, 2003). Therefore, *semiotics*, or the *science of signs*, focuses much deserved investigation on the basic building blocks of everyday modern life and communication: semiotics structure societal systems, construct identities, build public spheres, disseminate knowledge, map material and notional communities, and transmit ideologies. This empirical attention becomes especially important when considering health, wellbeing and life itself.

In the case of AIDS, across social work and the health sciences, semiotics and their analyses are overlooked as a site for theorising and intervention. The rapid formation and now dominance of the HIV industry materialised in an effort to cope with the intelligence of the virus. In prior days, medical doctors and dying patients provided a potent understanding of the virus and attendant technologies. Today, however, this industry is itself power, and is often only made apparent to nations and citizens through the mass circulation of health information in service of dominant notions of best practices, constructed by public authorities. Given this, the HIV industry can *do* many things – the most important of which is to brand, market and permeate the (social) world with what we know to be HIV. Quite crucially, this industry has the predominant power/privilege to mediate the relationship between HIV and the everyday person.

The Centers for Disease Control and Prevention (CDC) in the United States (US) (CDC, 2006, 2008, 2011) have published guidelines to re-/combat HIV, citing behaviour as the enduring principal risk factor. This is accompanied by other 'complex factors' that induce risk, such as an ageing MSM population, complacency, lack of experiencing real-time death by AIDS, stigma, homophobia and substance abuse. These factors are positioned as common-sense reasons for the seeming inadequate self-policing of individuals and communities to adopt recommended preventive technologies – and thus control the pandemic.

Accordingly, the CDC (2012) has recommended citizens to 'be smart about HIV': get facts, reduce one's risk, get tested and start talking about HIV. Guided by the National HIV/AIDS Strategy (NHAS; ONAP, 2010), the US has begun an aggressive structural focus on 'high-impact' HIV prevention, directing attention to cost-effective, feasible, scalable and impactful strategies. These efforts prioritise increased surveillance, expanded pre-exposure prophylaxis and testing for MSM, increased access to treatment and linkage to care, and the reduction of HIV stigma. These strategies continue to centralise around individual responsibilities, capacities and subjectivities – while at the same time, de-emphasising operative socioeconomic, environmental and other cultural factors that impact communities' abilities to prevent and/or cope with HIV. Incidentally, the HIV industry continues to be *less* accountable to the production and dissemination of knowledge, interventions and the neoliberal branding of the epidemic. And, structural changes that have the potential for greater impact and more institutionalised change at a population level are de-privileged and de-emphasised (Prado et al, 2013).

Given our express mission, social work is an optimal site to decentre the power/privilege of the HIV industry. Health promotion deserves increased critical analysis in order to apprehend the social forces that impregnate HIV and our communication. From a social work perspective, we can ask the long-overdue question of how *we*, privileged healthcare professionals, might in fact be contributing to the enduring epidemic. Within such a frame, the attention turns away from continuing to overburden targeted subjects, such as queer men and black and minority ethnic people, synonymising 'risk' with identity and perceived attendant (sexual) behaviours. Instead, this focus reorients the (clinical and research) gaze towards the operations of power/privilege, the processes of marginalisation, the production of inequality and the construction of risk within the environments in which various oppressed populations live.

As this chapter is being written in 2013, initiatives in the US are beginning to recognise language and culture as fundamental elements of health justice. The National Standards for Culturally and Linguistically Appropriate Services (CLAS) in Health and Health Care (OMH, 2013) are guidelines that are intended to advance health equity, improve service quality and help eliminate disparities by establishing a 'blueprint' to providing effective and respectful quality health services – responsive to diverse cultural health beliefs, practices, languages and health literacy. In particular, the CLAS standards foreground gender and sex/uality as imperative cultural aspects related to health, as well as provide a directive to partner with communities, conduct formative research and integrate culturally and linguistically appropriate content into healthcare. These standards reinforce the findings in this chapter that the development of communicative practices – and, therefore, the production of culture and health – require attention to all health professionals' knowledge-building, interventions and consequent health outcomes.

Practice aimed at making a difference in LGBT people's health and social outcomes

As one of the first social semiotic studies in social welfare, this project sought to intervene at the level of knowledge production about HIV through analysis of an exemplary semiotic site of mediated communication. The purpose herein is to interrogate how an object, like HIV, is made to become a subject by health and business professionals, and then obliged to discursively infect various subject positions, such as (young) queer men. This was accomplished by examining the production of discourse from the point of view of the object of HIV itself, rather than from the point of view of 'risky' subjects.

Methodology

Harnessing a queer methodology (Perry-Argüello, 2008), media objects that give the virus life in discourse were systematically examined, apprehending how micro processes (that is, language, visual symbols) normalise meanings for macro social processes (that is, HIV prevention, social identities). The work is labelled *queer* as it assumes HIV is already in all of us – since HIV is also a matter of discourse, not just biology. The methodology at large is named *social semiotic*, yoking together critical commitments in social welfare, textual criticism and visual analysis. Pragmatically, this transdisciplinary approach blends two interrelated methodologies: critical discourse analysis (CDA; Fairclough, 2003) and social semiotics (SS; Kress and van Leeuwen, 2006). In tandem, CDA and SS liberate germane assumptions of what texts and signs are, and interrogate the dialectical relations between texts and contexts.

In the contemporary, increasingly globalising, consumer-oriented world, language is an important societal institution as much as a resource that can be harnessed to exert influence in social practices aligned with the dominant social (Fairclough, 1999). At its core, SS has a goal to uncover the hidden agendas of ideology at work in texts (Cameron, 2001). In this sense, ideology is not simply a descriptive account of values and beliefs; rather, ideology is viewed as 'representations of the world which establish and maintain social relations of power and dominance and exploitation' (Fairclough, 2003, p 9). Therefore, in this method, it is common to seek to reveal *processes* and demystify *how* certain representations are positioned to be *neutral* and *normal*, and through their repetition over time and across multiple texts, they are *naturalised* into the common-sense notions and the social order that are talked about and promoted to consumers. Moreover, it is assumed that texts are not haphazardly constructed nor their discourses random in ideological patterning; rather, they are constructed through the un-/conscious choices of the professionals who produce and promote them.

The case study presented here made *media* about HIV and young queer life a problem, that is, investigated their inherent discursivity (Perry-Argüello, 2008). In the case of HIV, the *process* of mediatisation makes the virus and our knowledge thereof intelligible, consumerable, and transmittable in everyday life. The post-structurally inspired suffix '*-isation*' connotes a critical analysis of the object being modified (Schulz, 2004), going beyond representation and instead tending to the *reproductions* of social meaning, from incipient idea through consumption. To public authorities, these processes of knowledge disseminate knowledge to the citizenry. For individuals and communities, these processes are means to advocate for services, contest knowledge and mobilise resistance. For critical researchers, due to the dialectical nature of semiotic resources (for example language) and social practice, these analytics set the well-intentioned practices of the HIV industry against the unequally distributed stakes of economic and social life, and therefore work to expose the inner workings of (bio-)power and the 'texturing' of social processes (Thurlow and Jaworski, 2006).

Critical case study: the mediatisation of HIV

The avid use of multiple media, saturation of technologies into diverse lifestyles, alarming rates of HIV re-/infection and a reciprocally penetrating relationship between media and sex/uality in the information age make a focus on prevention *through* media important for young people, especially those who are queer. Singular media prevention campaigns are limited in their effectiveness, resulting in minimal curbing of re-/infections (KFF, 2006). Instead, given the cultural salience of AIDS, everyday communication practices are a productive site for intervention.

Considered here was 'infotainment' media that seeks to create a 'new' lifestyle of young queer people. The media derive from the first two mass-marketed and widely available print publications for young queer people in North America. The infotainment genre symbolises more honed marketing practices focused on niche audiences, and signifies an increasing choice for citizens to consume media more resonant with their lifestyles. (For example, infotainment media has long existed for young women, such as *Seventeen*, *TeenVOGUE*). Consequently, infotainment can be regarded as a democratisation of media in that its circulation signifies people and social practices that have not been previously allowed or represented in the public sphere. It is simultaneously a validation of marginalised cultures and a reflexive construction of an audience through its very circulation (Fairclough, 1995).

Moreover, the consistency of this infotainment genre serves to build credibility and reliability, as well as normativises and obliges the consumers to view as *normal* the characteristics of *who* and *what* is the 'authentic' young sexual subject. Ironically, the genre denies (through un-/conscious omission) variations in thought, lifestyles and other social practices. Simply stated, the distinctive aesthetic of this genre is, at once, innovative and implicitly privileges a particular young lifestyle. For example, the chaotically stylised layout does not depict an *actual* diversity of content and a diverse gay community, rather it portrays an 'appearance of diversity' (Aiello, 2007); the heavy use of photographs of young people trends towards middle class, cisgender, white young men (see Photographs 17.1 to 17.3). Through the power of editorial and creative discretion, consumers receive both a stylised young sexual subject *alongside* indoctrination into a particular rendering of Queer life. This becomes even more powerful considering how few outlets exist for this audience.

Photograph 17.1: *Young Gay America (YGA)* cover page

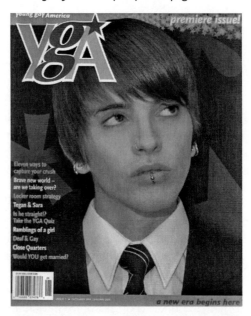

Photograph 17.2: *X Y* cover page

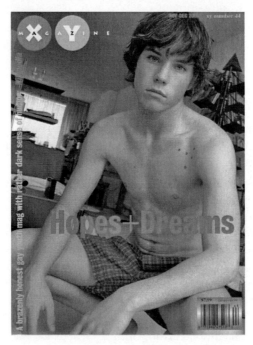

Photograph 17.3: Neoliberal subjects; prevention strategy: homonormative representation

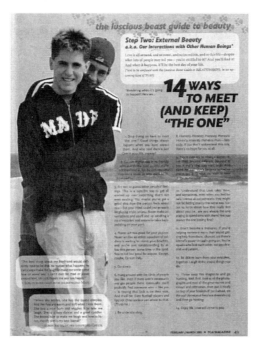

Parallel to the strength of this new, stylised sphere for young consumers, the social semiotic analysis revealed a number of discourses about HIV, generally categorised into representations and prevention. In the first case, these infotainment media mis-/represented HIV through an omission of 'HIV' itself, hyper-individualisation, and the simultaneous decontextualisation and recontextualisation of AIDS symbols. At baseline, the virus was largely absent linguistically and visually across the texts. Given their persuasive power, it would be reasonable to expect these texts to pay some attention to the pandemic, alongside other existing health content. The striking absence of HIV occurs in two ways: subtextually and patently. For example, in 'Letters to the Editor', a directive is made to the readers to 'play safely' (see Figure 17.1); it is never clarified *why* someone would need to 'play safely' nor how this would be achieved. When HIV does appear, however, the discourses privatise the virus, making it an individual rather than social problem; for example, literally locating it in one individual (see Photograph 17.4). Furthermore, the pandemic was decontextualised at large through an omission of history and politics. Common symbols, such as the red ribbon (see Figure 17.2) became recontextualised into icons for a new generation, sidelining recognition and concern for HIV.

Figure 17.1: Subtextual reference to HIV

> Please, everybody. XY loves you. Play safely. Be here for our future.

Figure 17.2: Recontextualising the AIDS ribbon

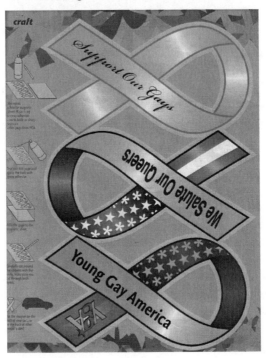

In terms of prevention, the infotainment media demonstrated an isolation of information, entrenched homonormativity and an omission of messaging. Little basic knowledge and techniques were offered related to HIV prevention. This sparse visualisation isolated HIV; quite simply, if readers wanted to find education about the virus, related symptoms and interventions, they would be hard pressed to do so. For example, it is *only* in *one* 'special issue' of *one* magazine edition that basic education is provided to readers about sexually transmitted infections, condoms, alcohol and drugs, among other co-factors. In the middle of this 'comprehensive' issue, a brief article discussed 23 directives for staying healthy, number 10 of which simply mandates: 'Get tested for HIV on a regular basis' (Nycum, 2000). This is one (of a few) clear instances across all these texts wherein readers are prompted explicitly to do anything with regard to prevention. Likewise, in lieu of common strategies (for example condoms), these media portrayed a sanitised, homonormative couplehood as the primary preventative tactic (see Photograph 17.3). Unfortunately, this idealised scene omitted messages that could engender sexual safety. Regardless of the amount or type of information, what is compelling to consider here is the inconsistency and omissions across these information media. These publications do a disservice to their consumers through generally excluding what is everyday best prevention practice that can promote health, as opposed to their liberal coverage of fashion or music. Yet again, when represented at all, HIV and its prevention are not integrated into other social practices.

Photo 17.4: Hyper-individualising HIV

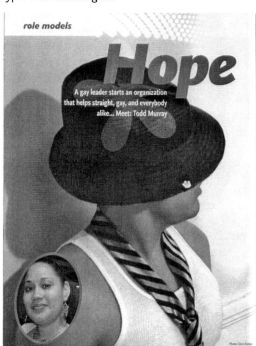

Within a critical paradigm, a number of important factors can be understood about young queer identity, culture, and HIV. The lifestyle presented within this infotainment media to the young readers *de-gays* AIDS and *de-AIDS* queer life (Perry-Argüello, 2008). HIV is removed from the operative concerns of the new young sexual subject: HIV is a condition of the Other, who is a vector of risk, versus the privileged, white, homonormative, cisgender neoliberal subject. Moreover, the 'brave new world' these media constructs is unfettered by AIDS:

apparently the virus does not circulate in this new world-making project. Given the representations described, silence can be viewed as the tie that binds, as HIV is practically rendered moot from the consumers' minds. Ironically, the authenticity authorised by these texts is one disconnected from a queer history. To embody the subject position represented within this media, one must perform an identity de-centred, destabilised and de-historicised from the exact material (for example the virus) and social phenomenon (for example the AIDS pandemic) that have defined in large part the contemporary queer counterpublic.

The young gay subject is further *de-AIDS'ed* by the lack of prevention practices suggested. This sanitised subject, compounded by the lack of substantive information on HIV, contributes to a prevention discourse that is something less than common sense, utilitarian, or less activist. Prevention is depoliticised, decollectivised and relegated to individual bodies and private behaviours not in the main of what is homonormatively queer. It appears that if a consumer follows the path to the new world as laid out by this infotainment, the consumer will be without need or want to prevent something like HIV, as it has been removed from (young) queer consciousness. Ultimately, these media seem unreliable resources for information about HIV prevention strategies.

Nevertheless, these media hold much power and have taken on the difficult job of networking a strangerhood of young queer people. There is no doubt they are both new brands and media resources; in fact, they are an aspirational achievement. By the act of addressing an *indefinite* audience, a potent moment in the social world manifests: the possibility to see representation, be represented and participate in mass circulation provides shape to the anonymous strangerhood of queer people that has *always* existed and will exist. All the while, this brave new world holds tension with the mainstream public spheres and that of the gay counterpublic. These texts do not authorise the natural order of young queer life; rather they show the fabrication of a lifestyle that sits at the intersections of identities *in progress*. Young queer people are nothing if not incomplete in their identities and self-identificatory practices. These texts deserve respect for *both* their triumphs and tribulations, and they deserve assistance in providing the basic tools to construct and grow the subjects and objects of whom they speak.

The work of this infotainment media is profoundly important, and as a site for prevention deserves more serious consideration by health professionals. At the same time, media professionals could work in conjunction with health professionals to provide information that may be more aligned with the pace and place of the virus. Most of all, critical language awareness (CLA; Fairclough, 1999) is a practical skill that should be emplaced in the arsenal of best practices when working with young queer counterpublics. CLA is one way to more effectively navigate the media-saturated existence these young people live. CLA works to appreciate communication as *mediatised*, acquiring and implementing critical skills that deconstruct mediated communication set in the context of organising social structures and ideologies. In the current era of neoliberalism, economy is based less on materiality but increasingly on the cultivation, control and consumption of information and knowledge (Fairclough, 1999). Empowering consumers to become critically aware of communication provides indispensable intellectual resources for reflexivity to discern cultural norms, expectations and social identities. Most importantly, critical awareness of the institution of media affords consumers access to the intellectual and material resources needed to re-/negotiate discourses, which is also a transferable skill that enables people to negotiate their local environments, especially where the risk of HIV may lie.

Implications for the field

This work contributes to social welfare in a number of ways. First, theoretically, an attempt was made to disturb the tendency in health research to naturalise and neutralise post-/positivist inquiry. This project calls into question positivism's meaning-making power/privilege and consolidated predictive abilities. The most joyous yet annoying quality of queer is its tendency to, among other abilities, infect the normative.

Second, these studies refute the tacit assumption that what we need in the HIV pandemic is better (top-down) communication. With the CDC's call for enhanced prevention and CLAS's mandate for linguistically sensitive services, new perspectives on communication are imperative. The messages in the public sphere have not stuck in the ways strategised; this is due, in part, to the agency of individuals, but it is certainly also due to the 'social distance' between privileged professionals and their targeted populations (Brown, 1995). Health promotion does not exist apart from operative social meanings and norms: signs are motivated by the practices that animate them. These studies foreground that signs are *already* imbued with and in-service of ideologies. How effective these ideologies are in curtailing the pandemic remains in question. Necessarily, this author, researchers, practitioners, HIV itself and citizens do not reside outside contemporary neoliberalism. We cannot! Instead, this project exemplifies how meaning, under the constraints of the modern political economy, can be renegotiated. Moreover, it evidences how texts and communicative strategies can be reworked and meaning renegotiated.

Third, the analysis foregrounds that there is no fundamental quality that makes HIV gay; no germane attribute to queerness that weds it to HIV. There is, however, a naturality to HIV that relates it to queerness: the viral processes of HIV rally against the functioning of the body; queerness finds mobility in the socially aggravating performative experience through the body. Both processes infect the social body, working against normativising forces, which in turn poses risk in modern life and necessitates a need for (hegemonic) prevention to protect the social order. Accordingly, since both queer and HIV are given social life through discourse, attention to language and visual culture is imperative.

Fourth, countering normativising forces requires self-reflexivity. This is no easy task and is not a finite outcome to validate ideologies and practice. Rather, it is an indefinite lens through which to continually gauge and interrogate the often-unquestioned embodied and lived experiences that pervade our personal and professional worlds. For those with expert power/knowledge, this aspect of labour is essential. Self-reflexivity is the conscious commitment to measure the intentions and implications of our work against the unequal stakes of political economies and their attendant social conditions. One way among many to foster such self-reflexivity is through transdisciplinary work. HIV has shown that it can inhabit and ravage various spaces: quite queerly, HIV is a good example of how strategies can be reworked and effect change.

Overall, the most important implication from this study is one of time. In the race to out-manoeuvre HIV, the stakes of the game (that is, life and death) are left sidelined. For queer people, the networking of semiotics is essential for their own networking – to be given life, made visible, performative, intelligible and to be allowed to speak their name. For queer counterpublics, semiotic resources do not function simply to make sex happen, inflected with the chronic risk of HIV infection. Rather, semiotic resources produce the space that makes the world possible for queer to have existence. For all the sign-making done upon them, semiotics are most critically a world-making project. The risk of HIV only makes that mission more vital: objects, as well as subjects, are deserving of social justice.

What we know about this already
• Queer men persist to endure disproportionate rates of HIV.
• Queer populations are more accurately understood as counterpublics.
• The contemporary world has become semioticised and technologised, that is, dominated by discourse, multi-media and technology.

What this chapter adds
• It shows that the production of infotainment is co-extensive with the production of health disparities.
• Also that 'prevention fatigue' can be understood, instead, as a 'semiotic fatigue'.
• It emphasizes that products of professional labour are already imbued with and in-service of ideologies.

How this is relevant for social work and LGBT health inequalities
• HIV is an exemplar for infecting and inverting the normative: contemporary interventions require transdisciplinary approaches.
• Self-reflexivity is a critical quality for ethical and effective practice.
• Critical communication studies are under-utilised in social work; this is one of the first studies to deploy CDA and SS in social welfare.

References

Aiello, G, 2007, 'The appearance of diversity: Visual design and the public communication of EU identity', in J Bain and M Holland (eds), *European Union identity: Perceptions from Asia and Europe*, 147–81, Baden-Baden, Germany: Nomos

Appadurai, A, 1996, *Modernity at large: Cultural dimensions of globalization*, Minneapolis, MN: University of Minnesota Press

Brown, M, 1995, 'Ironies of distance: An ongoing critique of the geographies of AIDS', *Environment and Planning D: Society and Space*, 13, 159-83

Cameron, D, 2001, *Working with spoken discourse*, London: Sage

CDC (Centers for Disease Control), 2006, 'Twenty-five years of HIV/AIDS – United States, 1981–2006', *MMWR*, 55, 21, 585-620

CDC (Centers for Disease Control and Prevention), 2008, *Estimates of new HIV infections in the United States: CDC HIV/AIDS facts*, Atlanta, GA: US Department of Health and Human Services

CDC, 2011, *CDC fact sheet: 30 years of HIV/AIDS*, Atlanta, GA: U.S. Department of Health and Human Services

CDC, 2012, *CDC fact sheet: HIV among gay and bisexual men*, Atlanta, GA: US Department of Health and Human Services

Fairclough, N, 1995, *Media discourse*, London: Edward Arnold

Fairclough, N, 1999, 'Global capitalism and critical awareness of language', *Language Awareness*, 8, 2, 71-83

Fairclough, N, 2003, *Analysing discourse: Textual analysis for social research*, London: Routledge

Foucault, M, 1978/1990, *The history of sexuality, Vol 1: An introduction*, New York, NY: Vintage Books

Foucault, M, 1985/1990, *The history of sexuality, Vol II: The use of pleasure*, New York, NY: Vintage Books

Foucault, M, 1986/1990, *The history of sexuality, Vol III: The care of the self*, New York, NY: Vintage Books

KFF (Kaiser Family Foundation), 2006, *Evolution of an epidemic: 25 years of HIV/AIDS media campaigns in the U.S.* (#7515), Julia Davis (ed), Menlo Park, CA

Kress, G and van Leeuwen, T, 2006, *Reading images: The grammar of visual design*, London: Routledge

Nycum, B, 2000, 'How to stay healthy and live longer', *XY survival guide: Everything you need to know about being young and gay*, 1, 60

OMH (Office of Minority Health), Think Cultural Health (OMH), 2013, *National standards for culturally and appropriate services in health and health care: A blueprint for advancing and sustaining CLAS policy and practice*, Washington, DC: US Department of Health and Human Services

ONAP (Office of National AIDS Policy, 2010, *National HIV/AIDS Strategy for the United States*, Washington, DC: The White House

Perry-Argüello, T, 2008, *Contagious communication: The mediatization, spatialization, and commercialization of 'HIV'*, Unpublished doctoral dissertation, Seattle, WA: University of Washington

Prado, G, Lightfoot, M and Brown, CH, 2013, 'Macro-level approaches to HIV prevention among ethnic minority youth: state of the science, opportunities, and challenges', *American Psychologist*, 68, 4, 286-99

Schulz, W, 2004, 'Reconstructing mediatization as an analytical concept', *European Journal of Communication*, 19, 1, 87-101

Thurlow, C and Jaworski, A, 2006, 'The alchemy of the upwardly mobile: Symbolic capital and the stylization of elites in frequent-flyer programmes', *Discourse & Society*, 17, 1, 131-67

Warner, M, 2002, *Publics and counterpublics*, New York, NY: Zone Books

Conclusion

Kate Karban and Julie Fish

Introduction

This book set out to bring together a range of international contributions on social work's contribution to tackling lesbian, gay, bisexual and trans (LGBT) health inequalities and looking back over the chapters it is useful to summarise some of the key themes and issues that characterise and integrate the various contributions. These will be considered in the light of the overall aims and purpose of the book, recognising the extent to which these have been met and the inevitable limitations as well as the overall significance of the material. Pivotal to this conclusion is also the need to balance reflection on what has been written, with some thoughts for the future, acknowledging that this text is a snapshot at one point of a journey and that there is a long road ahead. The implications for future theory, practice, education and research will also be considered within an approach that does not rest on a simple linear trajectory but recognises the contradictory and dynamic nature of progress towards human rights and social justice for LGBT people.

LGBT health inequalities – looking back

A key contribution of social work to tackling inequalities rests in the importance of bearing witness to human rights abuses, injustice and resistance (Healy, 2001; Heinonen and Metteri, 2005; Gitterman and Germain, 2008/2013). The contents of the chapters in this book highlight some of the challenges affecting the health and wellbeing of LGBT people and the strengths and resilience that are demonstrated in the face of prejudice and inequality. In particular, a number of the chapters make a powerful contribution to making visible the invisible, challenging us to recognise the reality of oppression and prejudice experienced by LGBT people and the far-reaching consequences for health. The limited attention in the social work literature to certain aspects of LGBT experience is noted in relation to care-experienced young people in Northern Ireland (Carr and Pinkerton) and asylum seekers in England (Karban and Sirriyeh), and the absence of LGBT issues from social work in Italy is also explored by Nagy and Nothdurfter. From a Swedish perspective, Knutagård explores the hidden experiences of men who are raped by men, while the ways in which LGBT health inequalities in Canada are obscured by a 'utopian veneer' and fly 'under the radar of formalised policy structures' provides a context for Mulé's chapter. Also in Canada, Sansfaçon and Manning acknowledge the lack of legal protection for trans people and the need to support families with a gender-creative child or young person. It is also important to recognise that there is both a need for more knowledge, for example Ranade refers to the lack of research evidence regarding the health and wellbeing of LGBT communities in India, and also a need to increase the visibility of LGBT and queer experience in heteronormative societies.

At same time, the book offers evidence of resilience and transformative practice/action. The support offered by *Chicos Net* to Latino gay men in Canada (Betancourt) acts to combat social isolation, provide knowledge and promote empowerment. In the United States (US), the success of gay–straight alliances in some high schools is seen as offering a counterbalance to the prevailing heterosexist and cisgendered environment (Winter et al) and additionally the account of the LGBT Roundtable of San Joaquin County (Breshears and Leyva) illustrates the value of advocacy and involvement in education and training for older LGBT people. The book also offers a theoretical perspective, building on the overview set out in the introduction, with evidence of a continuing human rights perspective on health inequalities and its central role in social work.

Mental health/minority stress

The book's orientation to health inequalities focuses primarily on upstream factors influencing the overall health and wellbeing of LGBT communities, recognising the challenges of age, ability and experiences of care in addition to the particular issues facing groups such as asylum seekers and migrants. Specific health conditions and the 'downstream' factors that may influence health behaviours and access to healthcare are beyond our remit here. An exception to this is mental health, with one chapter focusing on service provision and social inclusion for LGB adults in Wales (Maegusuku–Hewett et al) and a chapter by Leyva addressing the mental health needs of LGBT older. A number of chapters integrate mental health and wellbeing issues, for example in relation to young people (Chapter Five) and asylum seekers (Chapter Eleven). The experiences related in these chapters highlight the fundamental link between mental health and human rights violations, including trauma, discrimination and abuse, all of which are acknowledged by the World Health Organization (Herrman et al, 2005). Additionally, the complex inter-relationship between mental and physical wellbeing underlie the slogan of 'no health without mental health' that underpins policies in England (HM Government, 2011) and elsewhere.

The concept of 'minority stress' (Meyer, 2003) is used by several authors in explaining the complex relationship between the lived experience of discrimination and stigma by LGBT people and poor health or emotional wellbeing. There is a particular concern that these negative experiences, whether first hand or through the media and family/societal attitudes may be 'internalised', especially by young people who may lack access to positive role models and affirming relationships within their day-to-day lives. This is recognised by Nagy and Nothdurfter in their example of responses to a young lesbian in care and also by Carr and Pinkerton in their discussion of LGBT young people. However, as these authors and Winter et al emphasise, it is essential to consider the ways in which young people are resilient and demonstrate positive coping strategies.

Minority stress is also considered by other contributors who, as in the introduction, recognise that while this adds an additional dimension to the social determinants of health, there must also be a balance in identifying strategies of survival and resilience. Chapters by Westwood et al and Almack et al explore how the cumulative effects of marginalised identity impact on older LGBT people's health and how social work interventions need to be based on recognising and respecting individual experience through the lifespan and in promoting social inclusion, to bring about positive outcomes. This theme of stress and resilience is also reflected in the experiences of LGBT asylum seekers (Karban and Sirriyeh) where the additional stress of being LGBT, including the fear of being discovered and/or returned to the country of origin, is compounded by other aspects of being an asylum seeker, both materially and emotionally. Karban and Sirriyeh also refer to an understanding of mental distress in asylum seekers that recognises the individual's experiences before, during and following migration.

Intersectionality

Throughout the book is recognition of the complexity of LGBT experiences and a need to challenge simplistic notions of fixed identity. Here identity is understood as fluid, nuanced and multifaceted:

identifying as lesbian, gay, bisexual or trans will be affected by gender, ethnicity, age and dis/ability, notions of 'class' and citizenship as well as different meanings and experiences of identity, desire and behaviours.

The implications for social work rest in seeking to recognise the unique experiences of an individual, together with an understanding of these broader categories and their intersections, for example the reality of being a black lesbian mother, a young trans person, an older bisexual man who requires care or a gay male asylum seeker from the Indian subcontinent. Crucially, as Fook (2002, p 84) points out, 'the politics of identity construction become integral in resisting and challenging domination'.

Mulé highlights how professional documents fail to move beyond one-dimensional notions of identity, obscuring the way in which sexual orientation and/or gender identity intersect with race, ethnicity, age, (dis)abilities, religion and class. This theme is also addressed by Maegusuku-Hewett et al, who report that focus group participants refer to the impact of multiple stigmatised identities, and the challenge of accessing mental health services with adequate Welsh-speaking services that are also LGBT-sensitive, further compounded by living in a rural area. Maegusuku-Hewett et al also remind us that, for LGBT people, experiences of migration may also be significant between rural and urban areas within, as well as between, countries. Experiences of migration are also a reflected in the chapter by Betancourt where it is evident that in the account of *Chicos Net*, masculinity and sexuality can only be understood in the context of Latino gay men who have migrated to North America.

Looking forward to the future: implications for practice, education and research

Each chapter offers important messages for the application of knowledge to social work practice, research or education, underpinned by professional ethics, values and principles. Central to this are linked notions of empowerment and partnership. Additionally, the need for critical, reflective and self-reflexive thinking is paramount.

Empowerment

The work of Freire (2000) is referred to by Betancourt, and Breshears and Leyva. For Betancourt, the sharing of experiences within *Chicos Net* is itself a key factor in empowering men who experience homophobia, migration issues and other racialised experiences in relation to dating, online cruising and body image. Similarly, Breshears and Leyva stress the value of 'power with', involving LGBT older people in an initiative to improve responses to health and care needs. Sansfaçon and Manning stress that the use of participatory action research is essential for the realisation of empowerment and advocacy in working with families with gender-creative children, recognising that such an approach is helpful for effecting change while simultaneously embedding social work values in research, enabling parents to be recognised as 'knowers' and involving them as co-researchers. Dunlap's chapter also explores the importance of inviting LGBT participants to engage in a collaborative research process, recognising their position as 'experts' on their lives and experiences, echoing the call of the people's health and service users' movements for 'nothing about us without us' (Davis, 2009, p 266). These approaches re-enforce the values and principles enshrined in the International Federation of Social Workers' (IFSW) commitment to human rights and social justice and in seeking to promote social change, problem solving in human relationships and the empowerment and liberation of people to enhance wellbeing.

Partnership working

Partnerships in practice and the fostering of intersectoral relationships are also a running theme throughout this text. This includes evidence of collaboration reflected in joint and multiple-authored chapters, with LGBT authors being joined by their straight collaborators and the involvement of different academic disciplines including contributors with sociology, political science, psychotherapy and socio-legal expertise alongside social work educators, researchers and practitioners. Links between research, social work education and practice provide the basis for Nagy and Nothdurfter's chapter while Maegusuku-Hewett et al emphasise the need to align policy and service provision to address gaps in service delivery, promoting inclusivity and involvement through the involvement of mental health service users and carers in their research.

Joined-up working between team and sectors is highlighted in several chapters in Part Two, relating to service design and practice development. This relates to the importance of developing 'systems of care' for LGBT young people described by Winter et al, the need for joined-up working to provide quality care for older LGBT people with complex care requirements (Westwood et al) and the development of inter-agency collaboration to support LGBT asylum seekers (Karban and Sirriyeh). Notwithstanding the limitations of the social determinants of health, as one of the conceptual frameworks presented in the introduction of this volume, it is clear that the complex nature of the range of factors that lead to poor health outcomes, including socioeconomic conditions and the broad range of structural inequalities and disadvantage, requires equally broad and coordinated responses.

Critical reflection/reflexivity

An essential aspect of addressing LGBT health inequalities in practice requires attention to dominant heterosexist and cisgender discourses that may be internalised and impact on practice. For Salzburg, this demands pedagogic practices that engage social work students in dialogue informed by critical reflection, immersing them in the narratives of LGBT lives. Drawing on narrative therapy and community practice, Salzburg offers a way forward that has the potential to support and enable students as they develop self-awareness and prepare for practice with LGBT individuals and communities. Similarly, Argüello argues for the necessity of self-reflexivity in practice that prompts critical awareness of personal and professional assumptions, intentions and outcomes regarding practice.

Strengths and limitations of this book

It is important to be realistic about the breadth and range of this volume and to acknowledge that there are significant gaps. In addition to the chapters here from Europe, North America and India, the original groundwork for this book included contributions from authors in Australia and South Africa and on the topic of the African diaspora, which unfortunately were not realised. However, this volume, with its range of contributors, offers important perspectives that may not often be evident in texts dominated by English-speaking authors.

The range of chapters provides a rich and diverse insight into the individual contributors' experiences of social work practice, education and research relating to the lives of LGBT people, recognising the unique policy, legislative and cultural environment in which these experiences are embedded. At the same time, the book enables the reader to draw out overarching themes and shared challenges, transcending national boundaries.

Looking forward

It remains to look forward and beyond into the future for LGBT communities. Addressing LGBT health inequalities is a continuing journey, requiring attention to the past as well as the future. It is clear from the contributions contained in this book, and as noted in the foreword, that despite many achievements, progress can be slow, patchy and sometimes contradictory. There is no straightforward linear account but a complex and multifaceted narrative of change. This can be seen during the brief lifetime of this book's development from proposal to publication, during which time LGBT communities have seen progress (equal marriage in the UK and in California) alongside increasing homophobia manifest and fuelled by, for example, the reversal of a court judgment to decriminalise same-sex relationships in India and the 'anti-propaganda' legislation and law banning same-sex adoption in Russia. Additionally, even in one country, as Breshears and Leyva point out in their chapter on the needs and experiences of LGBT older people, the experiences of LGBT people may vary significantly between San Francisco and the Central Valley, places less than 160 kilometres apart.

Overall, it is hoped that the book, with its various contributions, will offer new and creative ideas, to stimulate and inspire the continuing development of social work practice to address LGBT health inequalities informed by social justice and human rights. As Gary Bailey stated in the foreword to this book, 'there is work for us all to do'. Fundamentally this a shared commitment to human rights and social justice that is recognised by all of us, regardless of age, ethnicity, gender, sexuality, dis/ability, religion and citizenship, building on the voice of black lesbian feminist, Audre Lorde (1984, p 125), who challenged the view that 'racism is a Black women's problem ... and only we can discuss it'. Equally, social work's contribution to tackling LGBT health inequalities is not only the responsibility of those of us who identify as lesbian, gay, bisexual or trans but rests on all our shoulders.

References

Davis, A, 2009, 'Addressing health inequalities: the role of service user and people's health movements', in P Bywaters, E McLeod and L Napier, (eds) *Social work and global health inequalities*, Bristol: Policy Press

Fook, J, 2002, *Social work critical theory and practice*, London: Sage

Freire, P, 2000, *Pedagogy of the oppressed*, New York, NY: Continuum

Gitterman, A and Germain, C, 2008/2013, *The life model of social work practice* (3rd edn), New York, NY: Columbia University Press

Healy, L, 2001, *International social work: Professional action in an interdependent world*, Oxford: Oxford University Press

Heinonen, T and Metteri, A, 2005, *Social work in health and mental health*, Toronto: Canadian Scholars Press Inc

Herrman, H, Saxena, S and Moodie, R (eds), 2005, *Promoting mental health*, Geneva: WHO

HM Government, 2011, *No health without mental health*, London: Department of Health

Lorde, A, 1984, *The uses of anger: women responding to racism in sister outsider*, Freedom, CA: The Crossing Press Feminist Series

Meyer, IH, 2003, 'Prejudice, social stress, and mental health in lesbian, gay, and bisexual populations: conceptual issues and research evidence', *Psychological Bulletin*, 129, 5, 674–97.

Index